T0276084

Pharmacy Education in the Twenty First Century and Beyond

Pharmacy Education in the Twenty First Century and Beyond

Global Achievements and Challenges

Edited by

Ahmed Ibrahim Fathelrahman

Mohamed Izham Mohamed Ibrahim

Alian A. Alrasheedy

Albert I. Wertheimer

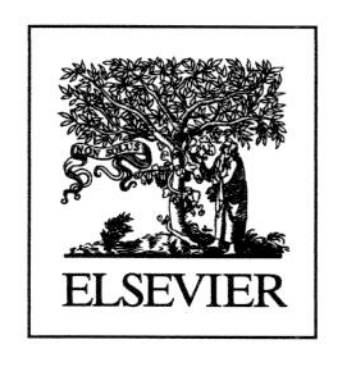

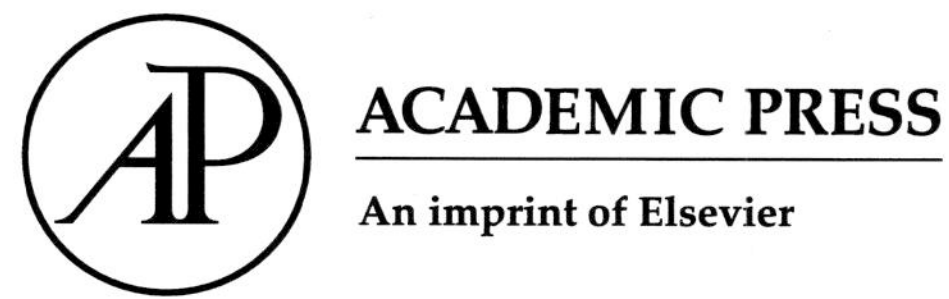

Academic Press is an imprint of Elsevier
125 London Wall, London EC2Y 5AS, United Kingdom
525 B Street, Suite 1800, San Diego, CA 92101-4495, United States
50 Hampshire Street, 5th Floor, Cambridge, MA 02139, United States
The Boulevard, Langford Lane, Kidlington, Oxford OX5 1GB, United Kingdom

Library of Congress Cataloging-in-Publication Data
A catalog record for this book is available from the Library of Congress

British Library Cataloguing-in-Publication Data
A catalogue record for this book is available from the British Library

ISBN 978-0-12-811909-9

For information on all Academic Press publications visit our website at https://www.elsevier.com/books-and-journals

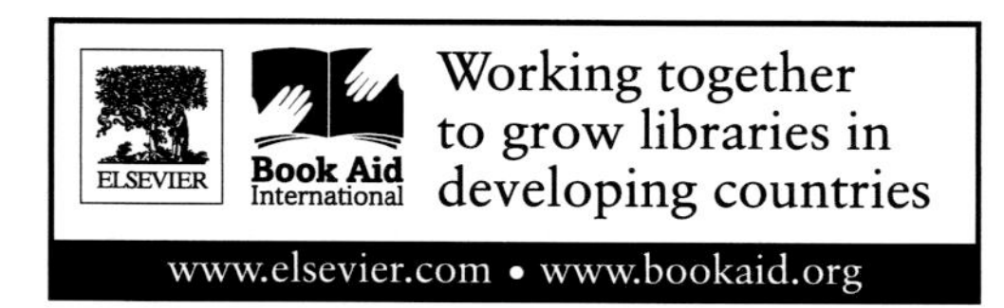

Publisher: John Fedor
Acquisition Editor: Erin Hill-Parks
Editorial Project Manager: Jennifer Horigan
Production Project Manager: Punithavathy Govindaradjane
Cover Designer: Mark Rogers

Typeset by SPi Global, India

Dedication

I dedicate this book to my dearest mother, wife, children, and the rest of my family, for their love and endless support. I also dedicate this book to all the colleagues with whom I studied or worked at Assuit University, Egypt; the Ministry of Health, Sudan; University of Science Malaysia (USM); and Qassim University and Taif University in Saudi Arabia.

Finally, I dedicate this book to all my students in Sudan and Saudi Arabia and to all those academic staff members who are interested in and devoted to the development of pharmacy education around the world.

Ahmed Ibrahim Fathelrahman

I dedicate this book to my parents, family, and professors.

Mohamed Izham Mohamed Ibrahim

I dedicate this book to all my family members and friends, for all their support and help. I dedicate the book to my wife Eman, for her constant support and love and for allowing me to have the time to spend long hours on my computer screen to finish this work.

I also would like to dedicate this book to all my teachers and professors who taught and guided me throughout my studies. I believe this is all because of their sincere efforts, dedication, and sacrifices.

I also would like to dedicate this book to all educators and health practitioners who have spent their lives helping and treating patients.

Alian A. Alrasheedy

This dedication is to my wife Joaquima, who permitted me to spend time on this endeavor and who also provided brilliant suggestions and critiques of my work. Thank you, Joaquima.

Albert I. Wertheimer

Contents

Contributors

Suhaj Abdulsalim
Unaizah College of Pharmacy, Qassim University, Qassim, Saudi Arabia

Patricia Acuña-Johnson
University of Valparaiso, Valparaiso, Chile

Abubakr A. Alfadl
Unaizah College of Pharmacy, Qassim University, Qassim, Saudi Arabia

Ahmad A. Almeman
Qassim University, Buraidah, Saudi Arabia

Alian A. Alrasheedy
Unaizah College of Pharmacy, Qassim University, Qassim, Saudi Arabia

Saleh A. Alrebish
Qassim University, Buraidah, Saudi Arabia

Claire Anderson
University of Nottingham, Nottingham, United Kingdom

Ahmed Awaisu
Qatar University, Doha, Qatar

Allah Bukhsh
Monash University Malaysia, Subang Jaya, Malaysia; University of Veterinary & Animal Sciences, Lahore, Pakistan

Maryam Farooqui
Unaizah College of Pharmacy, Qassim University, Qassim, Saudi Arabia

Ahmed Ibrahim Fathelrahman
College of Pharmacy, Taif University, Taif, Saudi Arabia

Mohamed Azmi Hassali
Universiti Sains Malaysia, Penang, Malaysia

Bhuvan K.C.
Monash University Malaysia, Subang Jaya, Malaysia

Maram G. Katoue
Kuwait University Faculty of Pharmacy, Kuwait City, Kuwait

Tahir M. Khan
Monash University Malaysia, Subang Jaya, Malaysia; University of Veterinary & Animal Sciences, Lahore, Pakistan

Nadir Kheir
University of Auckland, Auckland, New Zealand

Donald E. Letendre
The University of Iowa College of Pharmacy, Iowa City, IA, United States

Arijana Meštrović
Near East University, Nicosia, Cyprus; University of Split, Split, Croatia; Pharma Expert—Consultancy and Education, Zagreb, Croatia

Long C. Ming
KPJ Healthcare University College, Nilai, Malaysia; University of Tasmania, Hobart, TAS, Australia

Mohamed Izham Mohamed Ibrahim
College of Pharmacy, Qatar University, Doha, Qatar

David R. Mottram
Liverpool John Moores University, Liverpool, United Kingdom

Lisa M. Nissen
Queensland University of Technology, Brisbane, QLD, Australia

Abdirahman Osman
St George's Hospital Medical School, London, United Kingdom

Michael J. Rouse
Accreditation Council for Pharmacy Education (ACPE), Chicago, IL, United States

Terry L. Schwinghammer
West Virginia University School of Pharmacy, Morgantown, WV, United States

Ahmed Sherman
IPSA Medical Clinic and Pharmacy, London, United Kingdom

Judith A. Singleton
Queensland University of Technology, Brisbane, QLD, Australia

Derek Stewart
Robert Gordon University, Aberdeen, United Kingdom

Albert I. Wertheimer
College of Pharmacy, Nova Southeastern University, Ft. Lauderdale, FL, United States

Kerry Wilbur
Faculty of Pharmaceutical Sciences, The University of British Columbia, Vancouver, BC, Canada

CHAPTER

INTRODUCTORY NOTES: WHY DO WE NEED A BOOK ON PHARMACY EDUCATION?

1

Ahmed Ibrahim Fathelrahman*,[a], Mohamed Izham Mohamed Ibrahim[†]

College of Pharmacy, Taif University, Taif, Saudi Arabia, [†]College of Pharmacy, Qatar University, Doha, Qatar

INTRODUCTION

A quality and integrated academic workforce is important to prepare competent pharmacy graduates, as well as to produce new pharmacists for the workforce. The International Pharmaceutical Federation's Global Conference on Pharmacy and Pharmaceutical Sciences Education, held in Nanjing, China in 2016, laid out eight themes related to pharmacy education (International Pharmaceutical Federation (FIP), 2016). These themes provide international expectations on what an effective pharmacy education system should look like in order to meet local needs. Knowledge and education have fundamental values as means to improve health.

Pharmacy education in the 21st century has witnessed several important revolutionary changes in philosophy, orientation, and features, including:

1. A dramatic increase in the number of pharmacy education institutions worldwide involving both developed and developing countries, followed by tremendous growth in the number of pharmacy graduates (Al-Wazaify, Matowe, Albsoul-Younes, & Al-Omran, 2006; Fathelrahman, Ibrahim, & Wertheimer, 2016; International Pharmaceutical Federation, 2015; Marriott et al., 2008; Taylor, Bates, & Harding, 2004). Fig. 1 shows pharmacy education institutions in 15 developing countries.
2. An increase in the diversity of pharmacy programs, which differ in nature, scope, curriculum orientation, degrees offered, and length of study by regions, countries and institutions (Basak & Sathyanarayana, 2010; Bourdon, Ekeland, & Brion, 2008; Kheir et al., 2008; Marriott et al., 2008).
3. A global change in the scope of pharmacy practice from merely drug product orientation toward much more concern about patients and community health (Babar, Scahill, Akhlaq, & Garg, 2013; Nona & Wadelin, 1990). Countrywise, the degree of such change differs according to local needs, available resources, challenges, and public expectations. However, such change

[a]Part of the chapter was written while the author was working with College of Pharmacy, Qassim University, Buraydah, Saudi Arabia.

Pharmacy Education in the Twenty First Century and Beyond. https://doi.org/10.1016/B978-0-12-811909-9.00001-0

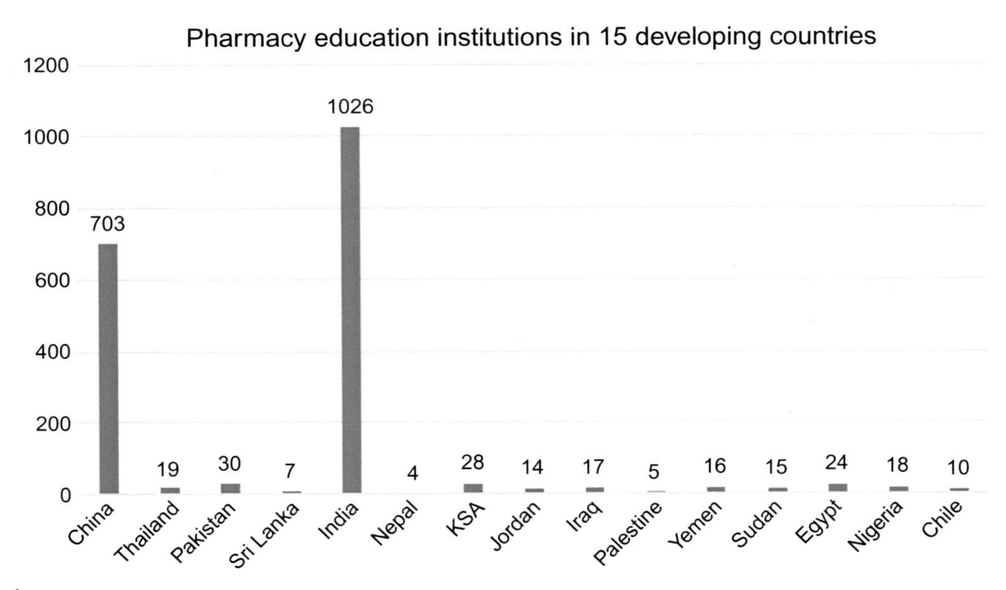

FIG. 1

Pharmacy education institutions in 15 developing countries.

From Fathelrahman, A. I., Ibrahim, M. I. M., & Wertheimer, A. (Eds.) (2016). Pharmacy practice in developing countries: achievements and challenges. *London: Academic Press an Imprint of Elsevier Science. ISBN: 0128017112, 9780128017111.*

requires reforms in pharmacy education, which involves changes in the nature of the subjects that should be taught to pharmacy students (Petit, Foriers, & Rombaut, 2008).

4. Advancements in technology—including information, communication, and educational technology—which make teaching easier, more effective, and more enjoyable than ever before but which require continuous training and updating to increase the capacity building of the institutions' infrastructures and academic staff (Brodie & Smith, 1985; Fox, 2011).
5. Better understanding of student learning, including learning styles, motivations for learning, and the effect and effectiveness of different teaching and assessment strategies on learning outcomes (Katajavuori et al., 2009; Newble & Cannon, 2002).
6. In the era of globalization, there is a global increase in private educational institutions' share, as opposed to government contributions, as a response to the increasing demand on pharmacy education and the huge gross of business orientation worldwide.
7. The worldwide growing concern about quality of education has called greater attention to new aspects of pharmacy education and has led to the domination of newer concepts like accreditation, leadership, capacity building, interprofessional education, e-learning, and continuing professional development (Austin & Ensom, 2008).
8. The global increase in political conflicts, wars, terrorism accidents, natural disasters, pandemic outbreaks, and unstable conditions, especially in the developing world, increases the gap between well-developed and poorer countries; this raises ethical issues related to the mismatch between supply and demand, disparities, and inequalities.

Readers should realize that this book is intended to cover major topics that have produced changes in pharmacy education. However, it has not been possible to cover all topics for several reasons, related to the nature of the particular topic, the availability of suitable literature on the topic, and the presence of experts in that field. The editors hope that other important topics can be covered in future editions of the book.

PHARMACY EDUCATION: TERMINOLOGY

A search of the literature related to pharmacy education (for example, simply searching through PubMed using the phrases "pharmacy education" and "pharmaceutical education" and the Boolean operator OR) revealed that "pharmaceutical education" was the predominant, or possibly even the only, terminology used in the literature before and during the 1950s to 1960s. The use of the term "pharmacy education" started to rise during the 1970s to 1990s, replacing the term "pharmaceutical education" gradually and becoming the dominating terminology after 2000. Thus, we can say that "pharmaceutical education" was the common terminology of the 20th century and "pharmacy education" is the terminology of the 21st century.

FROM MEDICAL EDUCATION TO PHARMACY EDUCATION

Medical education nowadays is a specialty that attracts the attention of educators and medical professionals who seek a new career in medical sciences. Although there is a growing pharmacy-related literature worldwide in this area in the form of research, published articles, and specialized journals, the term "pharmacy education" has not reached yet the stage of being a specialty in pharmacy similar to medical education. One day "pharmacy education" is going to grow and become an interesting stand-alone field of pharmacy-related disciplines, similar to pharmacoeconomics and pharmacoepidemiology, which were established between the 1960s and 1970s as newer fields of interest in pharmacy equivalent to health economics and epidemiology, respectively. The idea of writing a comprehensive book on pharmacy education came with an intention to make such area of specialization a reality.

PHARMACY EDUCATION: AN OVERVIEW OF THE LITERATURE

The literature on pharmacy education, including scholarly works such as books, book chapters, scientific papers, and technical reports, is still relatively limited compared to the literature on medical education. This is especially evident in the developing countries. Babar et al. conducted a bibliometric review of pharmacy education literature from low- to middle-income countries and concluded that there are few empiric publications in the area of pharmacy education (Babar et al., 2013). The following sections provide an overview of relevant literature.

BOOKS

1. *The pharmacist in public health: Education, applications and opportunities* by Hoai-An Truong, James L. Bresette, and Jill A. Sellers (Publisher: American Pharmacists Association, 2010)

2. *Pharmacy education: Teaching and research guide* by Desai, Kashappa Goud H. (Publisher: Anmol Publications, 2009)
3. *Pharmacy education at the University of Mississippi: Sketches, highlights and memories* by Mickey C. Smith (Editor) (Publisher: The Haworth Press, Inc., 2006)
4. *Pharmacy education: What matters in learning and teaching* by Lynne M Sylvia, Judith Barr (Publisher: Jones & Bartlett Learning, 2010)
5. *Promoting civility in pharmacy education* by Bruce A. Berger (Publisher: The Haworth Press, Inc., 2003)
6. *Pharmaceutical education in the Queen City: 150 years of service 1850–2000* by Michael A. Flannery and Dennis B. Worthen (Publisher: The Haworth Press, Inc., 2001)
7. *Multicultural pharmaceutical education* by Barry Bleidt (Editor) (Publisher: Taylor & Francis Group, 2013)
8. *Handbook for pharmacy educators: Contemporary teaching principles and strategies* by Noel Wilkin (Editor) (Publisher: The Haworth Press, 2000)
9. *Pharmacy education in Nigeria: Proceedings of the Pharmacy Curriculum Conference* by Fred B. Adenika (Publisher: Pharmacists Council of Nigeria, 2001)
10. *Pharmacy education and careers: The APhA resource book* (Publisher: American Pharmaceutical Association, 1988)
11. *Interdisciplinary education and practice in pharmacy: Expanding opportunities* by Janis P. Bellack (Publisher: Association of Academic Health Centers, 2002)

PEER-REVIEWED PHARMACY EDUCATION JOURNALS

The following are examples of peer-reviewed journals that focus primarily on pharmacy education.

1. ***American Journal of Pharmaceutical Education*** is the official publication of the American Association of Colleges of Pharmacy (AACP) founded in 1937. It is an open access journal that is issued 10 times per year (http://www.ajpe.org/).
2. ***Pharmacy Education*** has been published since 2001 with the endorsement and support of the International Pharmaceutical Federation (FIP), the World Health Organization (WHO), and UNESCO under the FIP-UNESCO UNITWIN program (http://pharmacyeducation.fip.org/pharmacyeducation).
3. ***Currents in Pharmacy Teaching and Learning*** is published by Elsevier. This journal maintains a particular focus in two major areas: pharmacy faculty development in the scholarship of teaching and learning and the scholarship of interprofessional pharmacy education (https://www.journals.elsevier.com/currents-in-pharmacy-teaching-and-learning).
4. ***Pharmacy*** is an international scientific open access journal on pharmacy education and practice published quarterly online by MDPI since 2013. Citations available in PubMed, full-text archived in PubMed Central from Vol. 3 (2015) (http://www.mdpi.com/journal/pharmacy).
5. ***INNOVATIONS in Pharmacy*** is a quarterly publication featuring case studies, clinical experiences, commentaries, idea papers, original research, review articles, and student projects that focus on leading edge, novel ideas for improving, modernizing, and advancing pharmacy practice, education, and policy. It is an open access journal published by the University of Minnesota since 2010 (https://pubs.lib.umn.edu/innovations/).

AN OVERVIEW OF THIS BOOK

The main features and aspects of this book are listed here.

- This book provides a brief overview of pharmacy education history by focusing only on the important milestones in this history.
- It is intended to be a useful guide for pharmacy educators who may want to inquire about the usefulness and the effectiveness of certain teaching or assessment strategies.
- It can be a guide for students who want to choose a particular program for their undergraduate or postgraduate study to best suit the future career they are planning.
- Based on available evidence, this book works on justifying why certain pharmacy programs attract students more than others, and why pharmacy educators prefer particular teaching strategies, assessment tools, or teaching styles.
- It provides options for the leaders of pharmacy colleges to choose the best approaches to improve and revise their programs based on worldwide experiences with regard to accreditation, leadership, capacity building, interprofessional education, legal aspects, and continuing professional development.
- It covers different types of education and learning, including undergraduate, postgraduate, continuing professional development, and self-learning.
- It illustrates different orientations of curricula, including classic and clinical-oriented curricula with descriptions of courses normally taught in each case.
- It describes and compares different degrees and qualifications that are offered worldwide, including entry-level to practice degrees (e.g., BSc(Pharm), BPharm, MPharm, PharmD), postgraduate qualifications (e.g., MClinPharm, DPharm), residency and fellowship programs, and Board certification.
- It describes and compares various teaching strategies used in pharmacy, such as team-based learning (TBL), problem-based learning (PBL), and interdisciplinary education.
- In all aspects mentioned here, the book highlights and discusses pros and cons as well as advantages and disadvantages.

RELATIONSHIPS BETWEEN CHAPTERS

It should be noted that, although each chapter has its own identity/scope and specific focus, some aspects are common or may overlap between one chapter and another, but these aspects have been addressed from a different perspective in each chapter.

For example, Chapter 2, "The Pharmacy Education: A Historical Perspective" by Derek Stewart and Donald Letendre includes some information about accreditation in the West. The authors covered such issues as part of the historical changes occurring in pharmacy education in the United States and Europe (i.e., historical perspective). However, Chapter 15 by Ahmed I. Fathelrahman and Michael Rouse is the main chapter focusing on quality and accreditation issues in pharmacy education. This chapter describes the terminology of quality and accreditation and other related terms, provides a review of the available evidence on the impact of accreditation on the quality of education, and describes some important accrediting bodies that work actively in the accreditation of pharmacy programs on an international level, besides other aspects. Chapter 13 by Nadir Kheir and Kerry L. Wilbur is on continuing professional development (CPD) and self-learning; it focuses mainly on continuing professional development but describes accreditation of the CPD programs, which is an issue not covered in Chapter 15.

Another example is Chapter 11 by Abubakr A. Alfadl on assessment methods and tools for pharmacy education, comprehensively covers the topic of assessment and evaluation in pharmacy education. Chapter 13 includes a short section on assessment of CPD needs and another section on CPD program assessment which cover the particular aspects of assessment that are relevant to CPD programs. Similarly, Chapter 12 by Maram Katoue and Terry L. Schwinghammer, titled "Competency-Based Pharmacy Education: An Educational Paradigm for the Pharmacy Profession to Meet Society's Healthcare Needs," covers issues like "assessing the learner's performance" and "selecting the assessment methods."

The readers may notice some other overlaps between chapters and they will discover that a certain chapter covers the particular topic heavily and extensively as a main focus, while other chapters touch only slightly on specific aspects of the topic. This makes reading the book as individual chapters, or collectively, convenient and easy for the readers.

ONE STYLE AND A DIVERSITY OF EXPERIENCES

Besides adherence to one writing style and format, the editors tried to be consistent in that every piece of information presented in this book must be evidence-based and supported by references, and claims must be supported by data and statistics as much as possible. However, the editors left space for the chapter authors to express their viewpoints and opinions and reflect their personal experiences in order to give the book a global taste and feel, especially since the editors and the contributing authors came from various regions representing 14 countries.

TARGET AUDIENCE

The audience for this book consists of:

- Pharmacy leaders in academia and practice
- Pharmacy educators
- Pharmacy practitioners
- Pharmacy students at both undergraduate and postgraduate levels
- Researchers interested in pharmacy practice and pharmacy education research
- Human resource departments in various pharmacy practice settings
- Other professionals who intend to learn from others

WHAT DOES THIS BOOK ADD?

Previous publications have focused primarily on particular aspects of pharmacy education or concentrated on pharmacy education in a certain country or institution. To our knowledge, this is the first comprehensive source on pharmacy education that covers most of the issues and aspects pertaining to the topic collectively in one document. The present book reflects the global view of pharmacy education. It has succeeded in reflecting the diversity of experiences in North America, Europe, Australia, Latin America, Asia, and the Middle East. The book takes the reader on a journey from ancient history, moving to the modern recent advances of the 21st century and ending in the future of pharmacy education, with both its beautiful dreams and its stressful challenges.

On behalf of the editors and contributing authors, we hope that the readers of this book will find an answer to a challenging question, an explanation of an ambiguous trend, a lesson they can learn from, a piece of information that can be used to solve a problem, a guide to undertake an action, or assistance in carefully setting a strategy or making a future plan.

Finally, the editors will be happy to receive valuable input, feedback and advice from you, the reader.

REFERENCES

Al-Wazaify, M., Matowe, L., Albsoul-Younes, A., & Al-Omran, O. A. (2006). Pharmacy education in Jordan, Saudi Arabia, and Kuwait. *American Journal of Pharmaceutical Education*, *70*(1), 18.

Austin, Z., & Ensom, M. H. (2008). Education of pharmacists in Canada. *American Journal of Pharmaceutical Education*, *72*(6), 128.

Babar, Z., Scahill, S. L., Akhlaq, M., & Garg, S. (2013). A bibliometric review of pharmacy education literature in the context of low- to middle-income countries. *Currents in Pharmacy Teaching and Learning*, *5*(3), 218–232.

Basak, S. C., & Sathyanarayana, D. (2010). Pharmacy education in India. *American Journal of Pharmaceutical Education*, *74*(4), 68.

Bourdon, O., Ekeland, C., & Brion, F. (2008). Pharmacy education in France. *American Journal of Pharmaceutical Education*, *72*(6), 132.

Brodie, D. C., & Smith, W. E. (1985). Implications of new technology for pharmacy education and practice. *American Journal of Health-System Pharmacy*, *42*(1), 81–95 (accessed by the author as abstract).

Fathelrahman, A. I., Ibrahim, M. I. M., & Wertheimer, A. (Eds.), (2016). *Pharmacy Practice in Developing Countries: Achievements and Challenges*. London: Academic Press an Imprint of Elsevier Science (ISBN: 0128017112, 9780128017111).

Fox, B. I. (2011). Information technology and pharmacy education. *American Journal of Pharmaceutical Education*, *75*(5), 86.

International Pharmaceutical Federation—FIP. (2015). *Global pharmacy workforce: Trends Report* (2nd ed.). The Hague: International Pharmaceutical Federation.

International Pharmaceutical Federation—FIP. (2016). In *Statements on pharmacy and pharmaceutical sciences education. Global Conference on Pharmacy and Pharmaceutical Sciences Education*. http://www.fip.org/nanjing2016/ (Accessed 6 November 2017).

Katajavuori, N., Hakkarainen, K., Kuosa, T., Airaksinen, M., Hirvonen, J., & Holm, Y. (2009). Curriculum reform in Finnish pharmacy education. *American Journal of Pharmaceutical Education*, *73*(8), 151.

Kheir, N., Zaidan, M., Younes, H., El Hajj, M., Wilbur, K., & Jewesson, P. J. (2008). Pharmacy education and practice in 13 middle eastern countries. *Journal of Pharmaceutical Education*, *72*(6), 133.

Marriott, J. L., Nation, R. L., Roller, L., Costelloe, M., Galbraith, K., Stewart, P., et al. (2008). Pharmacy education in the context of Australian practice. *American Journal of Pharmaceutical Education*, *72*(6), 131.

Newble, D., & Cannon, R. (2002). *A handbook for medical teachers*. New York, Boston, Dordrecht, London, Moscow: Kluwer Academic Publishers.

Nona, D. A., & Wadelin, J. W. (1990). Pharmaceutical education in the 21st century. *Journal of Pharmacy Practice*, *3*(2), 69–79.

Petit, P., Foriers, A., & Rombaut, B. (2008). The introduction of new teaching methods in pharmacy education—I. Lessons learned from history. *Pharmacy Education*, *8*(1), 13–18.

Taylor, K. M., Bates, I. P., & Harding, G. (2004). The implications of increasing student numbers for pharmacy education. *Pharmacy Education*, *4*(1), 33–39.

SECTION I

DEFINING PHARMACY EDUCATION

CHAPTER

THE PHARMACY EDUCATION: A HISTORICAL PERSPECTIVE

2

Derek Stewart*, Donald E. Letendre†

**Robert Gordon University, Aberdeen, United Kingdom, †The University of Iowa College of Pharmacy, Iowa City, IA, United States*

Pharmacy education within the western world has undergone tremendous and revolutionary changes when compared to the periods of history in which pharmacy practice was focused largely on compounding-related activities. Today many higher education institutions provide an array of undergraduate and postgraduate pharmacy programs, with graduates being awarded qualifications ranging from bachelor's degrees to doctorates. This chapter provides the reader with an overview of the key historical developments in pharmacy education in the West, covering Europe and the United States.

KEY DEVELOPMENTS IN EUROPE

Within Europe, commonly the Master of Pharmacy (MPharm), Bachelor of Science (BSc) or Bachelor of Pharmacy (BPharm) are the university-level qualifications leading to registration with a regulatory or professional body. Taking Great Britain as an example, the General Pharmaceutical Council (GPhC) is now the independent regulator for pharmacists, pharmacy technicians, and pharmacy premises. In relation to the education of pharmacists, principal functions of GPhC include setting standards for education, approving qualifications for pharmacists, and accrediting university education providers (General Pharmaceutical Council, 2016a). This is a sharp contrast to the situation in the 1800s: in 1841 the Pharmaceutical Society of Great Britain was established with several functions, including developing professional education and training. At that time, membership and examinations were entirely voluntary, conferring no title or indeed privileges. In 1852, the first Pharmacy Act empowered the Society to award the title of Pharmaceutical Chemist to those passing the examinations. There was little substantial change until 1904, when the first BSc in pharmacy was offered by the University of Manchester, and it wasn't until 1970 that only graduates of bachelor's programs could progress toward registration as pharmacists. In 2001/2, there was another fundamental change when the 4-year MPharm became the only route to registration. This change was driven to demonstrate harmonizing pharmacist education and training across the European Union community and in response to a UK Government–led enquiry on the future of pharmacy (General Pharmaceutical Council, 2016b). Today, many universities also now offer programs at postgraduate levels (e.g., MSc, PharmD), the most popular of which are related to aspects of clinical pharmacy and pharmacy practice. Within Great Britain, apart from the MPharm, only those university programs leading to registration as a pharmacist independent prescriber are regulated by the GPhC (General Pharmaceutical Council, 2016c).

Pharmacy Education in the Twenty First Century and Beyond. https://doi.org/10.1016/B978-0-12-811909-9.00002-2

KEY DEVELOPMENTS IN THE UNITED STATES

In the United States a similar dramatic change in pharmacy education and postgraduate training has taken place over the past 200 years (Hepler, 1987; Higby, 1997; Holland & Nimmo, 1999). The first college to train pharmacists in the United States was founded in 1821 as the Philadelphia College of Pharmacy (Pennsylvania). In the ensuing years the length of pharmacy education evolved from a 2-year academic degree (Graduate in Pharmacy, PhG), to 3 years (Pharmaceutical Chemist, PhC), to four- and then 5-year Bachelor of Science in Pharmacy (BSPharm) degrees, with the latter serving as a compromise to an earlier drive towards the implementation of a universal Doctor of Pharmacy (PharmD), which would not occur until almost 40 years later. Interestingly, the profession tinkered with an early version of professional doctoral education when some institutions offered a short-lived Doctor of Pharmacy (PharmD) degree in the early part of the 20th century. Moreover, in stark contrast to the rest of the country, a few programs in California decided to implement a 6-year PharmD in the late 1950s and early 1960s rather than compromise on a 5-year BSc education (Fink III, 2012).

Dramatic changes began to occur during the 1960s as new methods of drug delivery emerged and the early vestiges of clinical pharmacy services (e.g., drug information, patient consultation) began to take hold, especially in the larger teaching hospitals. And then in the 1970s and throughout the 1980s post-BSc PharmD programs began to take hold, helping to further drive education and training. By the late 1990s the nearly 80 accredited colleges of pharmacy in the United States had implemented or were in the process of implementing the PharmD as the entry-level degree for the profession. This action was the result of decades of deliberations and included perspectives offered by academicians, practitioners, national pharmacy professional associations, employers, and the Accreditation Council for Pharmacy Education (ACPE) (2016), the body that has responsibility for overseeing the accreditation of all US pharmacy educational programs.

KEY DRIVERS, ENABLERS, AND INFLUENTIAL FACTORS

A vast range of drivers, enablers, and factors has influenced the progress made in pharmacy education in the West. These key influences include: regulatory standards for education; advances in pharmacological, therapeutic, and technological innovation coupled with changing societal needs and expectations; national and international policy drivers; and evidence generated through high-quality, robust, and rigorous research. Each of these will now be examined in more depth, with key examples across the West. It must, however, be appreciated that there is a symbiotic relationship between education and practice with each informing, stimulating, and enhancing the other. There are many examples of educational developments preceding and anticipating changing regulatory standards, therapeutic and technological innovation, population needs, and policy.

ACCREDITATION OF EDUCATION PROGRAMS IN EUROPE

The most significant drivers are the standards required by the organizations and bodies accrediting university programs. As noted previously, these standards themselves are informed by developments and innovation in pharmacist education, and academics (and others) are involved in standard setting, review, and accreditation processes. In Europe, accreditation is conducted largely at the national level, with the GPhC being the accreditation body for programs leading to the award of MPharm in Great Britain (prior to 2007, this function was performed by the Royal Pharmaceutical Society of Great Britain). Accreditation is performed according to a rigorous and well-defined methodology, underpinned by standards, including *Future pharmacists: standards for the initial education and training of pharmacists in Great Britain*. Ten standards are described (see Table 1) and each standard includes criteria, required evidence, and advice on meeting the standard (General Pharmaceutical Council, 2011).

The final standard, *Outcomes*, lists 58 outcomes in areas of: expectations of a pharmacy professional (9 outcomes); implementing health policy (8); validating therapeutic approaches and supplying prescribed and over-the-counter medicines (10); ensuring that safe and effective systems are in place to manage the risk inherent in the practice of pharmacy and the delivery of pharmaceutical services (15); working with patients and the public (8); and maintaining and improving professional performance (8). Each outcome is mapped to Miller's pyramid of knows, knows how, shows how, does (Miller, 1990).

While this is the approach of GPhC, there are European requirements for the initial education and training of pharmacists which must be met, as described in Directive 2005/36/EC of the European

Table 1 Description of the 10 GPhC Accreditation Standards (General Pharmaceutical Council, 2011)

Standard	Description
Patient and public safety	There must be clear procedures to address concerns about patient safety arising from initial pharmacy education and training. Concerns must be addressed immediately
Monitoring, review and evaluation of initial education and training	The quality of pharmacy education and training must be monitored, reviewed, and evaluated in a systematic and developmental way
Equality, diversity, and opportunity	Initial pharmacy education and training must be based on principles of equality, diversity, and fairness. It must meet the requirements of all relevant legislation
Selection of students	Selection processes must be open and fair and comply with relevant legislation. Processes must ensure that students and trainees are fit to practice as students or trainees at the point of selection. Selection includes recruitment and admissions
Curriculum delivery and the student experience	The curriculum for MPharm degrees (and the preregistration scheme) must deliver the outcomes in Standard 10. Most importantly, curricula must ensure that students and trainees practice safely and effectively. To ensure this, pass criteria must describe safe and effective practice
Support and development for students	Students must be supported to develop as learners and professionals during their initial education and training
Support and development for tutors and academic staff	Anyone delivering initial education and training should be supported to develop in their professional role
Management of initial education & training	Initial pharmacist education and training must be planned and maintained through transparent processes that must show who is responsible for what at each stage
Resources and capacity	Resources and capacity are sufficient to deliver outcomes
Outcomes	Outcomes for the initial education and training of pharmacists

Parliament (European Parliament, 2005). Section 7, Article A4 requires evidence of formal qualifications, as a pharmacist shall attest to training of at least 5 years' duration, including at least: 4 years of full-time theoretical and practical training at a university or at a higher institute of a level recognized as equivalent, or under the supervision of a university; and 6-month traineeship in a pharmacy which is open to the public or in a hospital, under the supervision of that hospital's pharmaceutical department. Furthermore, the United Kingdom is a signatory to the *Bologna Declaration*, designed to harmonize higher education qualifications across Europe. Pharmacist education is covered within this declaration and, for those 29 countries in Europe which are also signatories, the outcomes from university pharmacist training will be at the same academic level (European Ministers of Education, 1999).

ACCREDITATION OF EDUCATION PROGRAMS IN THE UNITED STATES

As noted earlier, ACPE serves the body that has responsibility for overseeing the accreditation of all US pharmacy educational programs. Founded as the American Council on Pharmaceutical Education (ACPE) in 1932, the agency's name was changed to the Accreditation Council for Pharmacy Education in 2003. ACPE's *Standards 2016* comprises 25 standards (see Table 2) that must be met in order to achieve accredited status. Standards 1–4 are focused on educational outcomes and describe areas where programs can experiment and innovate within the didactic and experiential components of their curricula to meet the required outcomes. The structure and process needed to promote achievement of the educational outcomes are found in Standards 5–23. Finally, standards 24 and 25 are centered on assessment of the standards and other key elements of maintaining a quality academic program. Intertwined throughout the didactic elements of the pharmacy education is the requirement that students begin to apply what they learn. Hence, from the very beginning students are required to engage in *introductory pharmacy practice experiences* (IPPEs) and then progress to *advanced pharmacy practice experiences* (APPEs) in the latter stages of the program.

Germane to the purpose of this publication is ACPE's International Services Program (ISP), which was established in February 2011. The ISP was created to strengthen ACPE's ability to assist international stakeholders who seek guidance related to quality assurance and advancement of pharmacy education.

ADVANCES IN PHARMACOLOGICAL, THERAPEUTIC, AND TECHNOLOGICAL INNOVATION

Rapid developments in medicine preparation and availability have largely removed the need for compounding-related activities in pharmacy practice, with these occurring mainly within specialized hospital and industrial units. Furthermore, technological advances in pharmacy such as pharmacy robotics and scanning devices are likely to revolutionize practice toward an even greater clinical, patient-facing focus, hence acting as enablers of change (Lichtner, Venters, Hibberd, Cornford, & Barber, 2013). Altering population demographics along with their needs and demands for healthcare generally, and medicines specifically, have also markedly impacted and will continue to impact pharmacy practice and hence the educational requirements of pharmacists. Multimorbidity, "the co-occurrence of two or more chronic medical conditions in one person" (World Health Organization, 2008), in older people

Table 2 Description of the ACPE Accreditation Standards (Accreditation Council for Pharmacy Education, 2016)

Standard	Description
Section I: Educational Outcomes	
1	Foundational Knowledge
2	Essentials for Practice and Care
3	Approach to Practice and Care
4	Personal and Professional Development
Section II: Structure and Process to Promote Achievement of Educational Outcomes	
5	Eligibility and Reporting Requirements
6	College or School Vision, Mission, and Goals
7	Strategic Plan
8	Organization and Governance
9	Organizational Culture
10	Curriculum Design, Delivery, and Oversight
11	Interprofessional Education (IPE)
12	Pre-Advanced Pharmacy Practice Experience (Pre-APPE) Curriculum
13	Advanced Pharmacy Practice Experience (APPE) Curriculum
14	Student Services
15	Academic Environment
16	Admissions
17	Progression
18	Faculty and Staff—Quantitative Factors
19	Faculty and Staff—Qualitative Factors
20	Preceptors
21	Physical Facilities and Educational Resources
22	Practice Facilities
23	Financial Resources
Section III: Assessment of Standards and Key Elements	
24	Assessment Elements for Section I: Educational Outcomes
25	Assessment Elements for Section II: Structure and Process

is becoming the norm, being prevalent in almost two-thirds of individuals aged 80 years and over (Barnett et al., 2012; Ornstein, Nietert, Jenkins, & Litvin, 2013). Consequences of multimorbidity include increased use of health services, poorer quality of life, and high economic burden (Boyd & Martin Fortin, 2010; van den Bussche et al., 2011). UK data from 2014 highlight the use of medicines in older people, with one-fifth of those with two clinical conditions prescribed four to nine medicines, and one-tenth prescribed ten or more medicines; in those with six or more comorbidities, values were just under half (Payne et al., 2014). Data from the United States are similar in that, between 1999 and 2012, prescribing of five or more medicines increased from one quarter to just under one half of those aged 65 years and above (Dwyer, Han, Woodwell, & Rechtsteiner, 2010; Kantor, Rehm, Haas, Chan, & Giovannucci, 2015). This global trend requires pharmacists educated not for compounding but who are competent to optimize all aspects of medicine use.

NATIONAL AND INTERNATIONAL POLICY DRIVERS

National and international reports, strategies and policies for healthcare have also acted as key drivers in pharmacist education in the West. One notable driver in the United Kingdom was the Government-led *Nuffield Report* (*Nuffield Foundation Pharmacy Inquiry*) of 1986, the main conclusion of which was that "the pharmacy profession has a distinctive and indispensable contribution to make to health care that is capable of still further development" and that while pharmacists could play a "unique and vital role" in healthcare, their potential was not being realized (Nuffield Committee of Inquiry Pharmacy, 1986). The main recommendation was a transition from pharmacist involvement in the mechanics of dispensing to a much more clinically and patient-focused role. This report, along with other key developments including the landmark philosophy of *pharmaceutical care* described by Hepler and Strand (1990) and hospital-based clinical practice, was a key stimulus to the increased clinical focus for pharmacist training at undergraduate and postgraduate levels. Similarly, Government strategy and policy highlights the pharmacist role in areas of public health, caring for patients with long-term conditions, supporting self-care, and managing minor ailments to both enhance care and reduce pressures on the healthcare system (Department of Health, 2008): for example, within Scotland, the launch of *Prescription for Excellence: A Vision and Action Plan for the right pharmaceutical care through integrated partnerships and innovation* by the Scottish Government. The vision articulated within this document is that by 2023, "all pharmacists providing National Health Service (NHS) pharmaceutical care will be NHS accredited clinical pharmacist independent prescribers working in collaborative partnerships with medical practitioners who will continue to have overall responsibility for diagnosis (The Scottish Government, 2014). Independent prescribing by pharmacists (and other suitably trained health professionals) was introduced in 2006. Defined as "prescribing by a practitioner (e.g., doctor, dentist, nurse, pharmacist) responsible and accountable for the assessment of patients with undiagnosed or diagnosed conditions and for decisions about the clinical management required, including prescribing" (Department of Health, 2006), this allows pharmacist independent prescribers to prescribe, within their competence, the same range of medicines as doctors. University educational programs for pharmacist prescribers are regulated by the GPhC (General Pharmaceutical Council, 2016c). There are key implications for pharmacist education at all levels in order to realize the ambitions of *Prescription for Excellence*.

Throughout the United States and Canada, changes in pharmacy practice in recent decades have had an uncanny link to postgraduate residency training. In fact, key opinion leaders have suggested that the single greatest driver of practice change in North America has been the growth and development of residency training programs (Letendre, 1992; Letendre, Brooks, & Degenhart, 1995). First established as a means to address shortcomings in education that were required to practice in hospitals, residencies have evolved throughout the past 50 or more years from product production/drug delivery training programs to ones that require a broad range of experiences that serve to mimic the extensive breadth of practice elements that comprise contemporary pharmacy practice. Not surprisingly, the growth and changes that have occurred in residency training during this timeframe have coincided with the rapid progress that has been achieved through technological advances, the widespread introduction of clinical pharmacy services, emergence of specialization and Board certification, and increasingly greater adoption of concepts like "pharmacist interdependent prescribing" that recognize improved outcomes in patient care (Abramowitz, Shane, Daigle, Noonan, & Letendre, 2012). Clearly, the graduates of residency training, who now number in the tens of thousands, have undoubtedly become pharmacy's "disciples of change" throughout North America and have served to complement the tremendous advances witnessed in pharmacy education, practice, and applied clinical science.

ROBUST AND RIGOROUS RESEARCH EVIDENCE

Evidence generated through high-quality, robust, and rigorous research is also a major driver and enabler in progressive education. Healthcare is influenced greatly by evidence-based approaches to pharmacologically based therapeutics. Evidence-based approaches to pharmacy practice are emerging along with literature describing evidence of educational approaches themselves, all of which should influence student learning. The curriculum in the West is now vast and diverse, typically encompassing: learning based on experience that provides clinical and scientific education in a range of practices and procedures; interprofessional practice; demonstration of behaviors, attitudes, and values commensurate with professional practice; research integrating theory and practice; and reflection on learning and practice. The diversity is clear from the range of scientific fields that students must grasp and assimilate, ranging from traditional sciences to behavioral sciences and areas of pharmacy practice. Approaches to curriculum design are now much more comprehensive, robust, and rigorous and while there are many approaches, one commonly applied is the *Systems Approach to Curriculum Development*. The main paths in this approach are to: consider the target population characteristics and topic area; estimate the relevant existing skills and knowledge of learners; formulate objectives/learning outcomes; select appropriate instructional methods; operate the course or curriculum; and assess and evaluate (Brown, 1995). There is a great need to integrate the aspects of pharmaceutical sciences to clinical practice. Harden describes a ladder with 11 points on a continuum between the two extremes of isolation (integration is not explicitly facilitated and is left to students themselves) and transdisciplinary (the curriculum transcends the individual disciplines). While it may be unrealistic (and perhaps inappropriate) to have a course entirely transdisciplinary, it is no longer acceptable for students to learn science and practice in isolation (Harden, 2000). Cognizance must also be taken of how students learn, with consideration of those who are predominately: activists (love novelty, and will "try anything once"); reflectors (like to collect information and sift it); theorists (want to know the logic of actions and observations) and pragmatists (keen on ideas, bur want to try them out to see if they work) (Kolb & Kolb, 2005). Methods of course delivery and assessment in the West have also transformed radically from the traditional didactic lecture and examination as the norm. Approaches such as problem-based learning, team-based learning, experiential learning, interprofessional learning, and internships are now commonplace (Michaelsen & Sweet, 2011; Parsell & Bligh, 1998). The focus on the written examination as the sole method of assessment has shifted, with the assessments aligning to the learning outcomes and objectives and now also including objective structured clinical (performance) examinations, competency-based assessments, oral assessments, and assessment of internship performance. Many of these developments will be considered in later chapters.

CONCLUSION

In conclusion, pharmacy education in the West has undergone transformational change as a result of very many different and interacting enablers, drivers, and changes. These influences are likely to continue to place demands on educators to ensure that programs prepare students for the ever-changing world of pharmacy practice.

REFERENCES

Abramowitz, P. W., Shane, R., Daigle, L. A., Noonan, K. A., & Letendre, D. E. (2012). Pharmacist interdependent prescribing: a new model for optimizing patient outcomes. *American Journal of Health-System Pharmacy, 69*, 1976–1981.

Accreditation Council for Pharmacy Education (ACPE). (2016). *Accreditation standards and key elements for the professional program in pharmacy leading to the doctor of pharmacy degree.* Chicago, IL: ACPE-accredit.org.

Barnett, K., Mercer, S. W., Norbury, M., Watt, G., Wyke, S., & Guthrie, B. (2012). Epidemiology of multimorbidity and implications for healthcare, research, and medical education: a cross sectional study. *Lancet, 380*, 37–43.

Boyd, C., & Martin Fortin, M. D. (2010). Future of multimorbidity research: how should understanding of multimorbidity inform health system designs? *Public Health Reviews, 32*, 451–474.

Brown, J. D. (1995). *The elements of language curriculum: A systematic approach to program development.* Boston, MA: Heinle & Heinle Publishers. 02116.

Department of Health. (2006). *Improving patients' access to medicines: a guide to implementing nurse and pharmacist independent prescribing within the NHS in England* [online]. London: UK Department of Health. Available from: http://webarchive.nationalarchives.gov.uk/+/www.dh.gov.uk/en/PublicationsandStatistics/Publications/PublicationsPolicyandGuidance/DH_4133743 [Accessed December 2016].

Department of Health. (2008). *Pharmacy in England: building on strengths—delivering the future (white paper).* Available on-line at: https://www.gov.uk/government/uploads/system/uploads/attachment_data/file/228858/7341.pdf [Accessed December 2016].

Dwyer, L. L., Han, B., Woodwell, D. A., & Rechtsteiner, E. A. (2010). Polypharmacy in nursing home residents in the United States: results of the 2004 National Nursing Home Survey. *The American Journal of Geriatric Pharmacotherapy, 8*(1), 63–72.

European Ministers of Education. (1999). *Bologna Declaration (Joint declaration of the European Ministers of Education).* Available at: http://www.ifa.de/fileadmin/pdf/abk/inter/ec_bologna.pdf. [Accessed December 2016].

European Parliament. (2005). Directive 2005/36/EC of the European Parliament and of the Council on the recognition of professional qualifications. *Official Journal of the European Union L.* 255/22.

Fink, J. L., III. (2012). *Pharmacy: a brief history of the profession. In The student doctor network.* Available at: https://www.studentdoctor.net/2012/01/pharmacy-a-brief-history-of-the-profession/. [Accessed December 2016].

General Pharmaceutical Council. (2011). *Future pharmacists. Standards for the initial education and training of pharmacists.* Available from: https://www.pharmacyregulation.org/sites/default/files/GPhC_Future_Pharmacists.pdf. [Accessed December 2016].

General Pharmaceutical Council. (2016a). Available from: https://www.pharmacyregulation.org/ [Accessed December 2016].

General Pharmaceutical Council. (2016b). *Historic qualifications leading to eligibility to be admitted to the Register and to Membership of the (Royal) Pharmaceutical Society of Great Britain.* Available from: https://www.pharmacyregulation.org/sites/default/files/Historic%20qualifications%20g.pdf [Accessed December 2016].

General Pharmaceutical Council. (2016c). *Pharmacist independent prescribing programme—Learning outcomes and indicative content*. Available from: https://www.pharmacyregulation.org/education/pharmacist-independent-prescriber. [Accessed December 2016].

Harden, R. M. (2000). The integration ladder: a tool for curriculum planning and evaluation. *Medical Education*, *34*(7), 551–557.

Hepler, C. D. (1987). The third wave in pharmaceutical education: the clinical movement. *American Journal of Pharmaceutical Education*, *51*, 369–385.

Hepler, C. D., & Strand, L. M. (1990). Opportunities and responsibilities in pharmaceutical care. *American Journal of Hospital Pharmacy*, *47*(3), 533–543.

Higby, G. J. (1997). American pharmacy in the twentieth century. *American Journal of Health-System Pharmacy*, *54*, 1805–1815.

Holland, R. W., & Nimmo, C. M. (1999). Transitions, part 1: beyond pharmaceutical care. *American Journal of Health-System Pharmacy*, *56*, 1758–1764.

Kantor, E. D., Rehm, C. D., Haas, J. S., Chan, A. T., & Giovannucci, E. L. (2015). Trends in prescription drug use among adults in the United States from 1999 to 2012. *JAMA*, *314*(17), 1818–1830.

Kolb, A. Y., & Kolb, D. A. (2005). Learning styles and learning spaces: enhancing experiential learning in higher education. *Academy of Management Learning & Education*, *4*(2), 193–212.

Letendre, D. E., Brooks, P. J., & Degenhart, M. L. (1995). The evolution of pharmacy residency training programs and corresponding standards of accreditation. *Pharmacy Practice Management Quarterly*, *15*(2), 30–43.

Letendre, D. E. (1992). Reflections on the future of pharmacy residency programs: an ASHP perspective. *American Journal of Pharmaceutical Education*, *56*, 298–300.

Lichtner, V., Venters, W., Hibberd, R., Cornford, T., & Barber, N. (2013). The fungibility of time in claims of efficiency: the case of making transmission of prescriptions electronic in English general practice. *International Journal of Medical Information*, *82*(12), 1152–1170.

Michaelsen, L. K., & Sweet, M. (2011). Team-based learning. *New Directions for Teaching and Learning*, (128), 41–51.

Miller, G. E. (1990). The assessment of clinical skills/competence/performance. *Academic Medicine*, *65*(9), S63–7.

Nuffield Committee of Inquiry Pharmacy (1986). A Report to the National Foundation. Available from: http://hansard.millbanksystems.com/lords/1986/jun/04/pharmacy-nuffield-foundation-report [Accessed December 2016].

Ornstein, S. M., Nietert, P. J., Jenkins, R. G., & Litvin, C. B. (2013). The prevalence of chronic diseases and multimorbidity in primary care practice: a PPRNet report. *Journal of the American Board of Family Practice*, *26*, 518–524.

Parsell, G., & Bligh, J. (1998). Interprofessional learning. *Postgraduate Medical Journal*, *74*(868), 89–95.

Payne, R. A., Avery, A. J., Duerden, M., Saunders, C. L., Simpson, C. R., & Abel, G. A. (2014). Prevalence of polypharmacy in a Scottish primary care population. *European Journal of Clinical Pharmacology*, *70*(5), 575–581.

The Scottish Government. (2014). *Prescription for Excellence, Edinburgh*. Available from: http://www.scotland.gov.uk/Topics/Health/Policy/Prescription-for-Excellence. [Accessed December 2016].

van den Bussche, H., Schön, G., Kolonko, T., Hansen, H., Wegscheider, K., Glaeske, G., et al. (2011). Patterns of ambulatory medical care utilisation in elderly patients with special reference to chronic diseases and multimorbidity—Results from a claims data based observational study in Germany. *BMC Geriatrics*, *11*, 54.

World Health Organization. (2008). *The World Health Report. Primary Health Care—Now more than ever*. New York: The World Health Organization. ISBN 978 92 4 156373 4.

FURTHER READING

Barrows, H. S. (1996). Problem-based learning in medicine and beyond: a brief overview. *New Directions for Teaching and Learning*, (68), 3–12.

Cope, C. P., Abuzour, A. S., & Tully, M. P. (2016). Nonmedical prescribing: where are we now? *Therapeutic Advances in Drug Safety*, *7*, 165–172.

Stewart, D., MacLure, K., & George, J. (2012). Educating non-medical prescribers. *British Journal of Clinical Pharmacology*, *74*, 662–667.

CHAPTER

PHILOSOPHY, THEORIES, MODELS, AND STRATEGIES IN PHARMACY EDUCATION: AN OVERVIEW

3

Mohamed Izham Mohamed Ibrahim
College of Pharmacy, Qatar University, Doha, Qatar

INTRODUCTION

Pharmacy education has a very important role in determining the quality of pharmacists who will work for the community in the future. It has the ability to transform the profession into a patient-centered one. Pharmacy education worldwide has undergone substantial evolution in recent years to develop professional pharmacy competences and to meet the changing roles of pharmacists in the healthcare setting.

Education is derived from the Latin word *educare* meaning “bring up”; *educere* meaning “bring out potential”; and *ducere* meaning “to lead” (Bass & Good, 2004). Education is a system through which society creates change, and it is a changing environment driven by the goals to improve students’ (learners’) educational experience. A great need exists for revolution and renovation in the education and training of pharmacy students, practitioners, researchers, and regulators due to the rapid and dynamic progress in healthcare, e.g., progress in medical technology and the development of new pharmaceuticals. Regardless of the workplace, pharmacists are required to develop their expertise, cope with rapidly increasing amounts of information, and assume important roles in patient care. The issue of globalization has also forced pharmacists to face challenges in healthcare and to meet the expectations of the public and other stakeholders. Introductory and advanced pharmacy practice is fundamental to future pharmacists’ education and training. There is a continuous pressing need for pharmacy colleges to continuously upgrade the quality of their education and training to produce the best pharmacy graduates. The minimum level of education that pharmacy colleges must provide to broaden students’ scope of practice includes a wide range of clinical, patient-centered, and public health promotion skills in areas such as medication therapy management, disease management, preventive health care, immunization therapy and wellness care. In addition to classroom coursework, pharmacists’ education should be experiential in nature, i.e., learning at practice sites such as hospitals, community pharmacies, primary health care settings, and outpatient clinics. Pharmacy colleges must shift the educational paradigm to align with the evolving role of the pharmacy profession. Highly demanding preparation is required to reach a professional status.

Pharmacy Education in the Twenty First Century and Beyond. https://doi.org/10.1016/B978-0-12-811909-9.00003-4

A well-rounded student is shaped by various factors, such as the quality of the college to which the student is admitted, the environment of the college or university at which the student lives and studies, the curriculum of the professional program attended, and the effectiveness of the teaching style and strategies experienced. The student's outcomes and impact on clients, e.g., patients and society, very much depend on these factors. In addition, pharmacy educators play a highly significant role in molding the student. Educators must have the required qualifications, be well trained and experienced, hold a certain specialization, and possess teaching knowledge and skills.

A few critical questions in relation to pharmacy education need to be addressed: Have pharmacy colleges reached a minimum standard that produces quality graduates? Is pharmacy college education focused on patient care and aimed at producing competent pharmacists who are prepared to collaborate with other healthcare professionals in maximizing the benefits from the use of medications? Do pharmacy colleges prepare students to accept responsibility and accountability for the overall care of the patient? Does a theory-practice gap appear in pharmacy professional education?

It is often described that students experience a gap between their academic learning at university or college and the realities of practice during their practicum in, e.g., schools and healthcare institutions.

PHILOSOPHY, THEORIES, AND MODELS IN EDUCATION

Education and learning are built from various philosophies, theories, and models. Educational philosophy is the application of different aspects of philosophy in education. Education is greatly affected by both the theoretical and practical aspects of philosophy, e.g., educational policies, curriculum, methods of teaching, educators, discipline, assessment, and behavior. The theories describe the ways in which adults assimilate knowledge, skills and attitudes. Education theory seeks to prescribe educational policy and practice. Models of teaching address the approaches in which learning environments and instructional experiences can be constructed, sequenced or presented (Joyce, Weil, & Calhoun, 2000). According to Maker (1982), a teaching-learning model is "a structural framework that serves as a guide for developing specific educational activities and environments". Education is the process of how we impart and transmit knowledge in human society. It is also about how we think, plan, and organize to accomplish that important task. It is simply a process to make individuals better people. In contrast, learning is defined as "a process that brings together personal and environmental experiences and influences for acquiring, enriching or modifying one's knowledge, skills, values, attitudes, behavior and world views" (UNESCO, n.d.). It involves relatively permanent changes in knowledge, skills, behavior, or attitudes resulting from recognizable psychological or social experiences (Burns, 1995; Seifert & Sutton, 2009). Learning theories are conceptual frameworks that explain how knowledge is assimilated, processed, and retained during learning.

What learning models and theories could be used by pharmacy educators to shape pharmacy students and produce high-quality graduates? Do the models and theories differ at various levels/years of schooling, disciplines (e.g., basic sciences, clinical), and degree programs (e.g., baccalaureate, master's, doctoral)?

Why should we consider learning theories? Learning theories are used to conceptualize pharmacy education system arrangement in the classroom and clinical training incorporated into pharmacy education. Understanding learning theories is important in pharmacy education; it supports academic institutions in providing a proper setting for learning, thereby increasing the education system efficiency and harmonization in education (Joyce et al., 2000). Learning theories have tried to deliver explanations about learning and their use in pharmacy education (Basavanthappa, 2009). By acknowledging the individual differences among learners and by understanding relevant theories, pharmacy educators could work towards providing effective activities and strategies in educational programs. Pharmacy professions need to employ the regular use of theories and clear reasoning in educational activities. According to Ormrod (1995), patterns of teaching reflect the main philosophical and psychological orientation into teaching and learning. They all have a concrete theoretical basis and describe the learning environment (Ormrod, 1995).

For student learning, models are used as tools; they are appropriate for application development, especially for students whose record of learning should be considered. Quinn (2007) mentioned that each model comprises all elements of teaching as well as the overall goal, partial goals, content, behavior, methods, knowledge evaluation, media, and prior knowledge of students. Learning also enables pharmacists to devise and learn more effective approaches to educating and treating patients and each other in partnership.

It is important to identify the theory that can inform practice. There is still gap between educators and practitioners. Several theories can guide educators' teaching practices; one theory is better than others in a particular context. The principles generated from these theories and models can provide assistance for pharmacy educators.

Theories of learning encompass a wide range of philosophical perspectives, and there are several such theories (Berkeley Graduate Division, n.d.). First, the three basic types of learning theories are behaviorism, cognitive constructivism (also known as cognitive information processing), and social constructivism (Joyce, Weil, & Calhoun, 2005). Table 1 outlines the differences in these learning theories.

BEHAVIORISM

Behaviorist teaching methods have proven most successful in areas where there is a "correct" response or easily memorized material. This is called book-type learning, and it assumes a student is essentially passive. According to this theory, learning is a change in behavior. Behaviors can be learned, unlearned, and relearned, and students are shaped through positive or negative reinforcement. This type of learning emphasizes rewards and punishments. It is effective in easing learning that involves defining and illustrating concepts, recalling facts, applying explanations, and automatically performing an identified method. This type of learning tends to focus on what the lecturer does rather than the student. The effectiveness of behaviorist training methods depends strongly on the student's motivation. The following are examples and applications of behaviorist learning theory:

1. Repetitive practice: e.g., memorizing a fact. Students will easily recall a fact the more they repeat it; often, students memorize material without understanding the reasoning or relationships involved.
2. Making rules: e.g., students need to be punctual and be at a 50-min class on time. The maximum absenteeism is 25%, and whoever exceeds that will be barred from the final examination. Students who are absent because of illness need to present a medical note.
3. Positive (i.e., reward) reinforcement: e.g., providing incentives to do more or to participate, such as giving bonus points or marks. Teachers provide praise as verbal reinforcement, such as saying "Excellent! Your studying really paid off. That's a good mark on your midterm test." Certain

Table 1 Differences in Learning Theories (Joyce et al., 2005)

	Behaviorism	Cognitive Constructivism	Social Constructivism
View of knowledge	Knowledge is a repertoire of behavioral responses to environmental stimuli	Knowledge systems of cognitive structures are actively constructed by learners based on preexisting cognitive structures	Knowledge is constructed within social contexts through interactions with a knowledge community
View of learning	Passive absorption of a predefined body of knowledge by the learner. Promoted by repetition and positive reinforcement	Active assimilation and accommodation of new information to existing cognitive structures. Discovery by learners	Integration of students into a knowledge community; collaborative assimilation and accommodation of new information
View of motivation	Extrinsic, involving positive and negative reinforcement	Intrinsic; learners set their own goals and motivate themselves to learn	Intrinsic and extrinsic; learning goals and motives are determined by both learners and extrinsic rewards provided by the knowledge community
Implications for teaching	Correct behavioral responses are transmitted by the educator and absorbed by the students	The educator facilitates learning by providing an environment that promotes discovery and assimilation/ accommodation	Collaborative learning is facilitated and guided by the educator; group work

behavior follows, and it is possible that the behavior will be repeated. Students who are active and provide correct or good answers are praised, and the quality of their projects/assignments is acknowledged. Students who win awards at oral and poster competitions are praised and acknowledged by the Dean. Students are listed on the Dean's list if they achieve a cGPA of 3.5 or above.

4. Negative (i.e., punishment) reinforcement: e.g., marks will be deducted if students submit an assignment after the deadline; plagiarized assignments are given a "0" mark.

Behaviorist instruction does not prepare learners for problem solving or creative thinking (The Peak Performance Center, n.d.). Students do what they are asked and do not take any initiative to improve things or change. Students are prepared for the recall of basic facts, the performance of tasks, or automatic responses.

COGNITIVISM

The second theory includes cognitivist teaching methods. The purpose is to assist students in integrating new information with their existing knowledge and to allow them to make the appropriate changes to their existing intellectual framework in order to accommodate that information. It concentrates on what occurs in the mind, such as thinking, understanding, organizing, consciousness, and problem solving. The student's mind works as a mirror that reflects new knowledge and skills. Information processing leads to understanding and retention. According to Dale (1996), 90% of students' retention of material is "what they say and do." It is important that students play an active role in looking for ways to understand and process information that they obtain and link it to what is already known and stored within their memory. It is not just a change in behavior. The following are examples and applications of cognitive learning theory related to teaching methods:

1. Classifying information: e.g., classifying types of processes or events (in pharmacy management classes, students must classify community pharmacy assets into tangible and intangible).
2. Linking concepts: e.g., masters and doctoral students need to build a research conceptual framework that links different concepts to establish their research hypotheses.
3. Organizing lectures in efficient and meaningful ways: e.g., in an integrated curriculum, teachers should organize their lectures, allowing students to link the different pharmacy disciplines and link basic knowledge and applied knowledge.
4. Providing real-world examples: e.g., when teaching the topic of quality of medicines, such as problems with substandard and counterfeit medicines, students will be provided with statistics and cases of the worldwide prevalence of counterfeit medicines, and they need to suggest steps to take to control the situation.
5. Discussion: e.g., students are given a clinical case of an inpatient, discuss the conditions and recommend treatment using the pharmaceutical diagnosis approach.
6. Problem solving: e.g., students are given a case and data set to be solved using statistical methods and SPSS software; students construct a line graph/correlation to illustrate information given in a clinical case; students are given a clinical case and use pharmacotherapeutic problem-solving methods, such as pharmaceutical diagnoses, that provide an organizational structure to the delivery of direct patient care responsibilities.
7. Providing analogies: e.g., explaining pharmacodynamics concepts to students, such as how drugs work in the body (the relationships among the drug, receptor, and signal); this can be explained using a lock-and-key metaphor.
8. Providing pictures and models: e.g., pictures and models make teaching and learning interesting in pharmacy. For instance, in teaching medicinal chemistry, using a model of the chemical structure with animation and visualization may help students grasp it better if they see a graphical/visual demonstration, or students may better understand physiological processes through the use of a diagram.
9. Creating mnemonics: e.g., making good research objectives based on SMART (**S**pecific, **M**easurable, **A**ttainable, **R**esearchable, **T**ime-bound) principles or using I ESCAPED CPR, which stands for **I**nteractions, **E**fficacy, **S**ide effects, **C**ontraindications, **A**llergies, **P**regnancy, **E**limination, **D**ose, **C**ompliance, **P**urpose, and **R**oute (Bruno, Ip, Shah, & Linn, 2012) as a patient-focused tool that offers a simple way to remember important things when evaluating patient drug therapy.

SOCIAL CONSTRUCTIVISM

Next is (social) constructivism. According to this theory, learning is not just about acquiring knowledge but about participating in an active, contextualized process of constructing knowledge. Individual experiences are important in constructing knowledge. The level of potential advancement is the level at which learning takes place. It encompasses cognitive structures that are still in the process of maturing. However, they can mature only under the guidance of or in collaboration with others. Constructivist theory challenges the belief that learning is something that can be delivered by an educator transferring facts or knowledge to a group of passive recipient learners. Based on this theory, knowledge, meaning, and understanding are actively constructed by learners through a process of development. They build on what they already know, and they change and adapt and invent ideas. In practical terms, in a classroom where teaching is carried out in alignment with constructivist theory, the educator's role is not to deliver facts. Rather, the educator must provide learners with stimuli and experience, which then allows them to pose their own questions, hypothesize, explore, predict, and investigate knowledge for themselves. By directing their own learning process, learners understand difficult concepts better. Educators should involve students in their learning in an active way, e.g., learning through interactions with other people, such as peers and preceptors (also called social learning). Educators should use relevant problems and group interaction, and they should give adequate time to students for in-depth examination of new experiences.

This theory focuses on preparing people to solve problems. Within this theory, outcomes are not always predictable because students are creating their own knowledge. Therefore, when the results always need to be consistent, this theory fails to work. Examples and applications in teaching methods are the following:

1. Case studies: e.g., clinical cases and presentations. The following is an example of a clinical problem-solving and clinical reasoning exercise: A student has to obtain the case of a patient, study the case, determine the desired clinical outcomes, identify/prevent/solve drug-related problems, prepare for a presentation and organize all the information collected from the patient and the patient's medical records (Onishi, 2008).
2. Research project: e.g., students develop a validated questionnaire in a final-year research project to gather information based on the study objectives.
3. Problem-based learning (PBL): PBL is a student-focused teaching approach. PBL can use clinical cases to stimulate inquiry, critical thinking, and knowledge application and integration related to pharmaceutical sciences, and clinical and administrative pharmacy topics. PBL can be used in lab-based sessions to encourage self-directed learning and active intellectual processes with small-group discussions assisted by facilitators to solve problems—for example, taking into consideration the solubility and isotonicity aspects of a pharmaceutical solution before dispensing it to a patient.
4. Small-group work: e.g., in a Pharmacy Management course, four to five students are grouped together and work on developing a pharmacy business plan for setting up a new community pharmacy. A well-planned assignment promotes collaborative, cooperative, active, and independent learning and facilitates the development of critical thinking, communication, and decision-making skills.
5. Simulations: e.g., using simulated patients during Objective Structured Clinical Examination sessions for a clinical case scenario. The sessions can be video recorded. Simulation-based learning can be the method to build up health professionals' knowledge, skills, and attitudes while protecting patients from unnecessary risk. Using a simulation model in a laboratory experiment imitates real-world activities and processes but in a safe environment; it is a form of experiential learning (Lateef, 2010).

6. Brainstorming: e.g., creating a session to generate ideas or find solutions to a problem, creating value-added services in a pharmacy, or determining how best to ensure access to quality medicines in a country, especially in rural areas.
7. Action learning: e.g., hospital pharmacy organizations face several challenges, i.e., internal and external pressures. The hospital financial budget is tight, and the pharmacy department is requested to cut costs but still provide quality and cost-effective services to clients. Action learning involves small groups of students working on real and complex problems, taking action, and resolving the problems.
8. Laboratory work: e.g., students extract a compound from a traditional plant in a pharmaceutical chemistry lab or prepare a paracetamol suspension in a pharmaceutical lab. Students can develop scientific reasoning abilities, understand the complexity of empirical work, develop practical skills, and improve their teamwork abilities (Gitomer & Zisk, 2014).
9. Experiential learning: e.g., pharmacy colleges incorporate experiential learning into all years of study with students working in pharmacy-based settings such as hospitals; it emphasizes the integration of science (i.e., what is learned in the university) and practice (i.e., what is and should be done in healthcare institutional settings). Students will participate fully in the pharmacy and all aspects of patient care (Boyter & Winn, 2015).
10. Role play: e.g., involving students in a smoking cessation training program or any pharmaceutical care activities. Students interact with an asthmatic patient who is also a chain smoker. This is a good approach to develop skills in active listening, problem solving, teamwork, effective communication, consultation, and knowledge acquisition (Rao, 2011).
11. Debate: e.g., involve students in debating about ethical issues in health and pharmacy. This is an approach where opposing arguments are put forward. It is also an effective way to introduce complex and controversial matters in pharmacy and health into teaching, to enhance learning, to understand the course content, and to engage in learning (Hanna et al., 2014).

In addition to these three basic theories, there are a few more theories that are important and applicable in pharmacy (Stanford University, n.d.).

EXPERIENTIAL LEARNING

Experiential learning is about learners experiencing things for themselves and learning from these experiences. Kolb (1984) proposed a four-stage model known as the experiential learning cycle. Learners modify their behavior after understanding and learning their experiences. The model is based on the idea that the more repeatedly learners reflect on a task, the more chances they have to modify and improve their efforts. This theory suggests that people will continue to repeat their mistakes without reflection. It involves four stages: the doing stage, the thinking stage (i.e., what learners have done), the planning stage (i.e., how learners will do it differently), and the redoing stage (i.e., based upon experience and reflection). Experiential learning theory is categorized under the domain of constructivism. It is the most applicable to the concept of an integrated pharmacy program. Learners are put in an interactive environment, work in a team, learn by doing and are involved in problem-solving activities such as internships, housemanship, practicums, studying abroad in an exchange program, and volunteering in a nonprofit organization for community service. This approach is also suitable for interprofessional education.

Example

Students are given a case of a female patient who experienced chest pain while driving her car. She was brought to the Accident and Emergency Unit, admitted to the Cardiology Critical Unit and later transferred to the cardiology ward. This case requires a collaborative care approach that involves at least a physician, pharmacist, nurse, respiratory therapist, and dietician. Pharmacy students need to complete the relevant assessments and interventions and intervene appropriately. They are expected to communicate, consult, and work with the health team as required.

ANDRAGOGY

Andragogy is about informal teaching (i.e., student-focused approaches that adopt discussion and group work). Andragogy is "the art and science of helping adults learn" (Knowles and Associates, 1984). Knowles provided seven guiding principles on how to teach learners who tend to be independent and self-directed to at least some degree. Self-directed learning can be viewed as a method of organizing teaching and learning in which the learning tasks are largely within the learners' control. Learners strive to become empowered to accept responsibility and to have personal autonomy and choice. Many positive characteristics have been identified as being associated with self-direction. Self-directed learning skills can be developed through, for example, critically appraising new information, identifying learners' gaps in knowledge and skills, and asking questions. Andragogy emphasizes what the student is doing and the student's experiences and knowledge; it is highly engaging and interactive. Moreover, this approach concentrates on learning from others' experience and knowledge. It is built on five assumptions about adult learning:

- Adults are independent and self-directing.
- Adults have accumulated a great deal of experience, which is a rich resource for learning.
- Adults value learning that integrates with the demands of their everyday life.
- Adults are more interested in immediate and problem-focused approaches.
- Adults are more motivated to learn by internal drives than by external ones.

Example

In a self-directed learning course, at the master's and doctoral levels, students should be independent and learn what they are supposed to learn. The supervisor will guide them and provide the skills and support to become a self-directed and confident adult learner. For postgraduate researchers, the supervisor will at least provide the scope and topic of the research. It is the role and initiative of the students to search for information through literature search, develop the study proposal and protocol, execute the study, interpret and discuss the findings, prepare their thesis, and defend their work. Students are responsible for achieving the required competencies.

ACTION LEARNING

Action learning is a process of learning by doing (IFAL, n.d.; McGill & Beaty, 2002). It focuses on solutions to real problems. Learning is a function of programmed knowledge (e.g., traditional instruction) and questioning insight. Group members learn through reflective action, thereby improving their learning capabilities to solve and manage problems (Han, Zhang, Zhan, et al., 2016). It is a process of continuous reflection and learning that is supported by colleagues, with the goal of completing the intended work. The characteristics of action learning are reflectivity, cooperativeness, and subjectivity.

Example

Pharmacy students, as volunteers, join the Red Crescent and WHO team during a natural disaster, e.g., an earthquake or tsunami. It involves real people in real time in an urgent and emergency situation. It interrelates the learning environment with the workplace (e.g., in an institutional setting or community setting).

PRAGMATISM

This theory places the student, rather than the educator, as the focus (Graduate School University of Leicester, n.d.). Learning is facilitated through promoting various activities, and the traditional educator-focused method is not viewed as effective. Using different delivery methods, blended with practical activities, will help reach the different learning preferences of various learners. Activities can be carried out using case studies, problem solving and discussion. This theory values action.

Example

Students are provided with a problem on medication adherence and are asked to provide solutions on how to address this matter. Medication nonadherence is a challenging issue in health and pharmacy. There are many strategies used to overcome it. Pragmatists try their ideas and suggest techniques in practice. These kinds of students always believe there is a better way to do a task.

SENSORY THEORY

It is suggested that learning occurs when the senses of touch, hearing, sight, smell, and taste are stimulated (Laird, 1985). According to Laird (1985), most of the knowledge (75%) possessed by adults is learned through seeing. Educators need to make the teaching sessions interesting and memorable, e.g., facilitating practical activities in labs, using videos, and linking theory to practice. Educators should make the sessions enjoyable (e.g., using a sense of humor) and interesting in order to help students remember the topics better. The more senses are stimulated, the more students will learn.

Example

Students' training and experiential learning are arranged to occur in community pharmacy settings. They need to be in a pharmacy for 4 weeks under the supervision of a pharmacy preceptor. Every day, students will observe and experience the practice of pharmacists in this setting. They will interrelate the knowledge obtained in the classroom and the real practice. They will use their relevant senses in the learning process.

HUMANISM

This approach (also known as facilitation theory) believes that learning is a personal act to fulfill potential and that humans have a natural inclination to learn. Learning will happen if the person delivering it acts as a facilitator. Facilitative educators are more able to listen to learners, especially regarding their feelings. They also pay as much attention to their relationship with learners as to the content of the course. Learners are urged to take charge of their own learning and offer much of the input for the learning through their insights and experiences. This approach relates to intrinsic rewards, i.e., self motivation and rewards.

Example

Courses include topics that are relevant to the students' daily living experience, such as awareness of drug abuse in the neighborhood.

Should educators adopt a certain style or teach in a certain way? The learning outcomes and effectiveness of one group or individual learner might not be similar to another. All relevant theories are important to understand. Educators need to consider the following aspects when deciding the types of strategies to use:

1. The student's level of knowledge
2. The thought-processing demands, and
3. The desired outcomes.

Educators need to take into account multiple perspectives of learning theory when designing programs for students to address the diverse demands when they become pharmacy practitioners.

LEARNING STAGES AND STYLES

Students learn in many different ways (University of Birmingham, n.d.) and tend to have preferred learning styles. According to Riding and Rayner (1998), students' learning styles depend on their personality, cognitive processes, and previous learning experiences. Their learning styles determine how students gather, filter, process, comprehend, interpret, organize, come to conclusions about, and retain information for further use. Learning preferences, according to Kolb (1981), can vary from time to time and from situation to situation. According to Rush and Moore (2010), matching learning styles with learning activities may improve learning performance within a specific setting. It is advantageous to consider a variety of methods when planning a module and to consider different learning styles for learning to be fully effective. Knowledge of learning styles and applications through a multisensory approach increases learning effectiveness.

Thus, it is important for educators to take this into consideration when planning curricula and modules so that a range of learning theories, stages, and styles can be taken into consideration.

KOLB'S MODEL

The different learning stages are explained by Kolb's learning cycle theory (Kolb, 1976), which considers knowledge, experience and skills acquired. There are four stages: feeling, watching, thinking, and doing (Fig. 1). According to Kolb (1985), students act differently at different stages, and various techniques could be used to support learning (Table 2).

Hudak (1985) stated that accomplishments and fulfillment through learning will be greater if educators match students with their desired instructional mode. Kolb (1985) further classified learning into several styles: feel and do (accommodating), feel and watch (diverging), think and watch (assimilating), and think and do (converging). Students who are accommodators emphasize utility, divergers stress interrelationships and connections, assimilators focus on theory and expertise, and convergers emphasize value and application (Austin, 2016).

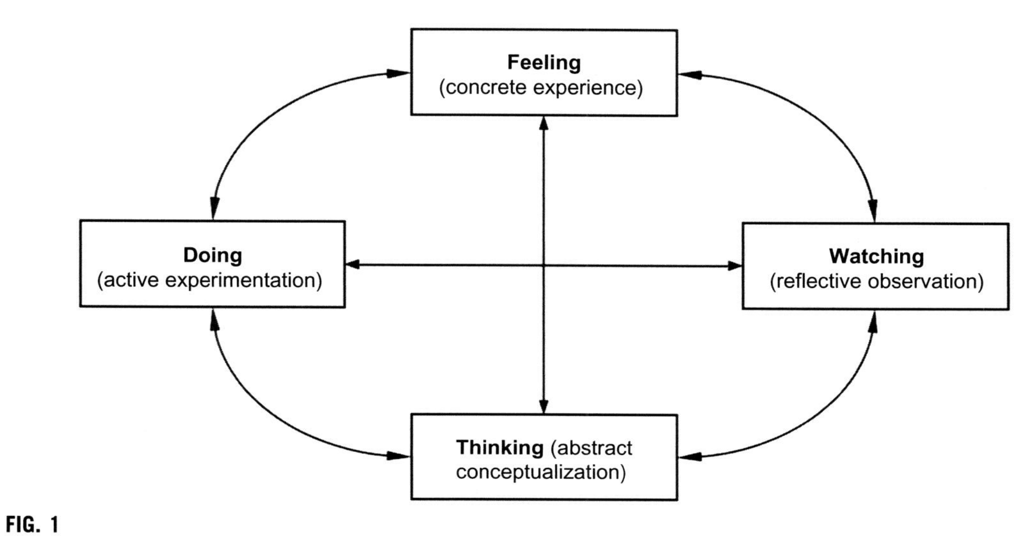

FIG. 1

Kolb's learning cycle (Kolb, 1985).

Table 2 Kolb's Learning Stage (Cycle) and Teaching Techniques (Kolb, 1981)

Learning Cycle	Activities	Teaching Techniques
Feeling stage (concrete experience)	Students are involved actively in new experiences; to learn, students must do	e.g., games/simulation, ice-breakers, problem solving, practical exercises
Watching stage (reflective observation)	Students reflect on their experiences and have open discussions with other students	e.g., journals, discussion, brainstorming
Thinking stage (abstract conceptualization)	Students must be able to form, reform, and process their ideas, take ownership of the ideas, and integrate their new ideas into sound and logical theories, i.e., learning from their experiences	e.g., projects, lecture, analogies
Doing stage (active experimentation)	Students use their knowledge to make decisions, solve problems, and test consequences in new conditions; student's needs are met if topics are taught in various ways; students consider how to put what they have learned into practice	e.g., projects, laboratory, case study, simulations

HONEY AND MUMFORD'S MODEL

In a variation of Kolb's model, Honey and Mumford (1992) proposed a model with another four styles: activists, reflectors, theorists, and pragmatists:

(i) Activists: these students learn best from activities where there are new problems and experiences.
(ii) Reflectors: these students get the most from learning activities where they are encouraged to observe and think over activities and have the opportunity to listen to/observe a group.

Table 3 Kolb's Four Types of Learning Behavior

Type of Student	Behavior	Question Asked by Learner	Type of Educator	Teaching Content
Type 1	Concrete and reflective	Why?	A motivator	Provide content relevant to their life and experience
Type 2	Abstract and reflective	What?	An expert	Provide content in a structured, organized, and rational manner
Type 3	Abstract and active	How?	A coach	Provide content that allows for hands-on experience and exercises
Type 4	Concrete and active	What if?	Does not interfere	Provide content with real life problems that allow self-directed solving

(iii) Theorists: these students learn best from doing things in organized situations with a clear aim, when they are required to understand and be involved in complex situations, and when they have time to explore the links and interrelations between ideas, events, and situations.

(iv) Pragmatists: these students learn best from activities where there is an obvious link between the subject matter and a problem set, practice techniques with coaching/feedback, and learn techniques that are applicable to the real world.

The more effective learning atmospheres contain all four of the following interdependent aspects: (1) learner-centered, (2) knowledge-centered (well-organized knowledge), (3) assessment-centered (ongoing evaluation for understanding), and (4) community-centered (community support and challenge) (Center for Teaching Vanderbilt University, n.d.). Learner-centered environments pay particular attention to the knowledge, skills, attitudes, and beliefs that learners bring to the educational setting. Knowledge-centered environments seriously consider the need to support students in learning the well-organized bodies of knowledge that help them acquire and adapt expertise. Assessment-centered settings offer numerous formal and informal opportunities for feedback focused on understanding, not memorization, to encourage and reward meaningful learning. Feedback is essential to learning, but feedback opportunities are often too uncommon in classrooms. Community-centered atmospheres foster norms for people to learn from one another and persistently attempt to improve. In such a community, students are urged to be active, constructive participants. Further, they are encouraged to learn from their mistakes. Intellectual solidarity encourages support, challenge, and teamwork. Kolb (1984) formed four types of learning behavior (Table 3).

VAK MODEL

From another perspective, Fleming and Baume (2006) classified learning styles as **V**isual learning, **A**uditory learning and **K**inesthetic learning, i.e., the VAK model. It is reported that up to 80% of individuals use the sense of sight (e.g., viewing and watching) as the primary learning style or modality. Educators can use visual strategies to enhance student learning (e.g., images, graphics). Around 10% of individuals learn by hearing, i.e., listening and speaking (e.g., lectures, group discussions, brainstorms) and between 25% and 50% of individuals are kinesthetic or hands-on learners, i.e., experiencing and doing (e.g., conducting experiment in the lab, role play, simulations).

4MAT SYSTEM

McCarthy (1997) introduced the 4MAT System that includes different learning styles from the VAK model. It suggests that there are four types of learners based on the left- and right-brain concepts (McCarthy, 1997):

Type 1 learners—imaginative learners (prefer feeling and reflecting).
Type 2 learners—analytical learners (prefer reflecting and thinking).
Type 3 learners—common sense learners (prefer thinking and doing).
Type 4 learners—dynamic learners (prefer creating and acting).

The concept of right- and left-brain learners is quite interesting. Both sides of the brain have different functions. The right brain is intuitive, random, and creative, while the left part is more analytical, systematic, and rational. Most people have a brain modality preference, and there is a relationship between brain modality and learning styles. It is reported that Type 1 and 4 learners use the right brain more (i.e., they are Problem Finding), while Type 2 and 3 learners use their left brain more (i.e., they are Problem Solvers). To be effective, educators should consider both sides of the brain.

Educators can use a more comprehensive approach to teaching if they can recognize the type of students, i.e., interpersonal, analytical, common sense, or dynamic, they are teaching. The 4MAT system is built on how individuals perceive and process reality, e.g., sensing/feeling or intuition, and rely on thinking through rationalization. The second aspect is processing reality. This involves the functions of watching and doing.

ASSESSMENT OF PHARMACY STUDENTS' LEARNING STYLES

There are several studies in pharmacy that have been carried out to assess students' learning styles.

Williams, Brown, and Etherington (2013) surveyed undergraduate pharmacy students in an Australian university and studied their learning styles using various tools. The findings showed that the learning styles most frequently preferred by pharmacy students were Intuitive, Feeling, Active-Reflective and Introverted, Assimilator, Judging (INFJ) and Extroverted, Intuitive, Feeling, Judging (ENFJ).

A study in Canada determined the learning styles of pharmacy practice residents and their faculty preceptors (Loewen & Jelescu-Bodos, 2013). The most dominant learning style among residents and faculty preceptors was assimilator; 93% were assimilators, convergers, or both. A follow up study was carried out by Loewen, Jelescu-Bodos, Yeung, and Lau (2014) to explore the learning styles of pharmacy residents as they transitioned from residency to practice. The findings illustrated changes in their learning style and showed no general direction of the change.

A study was conducted in the United States to evaluate the predominance of learning styles among pharmacy students (Teevan, Li, & Schlesselman, 2011) using the Index of Learning Styles. The findings demonstrated that sensory perception was the dominant style, followed by sequential understanding and then visual input. Another US study by Robles, Cox, and Seifert (2012) identified different learning styles using the Pharmacist's Inventory of Learning Styles (PILS) questionnaire among pharmacy students. Slightly more than half of the students reported assimilator as their dominant learning style. Crawford, Alhreish, and Popovich (2012) found that out of 299 students studied, the dominant style was assimilator, followed by converger. Novak, Shah, Wilson, Lawson, and Salzman (2006) conducted a study to evaluate students' learning styles before and after a PBL program. They found significant changes after students completed the PBL program.

Four studies were conducted in developing countries such as Malaysia and Brazil. John, Neoh, Ming, Hong, and Hassan (2016) used PILS to determine pharmacy students' learning styles in a public university. The dominant learning style preferred by the pharmacy students was assimilator, followed by converger. The findings were similar to those reported in the previous studies. In another Malaysian study, Aziz, Tey, Alwi, and Jet (2013) assessed the preferred learning styles of pharmacy students in another public university using Honey and Mumford's Learning Style Questionnaire (LSQ). They found that the most common learning style was reflector, followed by theorist, pragmatist, and activist. A third study in Malaysia applied the VAK Learning questionnaire to assess the learning-style preferences of first-year pharmacy students. The study found that students preferred visual learning and favored using images, pictures, colors, and maps to organize information and communicate with others (Saleem, Hassali, Ibrahim, Alrasheedy, & Aljadhey, 2015). A study was conducted in a Brazilian federal university to examine the learning styles of pharmacy students (Czepula et al., 2016). The authors used the LSQ and found out that the predominant style was pragmatist, followed by theorist, activist, and reflector.

Students who prefer to process information through reflection achieve greater academic success than those students who do not. Tsingos, Bosnic-Anticevich, and Smith (2015) suggest that effective learning aspects may involve reflection.

Based on all these studies, it is suggested that educators should take into consideration the learning-style preferences of undergraduate pharmacy students when developing curricula and evaluating teaching approaches, especially when planning, implementing, and evaluating education initiatives in order to create an effective, contemporary learning environment for their students. Learning is a process in which knowledge is created by the transformation of experience. The diversification in teaching approaches develops a wide scope of learning skills in students. The best possible method is to promote a balanced teaching methodology that fits the learning styles of all students.

INSTRUCTIONAL STRATEGIES

Instructional strategies are important in facilitating complex learning, either directly or indirectly. Instruction can be classified as educator-directed instruction (direct instruction) and student-centered models of learning (Seifert & Sutton, 2009). Each method of teaching is useful for certain purposes.

Educator-directed instruction programs are usually based on a mix of ideas from behaviorism and cognitive theories of learning. Students still have responsibility for working and expending effort to comprehend new material. Educators structure lessons in a straightforward, sequential manner. Educators obtain students' attention, reinforcing correct responses, providing corrective feedback, and practicing correct responses. Some teaching strategies that could be used by the educators are lecturing, discussion, questioning, demonstration, recitation, practice and drill, review, and audiovisuals.

For student-centered instructional models, the responsibility for directing and organizing learning is shifted from the educator to the student, but not completely. The educator still partly holds organizational and leadership responsibilities. Examples of strategies are independent study and self-reflection.

As educators, how would we like our students to think? Do we know the ways our students think? Do our students think critically? Are they creative thinkers? Are they able to solve problems; in other words, are they skillful problem solvers? The choices of instructional strategies will depend on forms of thinking. Each strategy encourages certain forms of learning and thinking that have distinctive educational aims. The forms might work synergistically with each other to achieve educational purposes.

There are three forms of thinking that are usually used in classrooms: (1) problem solving, (2) creative thinking, and (3) critical thinking. Problem solving is "the act of defining a problem; determining the cause of the problem; identifying, prioritizing and selecting alternatives for a solution; and implementing a solution" (American Society for Quality, 2017). There are four basic steps in problem solving: define the problem, generate alternative solutions, evaluate and select an alternative, and implement and follow up on the solution. Problem solving is an activity in which a best value is decided for an unknown, which is subject to a set of restrictions. Bloom's Taxonomy classifies and identifies six problem-solving skills: knowledge (define the problem), comprehension (understand the problem and analyze the situation), application, analysis, synthesis, and evaluation (determine actions to be taken to introduce the solution into the workplace) (University of Michigan, n.d.).

Creative thinking means thinking about new things or thinking in new ways. It is about thinking outside the box. It can be about an object, a skill, or an action. These objects, skills, and actions should be something strange, new, and valued. Creative students can devise new ways to carry out tasks, solve problems, and meet challenges. Creative thinking involves specific thought processes that improve the ability to be creative and generate new ideas. Creative students will maximize their ability to think of new, original, diverse, and elaborate ideas (Infinite Innovations, n.d.). Students who are creative thinkers adopt multiple perspectives of a problem and normally do not use standardized formats for problem solving. Creative thinking is also called divergent thinking. Torrance (1992) and Kim (2006) defined it as ideas that are open-ended and result in many directions. It is triggered by open-ended questions with many possible answers. Students, prior to engaging in this thinking, should have already acquired knowledge about the subject. Divergent thinking strongly depends on convergent thinking that is focused, logical reasoning about ideas, and experiences that lead to specific answers.

National Council for Excellence in Critical Thinking (1987) defined critical thinking as "the intellectually disciplined process of actively and skillfully conceptualizing, applying, analyzing, synthesizing, and/or evaluating information gathered from, or generated by, observation, experience, reflection, reasoning, or communication, as a guide to belief and action." It is a disciplined thinking that is clear, rational, open-minded, and informed by evidence (Dictionary.com, n.d.). Critical thinking can be seen as having two components: (1) a set of information and belief generating and processing skills, and (2) the habit, based on intellectual commitment, of using those skills to guide behavior. Someone with critical thinking skills is able to do the following: (Lau and Chan, n.d.) (1) understand the logical links between ideas; (2) determine, construct, and assess arguments; (3) identify irregularities and common mistakes in reasoning; (4) solve problems systematically; (5) identify the relevance and importance of ideas; and (6) reflect on the justification of one's own beliefs and values. Students use metacognition to think critically, i.e., the strategies for thinking about thinking and for monitoring the success and quality of one's own thinking. More precisely, it refers to the processes used to plan, monitor, assess one's understanding and performance, and make changes to one's own learning behaviors (Cambridge International Examination, n.d.). Metacognition includes a critical awareness of (a) one's thinking and learning, and (b) oneself as a thinker and learner (Center for Teaching Vanderbilt University, n.d.).

WHAT IS NEXT?

Can pharmacy colleges be vessels of transformative leadership to make pharmacy students capable of making an impact on society? It is possible, and one way is taking a multidisciplinary approach, building the development of the right skills and values into the curriculum, and setting up programs in a way that allows substantial time for practical experience and asking partners who provide that experience to measure the impact.

What is the best way to teach the new generations of pharmacy students? Many of these individuals are multitasking. They expect positive outcomes, appreciate innovative teaching, work in teams, and prefer collaboration. For pharmacy educators, it is important to choose and use the right and best methods, such as developing mentoring relationships, providing direct and frequent feedback, clarifying expectations, and personalizing learning experiences.

Educators are also encouraged to use technology in their classroom, e.g., internet, podcasting, digital cameras, Smart Boards, computers, YouTube, blogging, social media, and educational software. Technology devices have replaced chalkboards, pencils, and overhead projectors in classrooms. Even the computers have gone through a significant revolution. Tablets, iPads and e-books are replacing textbooks, and smartphones have become a powerful tool. Technology has a positive impact in the education and learning process. It pushes the educational capabilities to new levels. It makes learning more interesting and enjoyable, especially for subjects that are "dry" and boring. According to Dale (1996), the highest average retention rate of new information learners retain after 24h is "teach others," at 90%, followed by "practice by doing," 75%, "discussion group," 50% (all are classified as participatory teaching methods), "demonstration," 30%, "audiovisual," 20%, "reading," 10%, and "lecture," 5% (all are classified as passive teaching methods). Thus, pharmacy educators should move towards hybrid learning (or mixed-mode instruction or blended learning). They should use multiple methods to deliver teaching materials, i.e., combining face-to-face interactions with online activities, flipped classrooms, online learning, open education resources, and technology integration.

There are many factors that affect adult learning that educators have to take into consideration for effecting teaching and quality outcomes. These factors include age, language background, degree of language literacy, cultural background, individual learning preferences and styles, emotional and psychological issues, motivation and personal condition and stressors (Moore & Sugarman, 2010). Learners learn best when they are actively engaged in their own learning; as Confucius, the Chinese philosopher and reformer, said, "I hear and I forget. I see and I remember. I do and I understand" (Moncur, n.d.). Students have different kinds of intelligence, and thus they learn in different ways. Pharmacy educators need to be familiar with the different learning theories, styles, and strategies to make teaching and learning effective with positive outcomes and impacts.

CONCLUSION

The purposes for higher education are to go further than transmitting knowledge and to help students develop cognitive structures, skills, strategies, and motivation for continued learning and problem solving. Selecting the best teaching and learning practice requires some understanding of the challenges and rewards of each of the previously described methods.

Students' behavior and learning are significantly influenced by their preferred learning modes. The appropriate learning strategies should match the students' preferred learning modes. Information that is accessed through students' use of their modality preferences shows an increase in their levels of comprehension, motivation, and metacognition. Different pharmacy disciplines and degree programs will require different learning models and strategies. We need to shift the focus from teaching to learning. Thus it is necessary for all educators and trainers to be aware of these different possible learning styles and to try to accommodate as many of them as possible when planning their instructional programs.

REFERENCES

American Society for Quality. (2017). *Problem solving.* http://asq.org/learn-about-quality/problem-solving/overview/overview.html.

Austin, Z. (2016). *Understand learning styles, improve your teaching.* http://aphameeting.pharmacist.com/sites/default/files/slides/Understand%20Learning%20Styles_Handout.pdf.

Aziz, Z., Tey, X. Y., Alwi, S., & Jet, C. N. (2013). Learning style preferences of pharmacy students. *The European Journal of Social and Behavioural Sciences*, 820–837. eiss:2301-2218.

Basavanthappa, B. T. (2009). *Nursing education.* New Delhi: Jaypee Brothers Medical Publishers (P) Ltd.

Bass, R. V., & Good, J. W. (2004). Educare and Educere: Is a balance possible in the educational system? *The Educational Forum*, *68*, 161–168. https://eric.ed.gov/?id=EJ724880.

Berkeley Graduate Division (n.d.). Overview of learning theories. http://gsi.berkeley.edu/gsi-guide-contents/learning-theory-research/learning-overview/.

Boyter, A., & Winn, P. (2015). *Experiential learning in the pharmacy degree.* http://www.enhancementthemes.ac.uk/docs/paper/experiential-learning-in-the-pharmacy-degree.pdf?sfvrsn=6.

Bruno, C. B., Ip, E., Shah, B., & Linn, W. D. (2012). A mnemonic for pharmacy students to use in pharmacotherapy assessment. *American Journal of Pharmaceutical Education*, *76*(1), 16. https://doi.org/10.5688/ajpe76116.

Burns, R. (1995). *The adult learner at work.* Sydney: Business and Professional Publishing.

Cambridge International Examination (n.d.). Getting started with metacognition. http://cambridge-community.org.uk/professional-development/gswmeta/index.html.

Center for Teaching Vanderbilt University (n.d.) How people learn? https://cft.vanderbilt.edu/guides-sub-pages/how-people-learn/.

Crawford, S. Y., Alhreish, S. K., & Popovich, N. G. (2012). Comparison of learning styles of pharmacy students and faculty members. *American Journal of Pharmaceutical Education*, *76*(10), 192. https://doi.org/10.5688/ajpe7610192.

Czepula, A. I., Bottacin, W. E., Hipólito, E., Baptista, D. R., Pontarolo, R., & Correr, C. J. (2016). Predominant learning styles among pharmacy students at the Federal University of Paraná, Brazil. *Pharmacy Practice*, *14*(1), 650. https://doi.org/10.18549/PharmPract.2016.01.650.

Dale, E. (1996). *Audio-visual methods in teaching.* New York: Dryden Press.

Dictionary.com. http://www.dictionary.com/browse/critical-thinking.

Fleming, N., & Baume, D. (2006). *Learning styles again: varking up the right tree!.* Educational Developments. SEDA Ltd. issue 7.4 Nov, 4–7. http://www.johnsilverio.com/EDUI6702/Fleming_VARK_learningstyles.pdf.

Gitomer, D., & Zisk, R. (2014). Laboratory work: Learning and assessment. *Encyclopedia of Science Education.* https://doi.org/10.1007/978-94-007-6165-0_198-2.

Graduate School University of Leicester (n.d.). Honey and Mumford: learning theories. http://www2.le.ac.uk/departments/gradschool/training/eresources/teaching/theories/honey-mumford.

Han, E.-H., Zhang, Y., Zhan, J.-G., et al. (2016). Advances in the application of action learning in nursing practice. *Chin Nurs Res. 3.* https://doi.org/10.1016/j.cnre.2016.06.010.

Hanna, L.-A., Barry, J., Donnelly, R., Hughes, F., Jones, D., Laverty, G., et al. (2014). Using debate to teach pharmacy students about ethical issues. *American Journal of Pharmaceutical Education*, *78*(3), 57. https://doi.org/10.5688/ajpe78357.

Honey, P., & Mumford, A. (1992). *The manual of learning styles* (3rd ed.). Maidenhead: Peter Honey.

Hudak, M. A. (1985). Learning styles inventory. In D. J. Daniel & R. C. Sweetland (Eds.), *Vol. 2. Test critiques* (pp. 402–410). Kansas City, MO: Test Corporation of America.

Infinite Innovations (n.d.). Definition: brainstorming. http://www.brainstorming.co.uk/tutorials/definitions.html.

International Foundation for Action Learning (IFAL) (n.d.). Where action learning comes from and where it's going. http://ifal.org.uk/action-learning/origins-of-action-learning/.

John, M. E., Neoh, C. F., Ming, L. C., Hong, Y. H., & Hassan, Y. (2016). Learning style preferences of undergraduate pharmacy students in a Malaysian public university. *Indian Journal of Pharmaceutical Education and Research*, *50*(3).

Joyce, B. R., Weil, M., & Calhoun, E. (2000). *Models of teaching*. Boston: Allyn and Bacon.

Joyce, B. R., Weil, M., & Calhoun, E. (2005). *Models of teaching. Trans Behrangi MR*. Tehran: Kamale Tarbiat.

Kim, K. H. (2006). Is creativity unidimensional or multidimensional? Analyses of the Torrance tests of creative thinking. *Creativity Research Journal*, *18*(3), 251–259.

Knowles, M.S. & Associates. (1984). *Andragogy in action: Applying modern principles of adult learning*. San Francisco: Jossey-Bass.

Kolb, D. A. (1976). *The learning style inventory: Technical manual*. Boston, MA: McBer & Co.

Kolb, D. A. (1981). In A. Chickering (Ed.), *Learning styles and disciplinary differences in modern American college*. San Francisco: Jossey-Bass.

Kolb, D. A. (1984). *Experiential learning: Experience as the source of learning and development*. Upper Saddle River, NJ: Prentice-Hall.

Kolb, D. A. (1985). Learning styles and disciplinary differences. In A. Chickering (Ed.), *The modern American college*. San Francisco: Jossey-Bass.

Laird, D. (1985). *Approaches to training and development*. Harlow: Addison Wesley.

Lateef, F. (2010). Simulation-based learning: Just like the real thing. *Journal of Emergencies, Trauma and Shock*, *3*(4), 348–352. https://doi.org/10.4103/0974-2700.70743.

Lau, J. & Chan, J. (n.d.). What is critical thinking? http://philosophy.hku.hk/think/critical/ct.php.

Loewen, P. S., Jelescu-Bodos, A., Yeung, J., & Lau, T. (2014). The effect of transitioning from residency to pharmacy practice on learning style. *American Journal of Pharmaceutical Education*, *78*(8), 147. https://doi.org/10.5688/ajpe788147.

Loewen, P. S., & Jelescu-Bodos, A. (2013). Learning styles and teaching perspectives of Canadian pharmacy practice residents and faculty preceptors. *American Journal of Pharmaceutical Education*, *77*(8), 163. https://doi.org/10.5688/ajpe778163.

Maker, C. J. (1982). *Curriculum development for the gifted*. Austin, TX: Pro-Ed.

McCarthy, B. (1997). A tale of four learners: 4MAT's learning styles. In *Vol. 54, no. 6. How Children Learn* (pp. 46–51).

McGill, I., & Beaty, L. (2002). *Action learning: A guide for professional, management & educational development*. London: Psychology Press.

Moncur, L. (n.d.). Quotation details. (Quotation #25848) http://www.quotationspage.com/quote/25848.html.

Moore, S., & Sugarman, J. (2010). Center for applied linguistics, Washington DC, USA. *Language Teaching*, *43*(4), 522–526. https://doi.org/10.1017/S0261444810000212.

National Council for Excellence in Critical Thinking. (1987). *Critical thinking*. http://www.criticalthinking.org/pages/defining-critical-thinking/766.

Novak, S., Shah, S., Wilson, J. P., Lawson, K. A., & Salzman, R. D. (2006). Pharmacy students' learning styles before and after a problem-based learning experience. *American Journal of Pharmaceutical Education*, *70*(4), 74.

Onishi, H. (2008). Role of case presentation for teaching and learning activities. *The Kaohsiung Journal of Medical Sciences*, *24*(7), 356–360.
Ormrod, J. E. (1995). *Educational psychology: Principles and applications*. New Jersey: Englewood Cliffs, Merrill.
Quinn, F. M. (2007). *Principles and practice of nurse education* (5th ed., (pp. 15–21). London: Nelson Thornes.
Rao, D. (2011). Skills development using role-play in a first-year pharmacy practice course. *American Journal of Pharmaceutical Education*, *75*(5), 84. https://doi.org/10.5688/ajpe75584.
Riding, R., & Rayner, S. (1998). *Cognitive styles and learning strategies: Understanding style differences in learning and behaviour*. London: David Fulton.
Robles, J., Cox, C. D., & Seifert, C. F. (2012). The impact of preceptor and student learning styles on experiential performance measures. *American Journal of Pharmaceutical Education*, *76*(7), 128. https://doi.org/10.5688/ajpe767128.
Rush, G. M., & Moore, D. M. (2010). Effects of restructuring training and cognitive style. *Educational Psychology*, *11*(3–4), 309–321. https://doi.org/10.1080/0144341910110307.
Saleem, F., Hassali, M. A., Ibrahim, Z. S., Alrasheedy, A., & Aljadhey, H. (2015). Learning styles of pharmacy undergraduates: experience from a Malaysian University. *Pharmacy Education*, *15*(1), 173–177.
Seifert, K., & Sutton, R. (2009). *Educational Psychology*. The Saylor Foundation. http://www.saylor.org/courses/psych303/.
Stanford University (n.d.). Tomorrow's professor postings—teaching and learning theories https://tomprof.stanford.edu/posting/1505.
Teevan, C. J., Li, M., & Schlesselman, L. S. (2011). Index of learning styles in a U.S. school of pharmacy. *Pharmacy Practice*, *9*(2), 82–87.
The Peak Performance Center (n.d.). Learning theories. http://thepeakperformancecenter.com/educational-learning/learning/theories/.
Torrance, E. (1992). *Torrance tests of creative thinking*. Bensenville, IL: Scholastic Testing Service.
Tsingos, C., Bosnic-Anticevich, S., & Smith, L. (2015). Does a learning style preference for processing information through reflection impact on the academic performance of a cohort of undergraduate pharmacy students? *Pharmacy Education*, *15*.
UNESCO (n.d.). Most influential theories of learning. http://www.unesco.org/new/en/education/themes/strengthening-education-systems/quality-framework/technical-notes/influential-theories-of-learning/#.
University of Birmingham (n.d.). Learning theories, stages and styles. https://intranet.birmingham.ac.uk/as/cladls/edudev/documents/public/ebl/journey/learning-theories.pdf.
University of Michigan (n.d.). Bloom's taxonomy. http://umich.edu/~elements/probsolv/open/blooms/index.htm.
Williams, B., Brown, T., & Etherington, J. (2013). Learning style preferences of undergraduate pharmacy students. *Currents in Pharmacy Teaching and Learning*, *5*(2), 110–119.

FURTHER READING

Armstrong, P. (n.d.). Bloom's taxonomy. Center for Teaching. Vanderbilt University. https://cft.vanderbilt.edu/guides-sub-pages/blooms-taxonomy/.
Knowles, M., Holten, E., III, & Swanson, R. (2005). *The adult learner* (6th ed.). Oxford: Butterworth-Heineman.
Rogers, C. R. (1983). *Freedom to learn for the 80s*. Columbus, OH: Charles Merrill.
Skinner, B. F. (1974). *About behaviorism*. San Francisco, CA: Knopf.
Vygotsky, L. S. (1978). *Mind and society: The development of higher mental processes*. Cambridge, MA: Harvard University Press.

SECTION

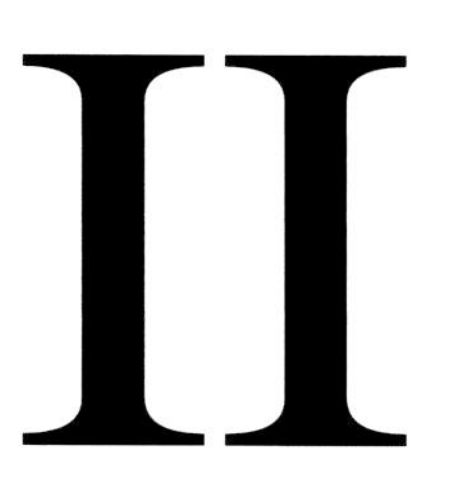

PHARMACY EDUCATION: BASIC ROLES AND CONTRIBUTIONS

CHAPTER 4

ROLE OF PHARMACY EDUCATION IN THE ADVANCEMENT OF PHARMACY PRACTICE: A WESTERN PERSPECTIVE

Ahmed Sherman*, Abdirahman Osman†

**IPSA Medical Clinic and Pharmacy, London, United Kingdom, †St George's Hospital Medical School, London, United Kingdom*

IMPORTANT FEATURES IN PHARMACY PRACTICE IN THE WESTERN WORLD

As the healthcare service evolves, pharmacy practice has grown to revolve around health advice and management. Patients often come to pharmacies not only for medication but also for professional advice and to manage their health. The pharmacist's involvement in primary care teams has also increased drastically. The team, once traditionally dominated by general practitioners (GPs), has and still is developing as a multidisciplinary practice. Pharmacists use their skills in managing patients taking medicines that require frequent monitoring, allowed by the development of prescription rights. Therefore, utilizing these varied healthcare professionals' skills ensures patients the best care possible; the main purpose of this team is to provide the local community with the best service in a time-efficient manner.

Pharmacy practice can vary over many different settings. In hospital pharmacy, pharmacists regularly attend ward rounds and are highly involved in the selection of treatment for patients. In addition, pharmacists can also work in the dispensary while prescribing. They have a variety of roles, ranging from the reviewing of drug charts to medication counseling. To do so, medicine reconciliation is of the utmost importance to avoid confusion and produce the best results. While monitoring patients, one must also evaluate the drug use of a patient, alongside reporting any adverse drug reactions. However, the most important role of pharmacists is to be able to apply their extensive evidence-based knowledge and provide specialist advice to GPs, nurses, and other healthcare professionals (Wassef & Moffit, 2014).

Among many other roles, the pharmacist's role in palliative care is on the increase in the Western world. The West's aging population has seen a growth in diseases that are no longer simply fatal, but that require long-term management and care. Therefore, palliative care pharmacists are an increasingly invaluable asset (Wassef & Moffit, 2014). These specialized pharmacists have a role as educators when interacting with patients and, especially, other healthcare professionals. This is because they are a source of expertise and knowledge for those individuals who do not specialize in the particular fields.

Pharmacy Education in the Twenty First Century and Beyond. https://doi.org/10.1016/B978-0-12-811909-9.00004-6

In the West, there has been a striking development in the world of healthcare; the roles of pharmacists will continue to expand and encompass more of the patient's management. Furthermore, pharmacists are playing critical roles in hospitals, primary care, and community pharmacies; their input will make patient care more efficient and less laborsome and decrease hospital admissions due to avoidable medicine and compliance issues. Thus this is helping free up hospitals to deliver better patient care, as outlined by the chief pharmaceutical officer. For pharmacists to deliver such a positive impact in the United Kingdom, this step in the right direction must be mirrored by the education system; academic pharmacy has and still is branching out, to equip future pharmacists with the skills and competency to provide the best care in all these healthcare settings.

ROLE OF PHARMACY EDUCATION IN THE ADVANCEMENT OF PRACTICE VIA PRODUCING COMPETENT PHARMACISTS

Just as a tree cannot survive without its roots, pharmacists cannot fulfill their professional and ethical responsibilities without a sound education. To produce competent pharmacists, it is important to develop two key characteristics: prospective pharmacists should be scholars and have an in-depth knowledge of medications, coupled with the drive to provide the best care possible to patients. To do so, pharmacists must develop and maintain commitment to care for patients, and empathy. Moreover, being a scholar also encompasses the ability to apply evidence-based practice and express ethical, professional, and social soundness.

The importance of focusing on academic pharmacy is increasing in modern healthcare, as the roles and responsibilities of pharmacists diversify in a range of different clinical settings. Having been involved in mainly compounding and manufacturing drugs in the past century, pharmacists are now more equipped to provide a more patient-centered approach and coach patients, working with them to provide the best possible care (Sosabowski & Gard, 2008). Therefore, courses are now based more on the interprofessional programs that are fundamental for integration of different healthcare professionals. As a result, pharmacists are in an environment where they can develop critical thinking, problem-solving skills and, most importantly, efficient teamwork (Toklu & Hussein, 2013).

As the need for a patient-centered approach becomes more and more apparent, the skill set of a pharmacist has to be expanded clinically. In particular, patient care skills are the most important and come from structured training and experience. Across the United Kingdom, a more clinically focused pharmacy degree is being established with clinical teaching placements, with a focus on quality management. Institutions like Birmingham University provide significant clinical placements in all 4 years of their course in community pharmacy and hospital pharmacy alongside primary care. Having understood that pharmacy education is a key foundation—alongside patient contact and experience—in producing competent pharmacists, it is also important to understand the implications that pharmacy education entails and their effects upon prospective students.

Recently, some UK universities have begun to offer a 5-year integrated MPharm degree. In this model, the preregistration training is integrated in the fifth year of the program. Prior to this proposal, the original course was 4 years long. Graduates were then required to undertake a 52-week preregistration training program to be registered as a pharmacist. University of Bradford was the first to run this course, and more recently the University of Nottingham and the University of East Anglia (Torjesen, 2016). This degree focuses on the importance of an integrated education alongside incorporating clinical practice to ensure that future pharmacists are confident and accept a more patient-centered approach. Data has shown that students from the integrated course at the University of Bradford have done better than the national average from 2002 to 2006, showing an increase of 5.8% in the average modules mark between the second and the final year for students doing the 5-year program compared with 0.7% for those doing the regular 4-year course (Torjesen, 2016).

ROLE OF PHARMACY EDUCATION CHAMPIONS AND KEY PLAYERS IN THE ADVANCEMENT OF PRACTICE VIA ACTING AS MODELS FOR PRACTICE AND VIA ESTABLISHING INITIATIVES

The Royal Pharmaceutical Society of Great Britain was split on September 2010 into the General Pharmaceutical Council (GPhC), which is responsible for regulatory function, and the Royal Pharmaceutical Society (RPS), which is responsible for the representative functions. The RPS membership is available to pharmacists, pharmacy students, and pharmaceutical scientists and provides many benefits for their academic pursuits (Royal Pharmaceutical Society, 2017a, 2017b).

The RPS supports its members in improving health outcomes for patients and society in general through professional development and support. The RPS is involved in improving the safety and efficacy of medicines by advancing pharmaceutical science and pharmacy practice, promoting professional practice and evidence-led patient care, and supporting continuing professional development (CPD). This is also done by increasing the public's awareness of the value pharmacists and other members provide in improving health outcome alongside supporting and shaping new models of care emerging in Great Britain and across the globe (Royal Pharmaceutical Society, 2016).

One of the major steps to advance pharmacy practice in the United Kingdom is prescribing rights. The GPhC, the independent regulator of pharmacists, pharmacy technicians, and pharmacy premises, plays a fundamental role in independent prescribing by certifying pharmacists as independent prescribers and accrediting the training programs of pharmacist independent prescribing at the UK universities. These GPhC-accredited independent prescribing programs give importance to the understanding of professional limitations, using diagnostic aids, and, most importantly, recognizing their responsibility as a healthcare professional (General Pharmaceutical Council, 2017).

Another major step to advance the professional training of pharmacists is the initiation of the professional doctorate (DPharm) in UK universities. The aim of this degree is to produce specialized pharmacists who can provide advanced care. Not only does this course develop the individual's communications skills, research skills, and leadership, it also helps in increasing the patient involvement and healthcare responsibilities. Consequently, these advances in education and training of pharmacists has helped to expand the roles of pharmacists in the United Kingdom.

ROLE OF PHARMACY PRACTICE RESEARCH CONDUCTED BY PHARMACY INSTITUTIONS IN ESTABLISHING THE EVIDENCE FOR THE EFFECTIVENESS AND SAFETY OF MEDICATIONS

By following evidence-based healthcare, healthcare professionals such as pharmacists are able to provide the best care possible to patients. The protocols and conducts that enable the pharmacists to carry out their role efficiently must have evidence for their effectiveness. In addition, the level of evidence provided for a particular decision-making process has to also be assessed.

Evidence-based pharmacy has an important principle to appreciate: the importance of assessing the care and satisfaction of the patient. More often than not, this is easier said than done. Therefore, providing pharmaceutical care that revolves around evidence-based pharmacy requires an education focused on skill development so pharmacists are able to adapt and deliver evidence-based care to patients. For example, in many chronic illnesses, the treatment involves multiple drug regimens and can become seriously complicated for patients. Therefore, an important task is ensuring that the effects of medicines are understood so that contraindications and harmful interactions with other medicines or conditions are made known. This is of the utmost importance to avoid any complications arising from drug administration in hospitals and other clinical environments. Therefore, this involves two distinct roles. One is conducting scientific and clinical research to investigate the efficacy and safety of medicines, including novel therapeutic agents. The other one is to train the future pharmacists in utilizing and applying the evidence in their practice.

Therefore, pharmacy practice research is fundamental to ensure the best patient health outcomes. Research is carried out to evaluate medications and their potential adverse effects or contraindications. In the following text, three examples of recent contributions of colleges of pharmacy in the United States, the United Kingdom, and Italy in conducting research related to the effects of medications are elaborated.

It is accepted worldwide that alcohol misuse causes many problems, ranging from societal to familial issues; as a result, it is an area of extensive research. The School of Pharmacy at the University of Southern California has investigated the use of moxidectin, an analogue of ivermectin, as therapy for alcohol use disorder. Even though the experiment was carried out on mice, the results display the potential for the use of moxidectin as pharmacotherapy for the treatment of alcohol use disorder. From this trial, the role of colleges of pharmacy can be appreciated, as their work can propel the world of pharmacy into being able to provide drugs for treating current health problems and diseases (Huynh et al., 2016).

Alongside finding novel therapeutics, pharmacy practice research is also important in modifying preexisting drugs for improvement. For example, myotonia is caused by a neuromuscular problem, which is characterized by the inability to relax skeletal muscle post–voluntary contraction. Myotonic patients are usually given sodium channel blockers to help with this problem, but many of them complain due to their low effectiveness and other varied reasons. In order to increase patient satisfaction, the University of Bari Aldo Moro in Italy has studied two newly synthesized derivatives of tocainide. From their results, the experiment suggests that these drugs have a better therapeutic index as they produce a use-dependent blockage of sodium channels. Reflecting upon this, the role of colleges of pharmacy can be crucial when evaluating patient satisfaction and leading the research to help in producing drugs with better efficacy (De Bellis et al., 2017).

Coupled with therapeutics is the importance of drug administration. Drug administration errors are varied as there are many different ways of going wrong, depending on the route of administration. The school of pharmacy in the University of London authored an article titled "Causes of intravenous medication errors." During an observation of 483 drug preparations and 447 administrations, a staggering 265 intravenous drug errors were made. Although mostly minor, these errors are associated with considerable harm. In order to improve upon these common errors, it is important to have a coordinated approach between pharmacists and other healthcare professionals (Taxis & Barber, 2003).

ROLE OF PHARMACY PRACTICE RESEARCH CONDUCTED BY COLLEGES OF PHARMACY IN EVALUATING THE OUTCOMES OF PHARMACEUTICAL SERVICES

A number of pharmaceutical services are provided within the NHS in the United Kingdom. One of these important services is the Medicine Use Review (MUR), aimed at improving safety, quality, and appropriate use of medicines. A number of colleges of pharmacy have researched the outcome of these medication reviews. A joint journal article written by authors from the school of pharmacy at Bradford University, University of Aberdeen, and University of Leeds has looked at the research evidence related to medication reviews and has summarized the evidence of effectiveness and also how these reviews may develop in the future (Blenkinsopp, Bond, & Raynor, 2012). They have stated that there is "good evidence" that medication reviews improve the risks of prescribing through the reduction of polypharmacy, use of more appropriate formulations, and better choice of medication (Blenkinsopp et al., 2012).

Another pharmaceutical service that impacts patient health outcomes is the New Medicine Service (NMS) implemented as an advanced service in October 2011. NMS is designed to improve compliance to therapy within the community for specific ailments: asthma/chronic obstructive pulmonary disease, type 2 diabetes, hypertension, and anticoagulant/antiplatelet treatment. Noncompliance has been linked to poor management of these long-term chronic conditions. Thus pharmacists within the community can play a vital role in supporting the management of these chronic conditions (Barber, Parsons, Clifford, Darracott, & Horne, 2004). To evaluate this service, researchers from the School of Pharmacy at the University of Nottingham have conducted a study on the NMS. They did a pragmatic, patient-level, parallel randomized controlled trial involving 504 participants across 46 pharmacies in England. Their findings suggested that NMS increased patient adherence to their new medication by 10% compared with normal practice (Elliott et al., 2016).

ROLE OF PHARMACY EDUCATION IN DOCUMENTING AND HIGHLIGHTING THE PAST AND CURRENT PRACTICES

Schools of pharmacy play an important role not only in teaching the current practice to the students, but also in highlighting some of the past practices to the students to learn the history of how the profession evolved. Moreover, as the practices change over time, schools of pharmacy across the Western world prepare pharmacy students for continuing professional development (CPD), which will be essential throughout their professional career. Pharmacy students are constantly coached on personal development planning (PDP), gaining confidence to self-assess and reflect on their practice in order to cultivate independent lifelong learners.

Once these students qualify as pharmacists, CPDs will provide them with competency in their area of practice and develop them further as professionals in their field of practice.

Among many past practices that have been documented, the thalidomide disaster is one that can be brought to attention. Thalidomide was a drug available from 1957 to 1962 for the treatment of morning sickness in early pregnancy. However, it was later found to have serious teratogenic effects, resulting in over 10,000 children born with severe congenital malformation (Vargesson, 2015). Therefore, while studying pharmacy at the university level, students are taught the effects medication can have during pregnancy and lactation. They are encouraged to consider potential harms and benefits in using these drugs prenatally and postnatally. This has also prompted the development of a more vigilant systematic testing of drugs before marketing them: considering differences in species sensitivity and toxicity manifestation, and taking into account the pharmacokinetics involved in pregnancy.

As an example of some current practices, some community pharmacies across the United Kingdom offer the Minor Ailments Scheme (MAS), which is locally commissioned by their Clinical Commissioning Group (CCG). The NHS England will be encouraging all CCGs across the United Kingdom to adopt similar schemes by April 2018 (Collins, 2016). In brief, the MAS is a scheme that allows pharmacists to provide advice and support for minor ailments and, where appropriate, supply medication for specific minor ailments. This is beneficial for those who would have otherwise visited their general practitioner (GP) for a prescription. Analysis carried out by the "Pinnacle Health Partnership of data" in 2015 on MAS, from 30 services and 473,327 patient consultations, found that 92% of patients would have gone to their GP if MAS was not available (Pharmaceutical Services Negotiating Committee, 2015). Thus pharmacy education plays a major role in highlighting these current practices and preparing students not only to be ready to enter the practice, but to be able to adapt to the changes and implement the new services and areas of practice in the future.

Therefore we can see how the implementation of such vital schemes across the United Kingdom and globally not only has the potential to reduce costs, but also affirms the expertise that the pharmacist can offer in improving patient satisfaction and care, alongside the role pharmacy education has played in achieving this.

THE NEED OF PHARMACY EDUCATION TO PREPARE THE GRADUATES TO MEET THE NEW AREAS OF PRACTICE

Colleges of pharmacy need to ensure that their graduates are prepared to have roles in the new areas of practice. For example, as community pharmacy continues to evolve, it is becoming more and more apparent that pharmacists are required to diversify their skills and begin to incorporate a more patient-centered approach as healthcare professionals. As a result of this future direction of healthcare, pharmacists are able to have more of a positive impact on public health, alongside being more involved in primary care access. In order for this to be more efficient, all healthcare professionals should have a better, more integrated way of working, especially with regards to the relationship between hospitals and the community. Alongside having a more integrated role in the community, pharmacists also have a responsibility with regards to optimizing medicines. This involves a range of roles from leading clinics for long-term conditions, to reviewing medicines for the purpose of avoiding hospital admissions and unnecessary usage of hospital resources (Smith, Picton, & Dayan, 2013). Hence, these skills and abilities need to be incorporated into the curriculum.

Among the aforementioned roles of pharmacists, it is also important to appreciate their roles in public health and primary care access. In public health, healthcare professionals focus on providing advice support, prevention programs and free information for the wider community. Pharmacists will be able to take part in many of these beneficial activities, such as education about sexual health and smoking cessation, in addition to being able to perform health checks and early detection of illness. Moreover, it is acknowledged that primary care plays a massive role in reducing hospital admissions and increasing patient satisfaction. One of the potential future roles of pharmacists would include dealing with minor ailments and out of hours' services, to improve primary care access (Smith et al., 2013).

As mentioned previously, the increasing roles of pharmacists require a more patient-centered approach. A positive step in this direction has been taken by NHS England, by the implementation of the Summary Care Records (SCR) in community pharmacy. SCRs are read-only materials available from the patients' interactions in a primary healthcare setting: for example, GPs. This record contains pertinent patient information centered around medications that have been prescribed to the patient, alongside other important information such as allergies, patient demographics and diagnoses. Initially, the summary care records were being utilized in the secondary care setting, before they were transitioned into primary care (Royal Pharmaceutical Society, 2017a, 2017b).

More recently, this system has been implemented in community pharmacies to improve patient satisfaction and safety. The two main benefits of this records summary are to add value to patient care alongside reducing prescribing errors. Feedback from community pharmacy users has highlighted that 18% of individuals who accessed the SCR have reported that the risk of a prescribing error had been avoided (Royal Pharmaceutical Society, 2015).

It is important to appreciate that the introduction of summary care records has been implemented as a result of its documented benefits. A study on the SCR by University College London and the Centre for Health Sciences at Bart's explored its use and confirmed its importance in reducing prescribing errors (Greenhalgh et al., 2010). However, it should be noted that the author commented on the subtlety of the benefits displayed, illustrating that the SCR, although being successfully integrated, should be coupled with other features to ensure quality care for patients.

Therefore, it is vital to acknowledge that the future of pharmacy will be geared toward the incorporation of technologies and software. With regards to other healthcare professions, technology has been able to augment and influence the clinical setting. For example, when looking at the production and the application of clinical tools, it is clear that their use can have economic benefit by accelerating cost savings (Thimbleby, 2013). The extent to which technologies will impact upon the field of pharmacy is where the discussion lies. Hence, the colleges of pharmacy need to ensure this component is covered well in the curriculum so that the graduates can engage in these new roles and advance the practice to further higher levels to meet the needs of society and the healthcare system.

CONCLUSION

As the role of pharmacists in healthcare diversifies, research and education in schools of pharmacy will become ever more vital. Interprofessional programs, which are becoming more common in the United Kingdom, have introduced students to their roles in the clinical settings much earlier in the course. This has the mammoth advantage of transitioning students into the multidisciplinary team and it also helps focus on the development of skills crucial for the profession. Research carried out by schools of pharmacy can revolutionize the evidence-based practice of modern pharmacists, highlighting the valuable relationship between pharmacy education and the continuing transformation of the pharmacy profession.

REFERENCES

Barber, N., Parsons, J., Clifford, S., Darracott, R., & Horne, R. (2004). Patients' problems with new medication for chronic conditions. *Quality and Safety in Health Care*, *13*(3), 172–175.

Blenkinsopp, A., Bond, C., & Raynor, D. K. (2012). Medication reviews. *British Journal of Clinical Pharmacology*, *74*(4), 573–580. https://doi.org/10.1111/j.1365-2125.2012.04331.x.

Collins, A. (2016). DH clarifies minister's comments on minor ailments funding. *Chemist and Druggist*. https://www.chemistanddruggist.co.uk/news/dh-clarifies-mowats-slip-minor-ailments-scheme.

De Bellis, M., Carbonara, R., Roussel, J., Farinato, A., Massari, A., Pierno, S., et al. (2017). Increased sodium channel use-dependent inhibition by a new potent analogue of tocainide greatly enhances in vivo antimyotonic activity. *Neuropharmacology*, *113*(Pt A), 206–216. https://doi.org/10.1016/j.neuropharm.2016.10.013.

Elliott, R. A., Boyd, M. J., Salema, N.-E., Davies, J., Barber, N., Mehta, R. L., et al. (2016). Supporting adherence for people starting a new medication for a long-term condition through community pharmacies: a pragmatic randomised controlled trial of the new medicine service. *BMJ Quality & Safety*, *25*(10), 747–758.

General Pharmaceutical Council. (2017). *Pharmacist independent prescribing programme—learning outcomes and indicative content.*

Greenhalgh, T., Stramer, K., Bratan, T., Byrne, E., Russel, J., & Potts, H. W. W. (2010). Adoption and non-adoption of a shared electronic summary record in England: a mixed-method case study. *British Medical Journal*, c3111.

Huynh, N., Arabian, N., Naito, A., Louie, S., Jakowec, M. W., Asatryan, L., et al. (2016). Preclinical development of moxidectin as a novel therapeutic for alcohol use disorder. *Neuropharmacology*, *113*(Pt A), 60–70.

Pharmaceutical Services Negotiating Committee. (2015). *PSNC briefing 045/15: analysis of minor ailment services data.*

Royal Pharmaceutical Society. (2015). *RPS, PSNC and Pharmacy Voice respond to SCR article in* Daily Telegraph.

Royal Pharmaceutical Society. (2016). *RPS Strategy 2016–2021.*

Royal Pharmaceutical Society. (2017a). *Student Membership.*

Royal Pharmaceutical Society. (2017b). *Summary Care Records—England.*

Smith, J., Picton, C., & Dayan, M. (2013). *Now or never: shaping pharmacy for the future.* Available at: https://www.rpharms.com/Portals/0/RPS%20document%20library/Open%20access/Publications/Now%20or%20Never%20-%20Report.pdf.

Sosabowski, M. H., & Gard, P. R. (2008). Pharmacy education in the United Kingdom. *American Journal of Pharmaceutical Education*, *72*(6).

Taxis, K., & Barber, N. (2003). Causes of intravenous medication errors: an ethnographic study. *Quality and Safety in Health Care*, *12*(5), 343–347. https://doi.org/10.1136/qhc.12.5.343.

Thimbleby, H. (2013). Technology and the future of healthcare. *Journal of Public Health Research*, *2*(3):e28 https://doi.org/10.4081/jphr.2013.e28.

Toklu, H. Z., & Hussein, A. (2013). The changing face of pharmacy practise and the need for a new model of pharmacy education. *Journal of Young Pharmacists*, *5*(2), 38–40.

Torjesen, I. (2016). Five years to success? *The Pharmaceutical Journal*, *296*(7887).

Vargesson, N. (2015). Thalidomide-induced teratogenesis: History and mechanisms. *Birth Defects Research Part C: Embryo Today: Reviews*, *105*(2), 140–156. https://doi.org/10.1002/bdrc.21096.

Wassef, C., & Moffit, K. (2014). Specialist roles in pharmacy. *The Pharmaceutical Journal*, 2014.

FURTHER READING

Keith, R. (2015). *Role of pharmacists is set to grow and grow.* [Blog post].

CHAPTER

ROLE OF PHARMACY EDUCATION IN THE ADVANCEMENT OF PHARMACY PRACTICE: AN EASTERN PERSPECTIVE

5

Suhaj Abdulsalim, Maryam Farooqui
Unaizah College of Pharmacy, Qassim University, Qassim, Saudi Arabia

INTRODUCTION

In a broad cultural and social context the Eastern world refers to countries from Asia, Africa, and eastern Europe. The concept of pharmacy practice is relatively new to the Eastern world; however, it has been recognized by the healthcare system gradually. Pharmacy education in the Eastern world has taken a shift from product-focused to patient-focused, recognizing the roles and responsibilities of pharmacists on the healthcare team. Pharmacists represent the third healthcare professional in the health work force, after medical doctor and nurse (Venkata, Kielgast, Udhumansha, & Airaksinen, 2016).

The profession of pharmacy has aimed to connect health sciences with basic sciences (Azhar et al., 2009). After the introduction of the concept of "pharmaceutical care" by Hepler and Strand in 1990 (Hepler & Strand, 1990), there was a paradigm shift in which the pharmacy profession became more responsible for achieving positive outcomes from drug therapy and promoting rational drug use (Rovers, 2003). Pharmacists are now seen as drug experts rather than as dispensers or chemists within a multidisciplinary healthcare team (Anderson et al., 2009).

The functional role of pharmacists may include compounding and dispensing of drugs, patient counseling, providing drug information, medication reviews, health promotion, pharmacovigilance, and promoting pharmaceutical care services. For the last few decades, pharmacy organizations have promoted pharmaceutical care as a standard patient care (Farris, Fernandez-Llimos, & Benrimoj, 2005). Clinical pharmacy has evolved with the provision of effective, safe, and economical drug therapy (Nagavi, 2004).

With the recognition of clinical pharmacy and the pharmaceutical care concept, many Eastern countries have expanded their pharmacy education curriculum into 5- to 6-year programs (Jamshed, Din Babar, & Masood, 2007). It is known that pharmacy education systems in most of the Eastern world are still facing problems, such as lack of resources, lack of qualified and well-trained staff, and outdated curricula, making implementation of pharmaceutical care more challenging. Despite these challenges, however, some of the

Pharmacy Education in the Twenty First Century and Beyond. https://doi.org/10.1016/B978-0-12-811909-9.00005-8

countries from the Eastern world have brought about drastic changes in their educational systems, which ultimately have made a huge difference in the pharmaceutical care in these countries.

IMPORTANT FEATURES OF PHARMACY EDUCATION IN THE EASTERN WORLD

Many of the Eastern world countries, such as India, Saudi Arabia, Lebanon, and Nigeria, have started PharmD programs, which is a patient-oriented program. Furthermore, traditional industry-based curricula have evolved to patient-oriented curricula in PharmD programs. The introduction of postgraduate programs such as master's degree and PhD in pharmacy practice is also an achievement of pharmacy education in Eastern countries.

A review of pharmacy education and pharmacy practice from 13 Middle Eastern countries concluded that there is a strong desire to advance the pharmacy practice (Kheir et al., 2008), which warrants collaboration with Western universities to improve the quality of education in the Eastern world. Pharmacy curricula in these countries are in a continuous phase of scrutiny to meet the accreditation requirements, locally and internationally.

Apart from biomedical, pharmaceutical, and clinical sciences, the PharmD curriculum is also designed to focus on education in humanities, behavioral sciences, and communication skills. Effective communication by pharmacists is essential to improve medication use and to ensure optimal therapeutic outcomes (McDonough & Bennett, 2006). Pharmacists can improve patient adherence to drug therapy through appropriate strategies, including patient counseling and education. For example, in India, patient information leaflets (PILs) prepared by pharmacists are reported to improve therapeutic outcomes among patients with chronic diseases (Suhaj et al., 2015).

The current curricula in Kuwait are designed to improve students' abilities to communicate more effectively, solve problems, make rational independent decisions based upon sound scientific reasoning, and create a caring attitude in their professional interactions with patients (Katoue, Awad, Schwinghammer, & Kombian, 2014). This balance in curriculum is especially needed to meet the standard of a pharmaceutical care model for the patient-centered approach. Pharmacy education aims to use a systematic approach to education that enables and supports a sustainable healthcare workforce (Anderson et al., 2009).

The changing face of pharmacy practice requires pharmacy graduates to be competent in critical thinking, problem-solving skills, and decision making. Students should be trained to create and apply new knowledge in the pharmaceutical, social, and clinical context. Furthermore, graduates must be trained to collaborate with other health professionals in order to enhance patients' quality of life through improved health (Toklu & Hussain, 2013). With this vision, some PharmD programs in Eastern countries are well incorporated with team-based learning (TBL) and problem-based learning (PBL) to enhance problem-solving skills and critical thinking, with a team-based approach. The ultimate aim is to produce pharmacists with a high level of knowledge and problem-solving skills (Ghayur, 2008). In order to improve the pharmacy graduate's soft skills, such as attitude, communication, leadership, work ethic, and time management, pharmacy curricula have incorporated role-plays, seminar presentations, and health awareness community-based projects.

A bibliometric review of literature on pharmacy education in low- and middle-income countries revealed that the Eastern world can build a world-class standard of pharmacy education by implementing or following key points, such as (1) introduction of tailored degrees such as PharmD or international standardization; (2) identify and address the barriers of professionalization; and (3) collaborate with Western countries (Scahill, Akhlaq, & Garg, 2013).

A coordinated and multifaceted effort to advance workforce planning, training, and education are needed in order to prepare an adequate number of well-trained pharmacists for the evolving roles of pharmacists (Anderson et al., 2011). For this reason, clinical training remains a prerequisite for most of the PharmD programs to obtain a license to practice and to ensure competent patient care.

Collaborative working between professionals is a key to quality care (McPherson, Headrick, & Moss, 2001); however, this is lacking in many Eastern countries because physician-centered healthcare systems still exist and are in practice (Sharma, Ladd, & Unnikrishnan, 2013). A randomized controlled study from India evaluated the effectiveness of a clinical pharmacist intervention program in COPD patients and concluded that health-related quality of life was improved significantly in the intervention group compared to the control group. The study also revealed that task-sharing to nonphysician healthcare professionals can improve the outcomes of patients, especially in a developing country like India (Suhaj, Manu, Unnikrishnan, Vijayanarayana, & Mallikarjuna Rao, 2016).

THE CONTRIBUTION OF PHARMACY EDUCATION TO THE ADVANCEMENT OF PHARMACY PRACTICE IN THE EASTERN WORLD

The International Pharmaceutical Federation (FIP) and World Health Organization (WHO) developed the "seven-star pharmacist" concept, which describes a pharmacist as an all-round caregiver, active communicator, decision maker, good manager, lifelong learner, good leader, teacher and researcher (World Health Organization, 1997). According to WHO, future pharmacists must possess specific knowledge, attitudes, skills, and behaviors in support of their roles.

The fundamental objective of pharmaceutical care is identification, prevention, and management of actual and potential drug-related problems and optimizing drug therapy (Strand, Cipolle, & Morley, 1992; Strand, Morley, Cipolle, Ramsey, & Lamsam, 1990). Low-income countries are not part of the development of the Pharmacy Education Action Plan (2008–2010) developed by FIP (Scahill et al., 2013). This creates a potential disconnect between what is proposed at the governance level and those that need to be engaged at the strategic and functional levels within low- and middle-income countries.

In a continuing effort to expand clinical pharmacy and pharmaceutical care services, pharmacy education in many Eastern countries has taken an initiative to move one step forward by introducing postgraduate studies in clinical pharmacy, social and administrative pharmacy, pharmacoeconomics, and pharmacovigilance. The curricula for these courses are developed keeping in view the global needs of pharmacy practice (Hadi, Ming, Leng, Shaharuddin, & Adam, 2010). Didactic lectures on identification and management of drug-related problems (DRP), drug evaluation (DE), and drug utilization review (DUR) enhanced the pharmacy student's skills to focus on evaluating and improving medication use, with a goal of achieving optimal patient outcomes (American Society of Health System Pharmacist (ASHP) Guidelines, 1998).

An Indian study in 2002 reported that clinical pharmacy services were implemented in India by 1997 with the collaboration of an Australian university and that development was rapid. Clinical pharmacy services were already implemented in some private teaching hospitals in India. Authors also revealed that the quality of these services was meeting the standards of the Western world and was promoting rational drug use (Parthasarathi, Ramesh, Nyfort-Hansen, & Nagavi, 2002). A PharmD program was introduced in India in 2008 by the effort of the Pharmacy Council of India (Ghilzai & Dutta, 2007).

A commentary on "A decade of pharmacy practice education in India" clearly implies some of the key insights or challenges faced in the Indian context, such as (a) profession of pharmacy practice is restricted to only university-based teaching hospitals; (b) regulatory agencies do not recognize the need for clinical pharmacists at the national level; (c) pharmacy practice graduates are moving to industry jobs such as pharmacovigilance or medical writing, as there is no post for clinical pharmacists in the public sector; (d) revision of topics based on industry needs (Basak & Sathyanarayana, 2010; Mangasuli, Rajan, & Khan, 2008). Overall, pharmacy practice education implemented in India needs rapid development in order for progress to occur.

Dib et al. reported that pharmacy practice in Lebanon is an integral part of healthcare (Dib, Saade, & Merhi, 2004). Lebanese American University (LAU) offers a PharmD program, which is the only program accredited by ACPE outside America. Most of the pharmacy schools in Lebanon are affiliated with Western universities. Consequently, implementation of pharmaceutical care is successful in Lebanon.

THERAPEUTIC DRUG MONITORING SERVICES

According to the American Society of Health-System Pharmacists (ASHP), clinical pharmacokinetics and therapeutic drug monitoring (TDM) skills are important to the pharmacists who provide pharmaceutical care services. Positive treatment outcomes of TDM include reduced morbidity and mortality, decreased duration of treatment, decreased length of hospitalization, and decreased adverse effects from drug therapy (ASHP Guidelines, 1998). Many of the Eastern countries started TDM centers to individualize the dosage in special cases, such as transplanted patients, pediatric infectious diseases, etc. For example, in India the first TDM center was a university teaching hospital-based establishment at Mumbai in the mid-1980s (Gogtay, Kshirsagar, & Dalvi, 1999).

In developing countries TDM services are provided either by major teaching or government hospitals or in the private sector (Gogtay et al., 1999). In Malaysia, TDM services were started in 1980 and currently nearly all major government hospitals are offering TDM services to their patients (Ab Rahman, Ahmed Abdelrahim, & Mohamed Ibrahim, 2013). Since TDM is one of the most sophisticated types of clinical service that definitely requires a pharmacist's expertise, TDM courses have been extensively included in the Malaysia pharmacy curricula at undergraduate and postgraduate levels.

DRUG AND POISON INFORMATION CENTER

Drug and poison information centers (DPICs) are aimed to provide drug- and poison-related information to the healthcare providers and to the general public. Several Eastern countries have established such services to provide indepth, evidence-based information via unbiased authentic sources.

The first drug information center in the world was university-based (i.e., the University of Kentucky, in the United States). Similarly, most of the drug and poison information centers established in Eastern countries are either university based or hospital based, after the implementation of pharmacy practice education (Fathelrahman, Ibrahim, & Wertheimer, 2016). These centers cater to the public's and other healthcare professionals' needs for adverse drug reactions (ADR) and poisoning. For example, in West Bank, Palestine, the only poison control and drug information center was established at An-Najah University. It offers free services of research, pharmaco-epidemiology, and poison-related issues to the public and health professionals (Sweileh, Al-Jabi, Sawalha, & Zyoud, 2009).

In Malaysia the first drug and poison center was established in 1982 at Universiti Sains Malaysia. The center started operating with a few teaching pharmacy staff after having some basic training on drug information. Within a period of 6 years, the center launched Integrated Drug & Poison Information Services (IDPIS) nationwide, with telecommunication services in Malaysia. Within a few years the established center had a drug and poison information unit, poison education and prevention unit, and toxicology laboratory unit. This university-based project was designated as a WHO Collaborating Centre for drug information in recognition of its contribution and services, among others, in the field of drug and poison information (National Poison Centre, University Sains Malaysia, 1998).

Currently, there is no standardized method to evaluate the quality of information provided by DPICs. However, some DPICs have adopted double-check systems to meet the quality standard (Chauhan, Moin, Pandey, Mittal, & Bajaj, 2013; George & Rao, 2005). Feedback from the requester or continuous monitoring and assessment using research, which can be guided by pharmacy colleges, or conducting an internal audit by a DI specialist, may all improve the quality of information provided by DPICs.

PHARMACOVIGILANCE PROGRAMS

National pharmacovigilance programs to monitor and prevent adverse drug reactions have been established by many Eastern countries and many of such centers have good collaboration with the WHO pharmacovigilance program and the Uppsala monitoring center.

In a collaboration with the Uppsala monitoring center, India established several regional and peripheral pharmacovigilance centers that contain enormous ADR data from the Indian population (Karim & Adnan, 2016). DPICs have been established in many states of India with the collaboration of WHO.

TOTAL PARENTERAL NUTRITION SERVICES

The purpose of total parenteral nutrition (TPN) services is to meet patient's nutritional needs when the digestive tract is nonfunctional. The nutritional support team usually requires a clinical pharmacist in the team, together with doctors, nurses, and nutritionists. TPN services are an important aspect of pharmacy practice. For a clinical pharmacist, a good command of TPN knowledge is desirable. Currently a number of hospitals in Eastern countries are offering TPN services to meet the nutritional demands of their patients. TPN services were first introduced in a Malaysian hospital in 1986, in a university-based hospital in Kelantan. Since then, the services have expanded and currently all major hospitals in Malaysia offer TPN services (Shamsuddin & Bahari, 1994).

NATIONAL DRUG FORMULARY DEVELOPMENT AND REGULAR REVISION

Another achievement of pharmacy practice education is regularly updated national drug formularies and essential drug lists in most of the countries. This enables the physician to select the drug from the available list based on rationality. The purpose of the formulary is to promote rational drug use (Academy of Managed Care Pharmacy, 2009; Loorand-Stiver, 2011).

MEDICATION THERAPY MANAGEMENT PROGRAMS AND PHARMACIST-MANAGED CLINICS

Implementation of clinical pharmacy activities in some of the teaching hospitals is another great achievement of pharmacy practice education in the Eastern world. This has helped to create the role of pharmacists as an integral part of the healthcare system.

Pharmacists started reviewing the medication charts of patients and resolving drug-related problems, improving the positive outcomes from medications (ASHP Guidelines, 2011). In Malaysia, pharmacist-managed medication therapy adherence clinics have been established since 2004, with the aim to improve the quality and safety of medication use (Alrasheedy, Hassali, Wong, & Saleem, 2017). Pharmacy-managed clinics such as anticoagulation clinics, TDM clinics, and individualized pharmacotherapy clinics have been found as an outcome of the advancement of pharmacy practice in some Eastern countries, such as Saudi Arabia (Al-jedai, Qaisi, & Al-meman, 2016). Pharmacy students in Eastern countries can be trained in performing various tasks such as antibiotic stewardship activities, clinical pharmacokinetics, anticoagulation monitoring and dose adjustments, individualized drug therapy management, and medication therapy management (McBane et al., 2015; Nuffer, Gilliam, Thompson, & Vande Griend, 2017).

EVOLVING ROLES AND FUTURE DIRECTIONS

INTERNATIONAL COLLABORATION TO EXCEL ACADEMIC AND RESEARCH EXCELLENCE

Academic and research collaboration with western institutions have improved the quality of pharmacy education in most of the Eastern countries. Currently, a number of pharmacy colleges in Malaysia, Saudi Arabia, and few other Eastern countries are collaborating with international universities. Such collaborations have provided pharmacy students with a chance to learn from qualified pharmacy academicians and researchers, and be exposed to well-established lab facilities, which sometimes is not possible in their local settings. Similarly, research collaboration via international funding (by FIP) has helped many postgraduate pharmacy students and teaching faculties to complete their research projects and training on topics such as antibiotic resistance and rational use of medicines, which has benefited pharmacy practice in the Eastern world (Vijayanarayana et al., 2014).

ADVANCEMENT IN INFORMATION TECHNOLOGY EDUCATION

During the last few decades there has been a tremendous growth in the medical literature, making retrieval of information more complex. Conventional resources such as textbooks and printed materials are replaced by electronic databases and mobile applications. The advantage of electronic, internet, or mobile-based resources is the easy and quick access to information. However, the pharmacist's informatics knowledge in this regard is critical. For this reason, the majority of pharmacy curricula have shifted their focus toward information technology (IT), in order to meet the pharmacist's needs in this area. This helps pharmacists to become acquainted with all drug information resources for quick response to DI queries, which makes them more efficient (Ghaibi, Ipema, & Gabay, 2015). The current practice requires the pharmacy curriculum to be well equipped with IT knowledge to meet future demands on pharmacists.

CLINICAL PRACTICE GUIDELINES

Unlike in Western countries, pharmacy practice in the Eastern world is still evolving and clinical practice guidelines (CPGs) are a relatively new concept. However, evidence-based practice has been started in many of the hospitals in the Eastern world where pharmacists are extensively involved in CPG development. This is one of the latest achievement of pharmacy practice. Pharmacy colleges have to rethink the inclusion of CPGs in their curricula (Brown, 2015).

ESTABLISHMENT OF DRUG AND THERAPEUTIC COMMITTEES/PHARMACY AND THERAPEUTIC COMMITTEE (PTC)

Many hospitals in Eastern countries have established drug and therapeutic committees (DTCs) and pharmacy and therapeutic committees (PTCs) after the implementation of pharmacy practice. However, the actual roles and responsibilities of such committees may not be as per the standards of ASHP (Cole et al., 2008). Traditional roles such as the development of a drug formulary and its periodic revision are achievements that have created good rapport between pharmacists and physicians.

HEALTH PROMOTION AND PUBLIC HEALTH SERVICES

Health awareness and promotion are among the major aspects of pharmacy practice. Monitoring blood pressure (BP) and blood sugar and holding public awareness camps on common diseases such as diabetes, hypertension, TB, and HIV have created a good image among the community. The public is more aware of pharmacists as medication experts rather than just retailers of medications (DiPietro Mager & Farris, 2016). Pharmacy students must be trained to handle different counseling aids, such as inhaler devices, insulin pens, etc. to improve patient counseling. Pharmacy students must be educated about medication adherence, possible intentional and unintentional reasons for nonadherence, and motivation strategies to improve medication adherence.

CONTINUING PHARMACY EDUCATION PROGRAMS

Continuing pharmacy education (CPE) programs have significantly improved the knowledge level of working pharmacists (Krska, 2004). Many were not regularly updating their knowledge once they were out of their colleges. After the implementation of pharmacy practice, many of the regulatory authorities made it compulsory for working pharmacists to update their knowledge by attending CPE programs.

CONCLUSIONS

The healthcare system is evolving rapidly around the globe, through consolidation, corporatization, and accreditation processes. The quality and safety of healthcare delivery plays a pivotal role in this scenario. Clinical pharmacists can catalyze the changes required in the healthcare sector in order to adapt to system evolution by collaborating with other healthcare providers. Over the last few decades, Eastern world has seen the development of pharmacy practice. The role of pharmacist has evolved from a product-oriented approach to patient-oriented care. Several developing countries have demonstrated the value of pharmacy practice education in various aspects of healthcare settings.

Challenges facing the Eastern world differ. Revising the existing curricula and incorporating more experiential education would definitely improve the current scenario of the pharmacy practice profession. Optimization of medication therapy and minimization of drug-related problems are some of the benefits of implementation of pharmacy practice that the Eastern world has experienced in recent years.

REFERENCES

Ab Rahman, A. F., Ahmed Abdelrahim, H. E., & Mohamed Ibrahim, M. I. (2013). A survey of therapeutic drug monitoring services in Malaysia. *Saudi Pharmaceutical Journal*, *21*(1), 19–24.

Academy of Managed Care Pharmacy. (2009). *Formulary management*. Retrieved from http://www.amcp.org/WorkArea/DownloadAsset.aspx?id=9788.

Al-jedai, A., Qaisi, S., & Al-meman, A. (2016). Pharmacy practice and the health care system in Saudi Arabia. *The Canadian Journal of Hospital Pharmacy*, *69*(3), 231–237.

Alrasheedy, A. A., Hassali, M. A., Wong, Z. Y., & Saleem, F. (2017). Pharmacist-managed medication therapy adherence clinics: The Malaysian experience. *Research in Social and Administrative Pharmacy*, *13*(4), 885–886.

American Society of Health-System Pharmacists. (1998). ASHP statement on the pharmacist's role in clinical pharmacokinetic monitoring. *American Journal of Health-System Pharmacy*, *55*(16), 1726–1727.

American Society of Health-System Pharmacists. (2011). The consensus of the pharmacy practice model summit. *American Journal of Health-System Pharmacy*, *68*(12), 1148–1152.

Anderson, C., Bates, I., Beck, D., Brock, T. P., Futter, B., Mercer, H., et al. (2009). The WHO UNESCO FIP pharmacy education taskforce. *Human Resources for Health*, *7*(1), 45.

Anderson, C., Brock, T., Bates, I., Rouse, M., Marriott, J., Manasse, H., et al. (2011). Transforming health professional education. *American Journal of Pharmaceutical Education*, *75*(2), 22.

Azhar, S., Hassali, M. A., Ibrahim, M. I. M., Ahmad, M., Masood, I., & Shafie, A. A. (2009). The role of pharmacists in developing countries: the current scenario in Pakistan. *Human Resources for Health*, *7*(1), 54.

Basak, S. C., & Sathyanarayana, D. (2010). Pharmacy education in India. *American Journal of Pharmaceutical Education*, *74*(4), 68.

Brown, D. L. (2015). Rethinking the role of clinical practice guidelines in pharmacy education. *American Journal of Pharmaceutical Education*, *79*(10), 148. https://doi.org/10.5688/ajpe7910148.

Chauhan, N., Moin, S., Pandey, A., Mittal, A., & Bajaj, U. (2013). Indian aspects of drug information resources and impact of drug information centre on community. *Journal of Advanced Pharmaceutical Technology & Research*, *4*(2), 84–93. https://doi.org/10.4103/2231-4040.111524.

Cole, S. W., May, J. R., Millares, M., Valentino, M. A., Vermeulen, L. C., Jr., & Wilson, A. L. (2008). ASHP guidelines on the pharmacy and therapeutics committee and the formulary system. *American Journal of Health-system Pharmacy*, *65*, 1272–1283.

Dib, J. G., Saade, S., & Merhi, F. (2004). Pharmacy practice in Lebanon. *American Journal of Health-system Pharmacy*, *61*(8), 794–795.
DiPietro Mager, N. A., & Farris, K. B. (2016). The importance of public health in pharmacy education and practice. *American Journal of Pharmaceutical Education*, *80*(2), 18.
Farris, K. B., Fernandez-Llimos, F., & Benrimoj, S. I. (2005). *Pharmaceutical care in community pharmacies: Practice and research from around the world.*
Fathelrahman, A. I., Ibrahim, M. I., & Wertheimer, A. I. (2016). *Pharmacy practice in developing countries: Achievements and challenges* (1st ed.). United Kingdom: Academic Press.
George, B., & Rao, P. G. (2005). Assessment and evaluation of drug information services provided in a south Indian teaching hospital. *Indian Journal of Pharmacology*, *37*(5), 315.
Ghaibi, S., Ipema, H., & Gabay, M. (2015). ASHP guidelines on the pharmacist's role in providing drug information. *American Journal of Health-System Pharmacy*, *72*(7), 573–577.
Ghayur, M. N. (2008). Pharmacy education in developing countries: need for a change. *American Journal of Pharmaceutical Education*, *72*(4), 94.
Ghilzai, N. M. K., & Dutta, A. P. (2007). India to introduce five-year doctor of pharmacy program. *American Journal of Pharmaceutical Education*, *71*(2), 38.
Gogtay, N. J., Kshirsagar, N. A., & Dalvi, S. S. (1999). Therapeutic drug monitoring in a developing country: an overview. *British Journal of Clinical Pharmacology*, *48*(5), 649–654.
Hadi, M. A., Ming, L. C., Leng, L. W., Shaharuddin, S., & Adam, A. (2010). Developing a practice-based master in clinical pharmacy program at the Universiti Teknologi MARA, Malaysia. *American Journal of Pharmaceutical Education*, *74*(2), 32d.
Hepler, C. D., & Strand, L. M. (1990). Opportunities and responsibilities in pharmaceutical care. *American Journal of Hospital Pharmacy*, *47*(3), 533–543.
Jamshed, S., Din Babar, Z. U., & Masood, I. (2007). The PharmD degree in developing countries. *American Journal of Pharmaceutical Education*, *71*(6), 125.
Karim, S., & Adnan, M. (2016). Pharmacy practice in India. In *Pharmacy practice in developing countries* (pp. 117–146).
Katoue, M. G., Awad, A. I., Schwinghammer, T. L., & Kombian, S. B. (2014). Pharmaceutical care education in Kuwait: pharmacy students' perspectives. *Pharmacy Practice*, *12*(3).
Kheir, N., Zaidan, M., Younes, H., El Hajj, M., Wilbur, K., & Jewesson, P. J. (2008). Pharmacy education and practice in 13 middle eastern countries. *American Journal of Pharmaceutical Education*, *72*(6), 133.
Krska, J. (2004). Drug formularies in Winfield AJ & RME Richards Pharmaceutical practice (*Ed*) (3rd ed.). *Published by* Churchil Livingstone, Edinburgh. 409–424.
Loorand-Stiver, L. (2011). *Hospital-based pharmacy and therapeutics committees: evolving responsibilities and membership.* Ottawa: Canadian Agency for Drugs and Technologies in Health.
Mangasuli, S., Rajan, S., & Khan, S. A. (2008). A decade of pharmacy practice education in India. *American Journal of Pharmaceutical Education*, *72*(1), 16.
McBane, S. E., Dopp, A. L., Abe, A., Benavides, S., Chester, E. A., Dixon, D. L., et al. (2015). Collaborative drug therapy management and comprehensive medication management—2015. *Pharmacotherapy: The Journal of Human Pharmacology and Drug Therapy*, *35*(4).
McDonough, R. P., & Bennett, M. S. (2006). Improving communication skills of pharmacy students through effective precepting. *American Journal of Pharmaceutical Education*, *70*(3), 58.
McPherson, K., Headrick, L., & Moss, F. (2001). Working and learning together: good quality care depends on it, but how can we achieve it? *Quality and Safety in Health Care*, *10*(Suppl 2), ii46–ii53.
Nagavi, B. G. (2004). Clinical pharmacy in India. In G. Parthasarathi, K. Nyfort-Hansen, & M. C. Nahata (Eds.), *A textbook of clinical pharmacy practice—Essential concepts and skills* (1st ed., pp. 1–8). Chennai: Orient Longmen.

National Poison Centre, Universiti Sains Malaysia. (1998). *WHO Collaborating Centre for Drug Information.* Retrieved from http://www.prn.usm.my/who_collaborating_centre.php.

Nuffer, W., Gilliam, E., Thompson, M., & Vande Griend, J. (2017). Establishment and implementation of a required medication therapy management advanced pharmacy practice experience. *American Journal of Pharmaceutical Education*, *81*(2), 36.

Parthasarathi, G., Ramesh, M., Nyfort-Hansen, K., & Nagavi, B. G. (2002). Clinical pharmacy in a south Indian teaching hospital. *Annals of Pharmacotherapy*, *36*(5), 927–932.

Rovers, J. P. (2003). *A practical guide to pharmaceutical care.* Washington, DC: APhA Publications.

Scahill, S. L., Akhlaq, M., & Garg, S. (2013). A bibliometric review of pharmacy education literature in the context of low- to middle-income countries. *Currents in Pharmacy Teaching and Learning*, *5*(3), 218–232.

Shamsuddin, A. F., & Bahari, M. B. (1994). In *Role of clinical pharmacist in nutritional support—experience in a teaching hospital 1st National Symposium on Clinical Nutrition, 28–30th March, Kuala Lumpur* (pp. 144–149).

Sharma, A., Ladd, E., & Unnikrishnan, M. K. (2013). Healthcare inequity and physician scarcity empowering non-physician healthcare. *Economic and Political Weekly*, *XLVIII*(13), 112–117.

Strand, L. M., Cipolle, R. J., & Morley, P. C. (1992). *Pharmaceutical care: An introduction.* Kalamazoo, MI: Upjohn.

Strand, L. M., Morley, P. C., Cipolle, R. J., Ramsey, R., & Lamsam, G. D. (1990). Drug-related problems: their structure and function. *DICP*, *24*(11), 1093–1097.

Suhaj, A., Manu, M. K., Mohapatra, A. K., Magazine, R., Rao, M. C., Unnikrishnan, M. K., et al. (2015). Development and readability assessment of patient information leaflets for chronic obstructive pulmonary disease. *Asian Journal of Pharmaceutical and Health Sciences*, *5*(2), 1237–1241.

Suhaj, A., Manu, M. K., Unnikrishnan, M. K., Vijayanarayana, K., & Mallikarjuna Rao, C. (2016). Effectiveness of clinical pharmacist intervention on health-related quality of life in chronic obstructive pulmonary disorder patients—a randomized controlled study. *Journal of Clinical Pharmacy and Therapeutics*, *41*(1), 78–83.

Sweileh, W. M., Al-Jabi, S. W., Sawalha, A. F., & Zyoud, S. H. (2009). Pharmacy education and practice in West Bank, Palestine. *American Journal of Pharmaceutical Education*, *73*(2), 38.

Toklu, H. Z., & Hussain, A. (2013). The changing face of pharmacy practice and the need for a new model of pharmacy education. *Journal of Young Pharmacists*, *5*(2), 38–40.

Venkata, S. P. R. M., Kielgast, P., Udhumansha, U., & Airaksinen, M. (2016). Public health and patient care aspects in Indian pharmacy curricula: a comparison with USA, Finland and Denmark. *Indian Journal of Pharmaceutical Education and Research*, *50*(1), 1–8.

Vijayanarayana, K., Sekhar, M. S., Surulivelrajan, M., Rajesh, R., Suhaj, A., Kumar, S. P., et al. (2014). Bridging pharmaceutical education. *Currents in Pharmacy Teaching and Learning*, *6*(5), 745–747.

World Health Organization. (1997). The role of the pharmacist in the health care system: Preparing the future pharmacist: Curricular development: Report of a third WHO consultative group on the role of the pharmacist, Vancouver, Canada, 27–29 August 1997.

CHAPTER

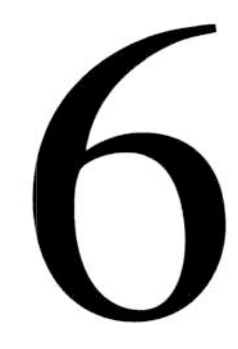

HOW PHARMACY EDUCATION CONTRIBUTES TO PATIENT AND PHARMACEUTICAL CARE

Ahmed Awaisu*, David R. Mottram†

**Qatar University, Doha, Qatar, †Liverpool John Moores University, Liverpool, United Kingdom*

THE INTRODUCTION OF PHARMACEUTICAL CARE AS A MODEL OF PHARMACY PRACTICE AND EDUCATION

The practice of pharmacy has undergone transformation over the past four decades, from being mostly concerned with the preparation and distribution (compounding/manufacturing and dispensing) of drug products, to a patient-centered and cognitive practice in which the roles of the pharmacist have evolved and expanded to include direct patient care activities and patient education. These practice changes have occurred primarily as a result of radical changes in healthcare systems, demographic changes in population, and advancements in drug discovery and technology, as well as political and economic forces modulating the healthcare system in many countries. These changes have meant expanding the roles and responsibilities of pharmacists as experts in drug therapy and medication safety. The transformation began with the development of clinical pharmacy services. This led to a number of similar models of practice, such as cognitive pharmacy services, pharmaceutical care, medicines management, medication use review, medication management services, and medication therapy management (Martín-Calero et al., 2004), all of which share similar philosophies and a common goal as per the definition of pharmaceutical care by Hepler and Strand (1990). In addition, most of these services describe similar practices and different countries use different terminologies. For instance, in the United Kingdom both *medicine management* and *pharmaceutical care* have been used to describe similar practices (Barber, 2001; Robert Gordon University, 2000).

Initially, there was a lack of clarity regarding the specific functions and responsibilities of a pharmaceutical care practitioner (Winslade, Strand, Pugsley, & Perrier, 1996). This fact resulted in confusion about what is considered and what is not considered to be pharmaceutical care (Martín-Calero et al., 2004). In particular, there have been controversies and debates on the concept and practice of clinical pharmacy as compared with pharmaceutical care, but the common goal of both is patient care. While clinical pharmacy is often considered as a discipline and a professional practice, pharmaceutical care is an emerging practice model (American College of Clinical Pharmacy, 2008; Hepler, 2004). Semantic comparisons show that clinical pharmacy and pharmaceutical care are compatible and mutually complementary ideas; although both concepts are incomplete, they support and complement each other (Hepler, 2004). It is believed that pharmaceutical care is a philosophy and model of practice

Pharmacy Education in the Twenty First Century and Beyond. https://doi.org/10.1016/B978-0-12-811909-9.00006-X

that is today embraced by the discipline of clinical pharmacy (American College of Clinical Pharmacy, 2008; Hepler, 2004). The developers of the definitions of pharmaceutical care intended it to be an extension of, not a substitute for, clinical pharmacy (Hepler, 2004). Regardless of these debates and controversies, pharmaceutical care is regarded as the maturation of pharmacy as a clinical profession by accepting its responsibility to minimize the incidence of preventable drug-related morbidities and mortalities (Hepler, 2004; Hepler & Strand, 1990; Hudson, Mc Anaw, & Johnson, 2007). The evidence of clinical, economic, and humanistic benefits of pharmaceutical care and other cognitive pharmacy services have been adequately demonstrated and widely published in the literature (Anderson, Blenkinsopp, & Armstrong, 2003; Beney, Bero, & Bond, 2000; Bernsten et al., 2001; Johnson & Bootman, 1995; Kennie, Schuster, & Einarson, 1998; Plumridge & Wojnar-Horton, 1998; Schumock et al., 2003; Touchette et al., 2014).

To assume the new roles of pharmaceutical care practice, pharmacists need to perform many different functions, including assessment, care planning, follow-up evaluation (monitoring), and documentation. These practice changes and new roles must be reflected in the curricula of schools and colleges of pharmacy around the world. Accordingly, the curricula of pharmacy degree programs for training pharmacists now incorporate content related to pharmaceutical care as a philosophy and new practice model. The curricula also expand to include new courses that provide the knowledge base and skills to practice pharmaceutical care, such as therapeutics, pathophysiology, patient assessment, and interpretation of laboratory data. As these new pharmacy graduates move into practice, the practice of pharmacy changes, to reflect the changes in education and knowledge base. Similarly, pharmacy educators, accreditation agencies, pharmacy professional bodies, and international pharmacy and health organizations, such as the International Pharmaceutical Federation (FIP) and the World Health Organization (WHO), play a significant role in ensuring the implementation of changes in pharmacy education for training new graduates and for continuing professional development of pharmacists who are already in practice. Other evolving areas of pharmacy practice include evidenced-based pharmacy, public health, medication safety including pharmacovigilance, and quality assurance of pharmaceutical care services. These changes in focus of pharmacy practice dictate that the pharmacy curriculum should change in parallel, in order for the pharmacy practitioners to be able to acquire new skills and knowledge (Van Mil, Schulz, & Tromp, 2004).

This chapter is primarily intended to provide insight into the evolution of patient and pharmaceutical care as a new model of practice and how pharmacy education contributes in these transformations around the world. The chapter also highlights research and scholarship in pharmaceutical care education.

PHARMACEUTICAL CARE AS A MODEL OF PHARMACY PRACTICE

The concept and practice of pharmaceutical care is now well established. The definition of pharmaceutical care, its historical development in practice, as well as its impact on patient care and health outcomes have been extensively discussed elsewhere. The discussions here will briefly dwell on the different meanings of pharmaceutical care and related practices and the historical milestones in its development to the present day, with a goal of transitioning to how pharmacy education contributed to its development and implementation.

Historically the concept of pharmaceutical care evolved in the 1970s when Mikeal and colleagues defined "pharmaceutical care" as analogous to "medical care" (Mikeal, Brown, Lazarus, & Vinson, 1975). Subsequently, Brodie (1981) and other researchers further developed the concept by including the patient's drug-related needs and provision of safe and effective drug therapy as important components of this care (Brodie, 1981). Clinical pharmacy was considered one of the most important developments in pharmacy education and practice during the 20th century and it promised to make pharmacy education patient-centered and to improve the quality of drug therapy in the society (Hepler, 1987, 2004). Further, it was proposed that the discipline of clinical pharmacy must be involved in research in order to contribute to the generation of new knowledge for the advancement of health outcomes and quality of life (American College of Clinical Pharmacy, 2008; Hepler, 1987, 2004).

A new era in pharmaceutical care emerged in 1990 through a publication by Hepler and Strand in which they clearly defined the concept of pharmaceutical care and described the opportunities, responsibilities, and the processes required in it (Hepler & Strand, 1990). These scholars defined pharmaceutical care as "the responsible provision of drug therapy for the purpose of achieving definite outcomes which improve a patient's quality of life" (Hepler & Strand, 1990). In this patient-centered and outcome-oriented practice, the pharmacist assumes direct responsibility for all the patient's drug-related needs and is held accountable for this commitment (Cipolle, Strand, & Morley, 1998). The philosophy of pharmaceutical care practice has as its core social responsibility, patient-centeredness, and caring through establishing therapeutic relationships to achieve definite outcomes that improve the patient's quality of life. As described by various scholars, the patient care process in pharmaceutical care comprises the following: establishment of a therapeutic relationship; assessment that includes identification of actual or potential drug therapy problem (DTPs); development of a care plan to resolve or prevent DTPs; and follow-up evaluation (i.e., continuous monitoring) to ensure the achievement of the desired outcomes or goals of therapy (Cipolle et al., 1998; Robertson, 1996; Strand, Morley, Cipolle, Ramsey, & Lamsam, 1990).

Several definitions of pharmaceutical care have emerged since the initial definition by Mikeal et al. (1975) and the popularized definition of the term by Hepler and Strand (1990). In addition, new terms and concepts of drug-related patient care such as medicine management, medication therapy management (MTM), and medication use review (MUR) continue to evolve. The Pharmaceutical Care Network Europe (PCNE) has recognized that over two decades after the definition by Helper and Strand, substantial confusion still exists about the definition of pharmaceutical care and its differentiation from other terms. While some believe that the practice of pharmaceutical care is a sole responsibility of the pharmacists, others believe that it is a shared responsibility between all healthcare providers (Allemann et al., 2014). It was interesting to note that the PCNE, a network of researchers in the field of pharmaceutical care in Europe, felt the need to redefine pharmaceutical care in 2013 through a review of the existing definitions of pharmaceutical care, moderated discussions, and consensus by a panel of experts (Allemann et al., 2014). Fourteen members of PCNE and 10 additional experts attended the moderated discussion. From their deliberations, 19 definitions of the term were identified and paraphrased using a standardized syntax (care provider, recipient, subject, outcome, activities). A consensus was reached on PCNE definition of pharmaceutical care as "the pharmacist's contribution to the care of individuals in order to optimize medicines use and improve health outcomes" (Allemann et al., 2014).

The evolution of pharmacy practice toward the pharmaceutical or patient care approach has occurred to varying degrees in different countries around the world. In concert with this, the definition of pharmaceutical care varies across the world due to differences in healthcare and pharmacy systems among different countries (Berenguer, La Casa, de la Matta, & Martin-Calero, 2004), with the definition by Hepler and Strand (1990) regarded as the most widely used of this practice model (Hepler & Strand, 1990). Despite this, the ultimate goal of pharmaceutical care of optimizing the outcomes of patient drug therapy and improving the patient's quality of life is uniformly accepted globally. There are several barriers to implementation of pharmaceutical care, which include problems in pharmacy education, skills, resources, and environment. New challenges emerge even in countries and places where pharmaceutical care is successfully implemented. These include, but are not limited to, shortage of human resources for health including pharmacists, increased burden of disease, increased healthcare costs, inefficient health systems, and changes in socioeconomic and political environments (Wiedenmayer et al., 2006).

As pharmacists assume responsibility for the outcomes of drug therapy in their patients, they undertake a variety of functions and services encompassing both traditional and new ones (Commission to Implement Change in Pharmaceutical Education, 1993b). Hence, pharmaceutical care is a revolutionary concept and forms the basis of pharmacy practice as clearly outlined in the evolving mission of pharmacy practice (Commission to Implement Change in Pharmaceutical Education, 1993b). Broadly speaking, the pharmacists use their skills and knowledge to identify potential and actual DTPs, resolve the actual DTPs, and prevent the potential for new problems (Cipolle et al., 1998; Hepler & Strand, 1990; Strand et al., 1990). The implementation of pharmaceutical care in practice requires some foundational knowledge and skills including the concepts of pharmaceutical care and its processes, pharmacotherapy, pathophysiology, pharmacology, and interpretation of clinical laboratory data, physical assessment, interviewing skills, communication skills, and documentation skills. Therefore, it is paramount to consider pharmaceutical care as a basic element of curriculum in undergraduate pharmacy degree programs and to strengthen several domains of skills and knowledge. Most importantly, as the profession of pharmacy shifted from being a product-oriented one to a patient-centered one, clinical training requirements and competency standards for pharmacy graduates have tremendously changed in many countries of the world. Traditionally, emphasis in pharmacy curricula has been on technical aspects of pharmacy instead of professional practice aspects (Wiedenmayer et al., 2006). Substantial curricular changes have been implemented in pharmacy education across the globe, as elaborated in the subsequent sections of this chapter.

THE EVOLUTION OF PHARMACY EDUCATION, TRAINING, AND EDUCATIONAL OUTCOMES TOWARD PATIENT-CENTERED AND PHARMACEUTICAL CARE PRACTICE

The need to introduce changes in the curricula of schools and colleges of pharmacy, including new content related to pharmaceutical care, has been evident over the past few decades in universities globally, despite variable results with respect to their implementation (Martín-Calero et al., 2004). These changes stem from the clarion call by the pharmacy profession for pharmacists to be prepared to effectively deliver pharmaceutical care in all healthcare settings, which will ultimately help patients make the best use of their medications. FIP statements of policy and professional standards stress that the changes in pharmacists' roles and pharmacy practice must be reflected in undergraduate pharmacy education and continuing education for pharmacists (International Pharmaceutical Federation, 2000, 2002).

The paradigm shift in pharmacy practice dictates the need for pharmacy curricula to shift from the traditional pharmaceutical sciences–based approach to a clinical-based approach; pharmacists should gain knowledge and expertise beyond pharmacology, pharmaceutics, pharmaceutical chemistry, pharmacognosy, and pharmacy administration. They need to know and apply the principles surrounding the activities necessary to manage drug therapy (Wiedenmayer et al., 2006) for achieving definite outcomes that will improve the patient's quality of life. Since the general consensus is that pharmaceutical care is the primary mission of the pharmacy profession, the linkage between the new roles and the curricula must ensure that the intended educational outcomes of pharmacy curricula are directly related or identical to the functions and responsibilities required of a pharmaceutical care practitioner (Newton, 1991; Winslade et al., 1996).

The change in pharmacy practice toward a patient care approach has occurred to varying degrees and at different paces in different countries globally, resulting in variabilities in pharmacy curricula in different countries. As these roles continue to evolve and expand, the need to increase pharmacists' direct patient care skills and knowledge base has resulted in changes in pharmacy curricula to incorporate new content (Awaisu & Pawluk, 2015). The curricular changes toward patient care are more evident in developed countries, such as those in North America and Europe, than in developing countries, with many schools in developing countries still using traditional pharmacy curricula that are largely product-oriented.

In 1990, the American Association of Colleges of Pharmacy (AACP) formed the Commission to Implement Change in Pharmaceutical Education (CCPE) with a broad responsibility of providing direction to evolving pharmacy education toward meeting the changing healthcare needs of the society. The CCPE developed views of the missions of the pharmacy profession and pharmacy practice, and ultimately a mission statement for pharmacy education. These three interrelated mission statements revolved around the idea of pharmaceutical care, now referred to as patient-centered care. The CCPE, therefore, developed a framework for changes in pharmacy education in the United States through four fundamental papers (Commission to Implement Change in Pharmaceutical Education, 1993a, 1993b, 1993c, 1993d). Background Papers I and II clearly outlined the significant changes in pharmacy practice and the proposed changes in pharmacy education that were necessary to accommodate those practice changes. These papers and the recommendations thereof were accepted by the AACP, thereby demonstrating pharmacy educators' recognition of the proposed changes. Pharmacy degree programs in developed countries implement and emphasize outcome-based education with a focus on student's learning outcomes as their centerpiece (Bruce, Bower, Hak, & Schwartz, 2006). Outcome-based professional pharmacy education frameworks advocate that course learning objectives should be mapped against program learning outcomes and designed to meet certain competency standards. In addition, increased emphasis has been placed on outcomes assessment as a means for documenting success and programmatic quality in accreditation standards (Bruce et al., 2006; Wadelin, 2003). The principal mission of pharmacy education is to maintain a dynamic curriculum that included a strong liberal arts education and foundation in various aspects of pharmacy necessary to prepare graduates to provide optimal pharmaceutical care (Bradberry et al., 2007; Commission to Implement Change in Pharmaceutical Education, 1993a, 1993b, 1993c, 1993d). Educators should continually refine courses in terms of content and delivery in order to achieve the designated educational outcomes of the program.

The educational outcomes of evolving curricula should be determined and clearly defined. These educational outcomes are used as frameworks that integrate science, ethics and professionalism, and interprofessional education across the major headings of pharmaceutical care, public health, and other emerging aspects of pharmacy practice (Wiedenmayer et al., 2006). In alliance with this, accreditation standards, professional bodies, and pharmacy academia in North America require the curricula of entry-to-practice professional degree programs in pharmacy to be outcome-based (Accreditation Council for Pharmacy Education, 2011; American Association of Colleges of Pharmacy (CAPE), 2013; Association of Faculties of Pharmacy of Canada, 2010). The AACP Center for the Advancement of Pharmacy Education (formerly known as the Center for the Advancement of Pharmaceutical Education) (CAPE), created the CAPE 2013 Educational Outcomes, which are primarily intended to be the target toward which the evolving pharmacy curriculum should be aimed. The CAPE 2013 Educational Outcomes represent the fourth revision of the outcomes, preceded by CAPE 2004, CAPE 1998 and CAPE 1992. The outcomes were developed to guide curricular discussions, curricula planning, delivery, and assessment within pharmacy academia (American Association of Colleges of Pharmacy, 1998; American Association of Colleges of Pharmacy (CAPE), 2013; Medina et al., 2013). The CAPE 2013 Educational Outcomes include four broad domains (foundational knowledge, essentials for practice and care, approach to practice and care, personal and professional development), 15 subdomains, and examples of learning objectives (Medina et al., 2013).

In Canada, the Association of Faculties of Pharmacy of Canada (AFPC) formed the AFPC Task Force on Educational Outcomes, charged with the responsibility of developing educational outcomes for all first professional degree programs in pharmacy in Canada in 2008, and completed their work in 2010 (Association of Faculties of Pharmacy of Canada, 2010). The Task Force developed one set of educational outcomes for all entry-to-practice pharmacy degree programs in Canada, regardless of the degree offered (Entry-level PharmD or Bachelor of Science in Pharmacy). The 2010 revised educational outcomes were developed based on an overarching goal of graduating pharmacists as Medication Therapy Experts, which requires graduates to integrate knowledge, skills, and attitudes from seven educational outcomes (Care Provider, Communicator, Collaborator, Manager, Advocate, Scholar, and Professional) (Association of Faculties of Pharmacy of Canada, 2010).

In a similar transformation in Europe, in 1999, the European Association of Faculties of Pharmacy (EAFP) through the Task Force for Implementing Pharmaceutical Care into the Curriculum proposed a shift in the structure and content of pharmacy degree programs from laboratory-based sciences to practice and clinical sciences (Tromp, 1999). The Task Force concluded that pharmaceutical care modules in Europe should be mandatory for all pharmacy students, should focus on certain patient groups or disease states, should integrate knowledge and skills, and should be taught through didactic (classroom) and experiential training (practice settings) (Tromp, 1999). The process of curriculum change could vary in different European countries depending on the stakeholders and healthcare systems. In a review of European developments in pharmaceutical care concepts and their implementation, teaching, and research, van Mil et al. stressed that if pharmacists are to provide pharmaceutical care, it will be necessary for European universities to customize their curricula and to equip pharmacy graduates with the skills and knowledge needed for delivering pharmaceutical care (Van Mil et al., 2004).

The FIP, in a broad-based collaborative partnership with WHO and United Nations Educational, Scientific and Cultural Organization (UNESCO), spearheaded the development of a holistic and comprehensive pharmacy education and workforce action to support and strengthen local, national, and regional efforts through its Global Pharmacy Education Action Plan 2008–2010 (Anderson et al., 2008). The aims of the Action Plan were to develop evidence-based frameworks that will facilitate the development of pharmacy and higher-education capacity to enable the sustainability of a competent pharmacy workforce relevant to the needs of the society and that is appropriately prepared to provide optimal pharmaceutical services. The Action Plan encompassed four broad domains: vision for pharmacy education, competency framework for pharmaceutical services, quality assurance, and academic and institution capacity (comprising workforce and infrastructure) (Anderson et al., 2008).

The FIP-WHO-UNESCO task force recognized that an essential need exists to have a shared vision for pharmacy education and a process for building collective action and momentum to develop quality education (Anderson et al., 2008). The joint task force believed that a "one-size fits all" educational model or system was neither feasible nor desirable. Therefore, the consultation stressed the need for education development geared toward local needs. However, the task force recognized the need for focusing efforts toward areas where global collective activity would be beneficial through harnessing opportunities for global exchange and sharing of experiences in education development.

It is worthwhile to recognize that the educational changes that are needed require not only curricula revision and restructuring, but also a significant commitment to capacity building and faculty development to prepare educators to train pharmacy graduates who will be competent in the delivery of pharmaceutical care and meet the new demands of society (Anderson et al., 2008; Wiedenmayer et al., 2006). We must also recognize that the nature and intensity of didactic and experiential learning currently included in pharmacy curricula varies across countries, in part due to constraints on resources.

It is clear that pharmacy programs should develop and evaluate practice models that could be used within evolving healthcare environments (Tromp, 1999). Delivery of effective pharmaceutical care requires not only knowledge recall, but several other skills, including, but not limited to, communication and problem-solving skills. Hence, innovative teaching strategies and pedagogies are needed to adequately prepare future graduates for patient-centered practice (Caldwell, Sexton, Green, & Farrar, 2001). The use of active learning strategies such as problem-based learning (PBL) and case-based learning (CBL) has been introduced in pharmacy education in several countries.

In conclusion, the important considerations when introducing new courses into the curriculum include ensuring clearly defined learning outcomes, course content, use of innovative teaching methods, teaching-learning resources (i.e., infrastructure), learners' assessment, course evaluation, and quality assurance (Anderson et al., 2008; International Pharmaceutical Federation, 2009).

THE ROLE OF PHARMACY CURRICULA AND CONTINUING PROFESSIONAL DEVELOPMENT IN ADVANCING THE PHARMACEUTICAL CARE PRACTICE MODEL

In order to develop sound educational principles, there is a need for clear articulation of a model of practice. Therefore, any reform of pharmaceutical care curricula should explicitly describe the functions and responsibilities required of the pharmaceutical care practitioner (Newton, 1991). Undoubtedly, pharmacy education has greatly contributed to the pharmacy practice advancements that we have witnessed globally over the last several decades. This has resulted in the development of effective patient care practitioners with appropriate skills, knowledge, and competencies to provide optimal pharmaceutical care and to advance health outcomes (Raman-Wilms, 2012). Healthcare in general and pharmacy practice in particular have advanced through innovation and excellence in education, research, and service development. Pharmacy schools and accreditation agencies in all regions of the world have developed new competencies and implemented changes in pharmacy education, albeit with variable extents of implementation (Martín-Calero et al., 2004).

A review of the pharmacy education literature revealed that there are several landmark articles from different countries describing the evolution of pharmacy education. However, many of these are general in nature and do not provide details about the curricula content and syllabi. For example, in 2008, The *American Journal of Pharmaceutical Education* (AJPE) published a themed issue called "International Pharmacy Education Supplement" (Fielding, Brazeau, & Wasan, 2008). This special series was designed to provide greater insight into the current developments, issues, and challenges facing pharmacy education and practice world-wide and how countries tackle them. The articles were related to aspects of pharmacy education and practice development from Australia (Marriott et al., 2008), Canada (Austin & Ensom, 2008), China (Ryan et al., 2008), France (Bourdon, Ekeland, & Brion, 2008), the Middle East (Kheir et al., 2008), and the United Kingdom (Sosabowski & Gard, 2008). Similar articles from other countries have included: Jordan/Saudi Arabia/Kuwait (Al-Wazaify, Matowe, Albsoul-Younes, & Al-Omran, 2006), India (Basak & Sathyanarayana, 2010), Yemen (Al-Worafi, 2014), United Arab Emirates (Sarheed, Al-Azzawi, & Nagavi, 2014), China (Hu et al., 2014), and Palestine (Hamouda, Al-Rousan, & Alkhateeb, 2015). In general, similar challenges and concerns were expressed in these articles. However, the authors did not provide in-depth description of topics in the curricula and the place of pharmaceutical care education. We therefore sought to determine published literature that is specific to pharmaceutical care education within pharmacy curricula.

Our scoping review of published literature revealed some details of curricula design relating to pharmaceutical care education, including many studies that reported on the knowledge, attitudes, and perceptions of pharmacy students and pharmacists relating to pharmaceutical care teaching and practice. From this evidence base, we wish to highlight some of the key global developments in teaching pharmaceutical care using examples from different regions. We conducted a scoping review of this literature and have summarized the key findings here.

Pharmacy schools in North America have long incorporated pharmaceutical care content into their curricula. The reports of the CCPE on implementation of changes in pharmacy education significantly influenced the curricular design of pharmaceutical care education in the United States (Commission to Implement Change in Pharmaceutical Education, 1993a, 1993b, 1993c, 1993d). Shortly after these reports, the curricula of numerous universities in the United States and Canada, including Minnesota, Florida, Butler, Virginia Commonwealth, Washington State, Toronto, British Columbia, Alberta, and several others, were modified (Chambers, Schmittgen, & Allen, 2000; Cipolle et al., 1998; Isetts, 1999; Kassam, 2006; Kennedy, Ruffin, Goode, & Small, 1997; Perrier, Winsdale, Pugsley, Lavack, & Strand, 1995; Robertson, 1996). In concert with this, the 2006–07 AACP Academic Affairs Committee (Bradberry et al., 2007) conducted an environmental scan of the changes that have happened in academia in the United States from a pharmacy curricular perspective since the original Background Papers from the Commission to Implement Change in Pharmaceutical Education, formed in 1989 (Commission to Implement Change in Pharmaceutical Education, 1993a, 1993b, 1993c, 1993d). The report provided a reflection and overview of the impact of the reports on curricular transformations toward patient-centered care in the United States. The Committee felt that the academic pharmacy has done well in terms of curricular reforms to meet the mission of pharmacy education and pharmacy practice toward patient-centered care. However, areas for improvement were identified for which the authors provided appropriate recommendations (Bradberry et al., 2007). Around the early to mid-1990s, Perrier and colleagues at the Faculty of Pharmacy, University of Toronto designed and implemented a pharmaceutical care–based curriculum that provided pharmacy students with the knowledge and skills to deliver pharmaceutical care (Perrier et al., 1995; Winslade et al., 1996). The process involved logical and systematic development of a pharmaceutical care practice model that resulted in a pharmaceutical care curriculum with an explicit description of the curricular content, educational processes, and assessment techniques required to achieve the specific educational outcomes (Perrier et al., 1995). The interrelationship between these components is illustrated in Fig. 1. New courses related to pharmaceutical care were introduced in professional years II to IV, in some cases using a PBL approach. The University of British Columbia and that of Alberta have equally introduced pharmaceutical care content in their syllabuses.

Universities in the United Kingdom including, but not limited to, Liverpool, Brighton, and Robert Gordon Universities incorporated pharmaceutical care teaching in their schools of pharmacy syllabi (Caldwell et al., 2001; James, Nastasic, Horne, & Davies, 2001; Robert Gordon University, 2000).

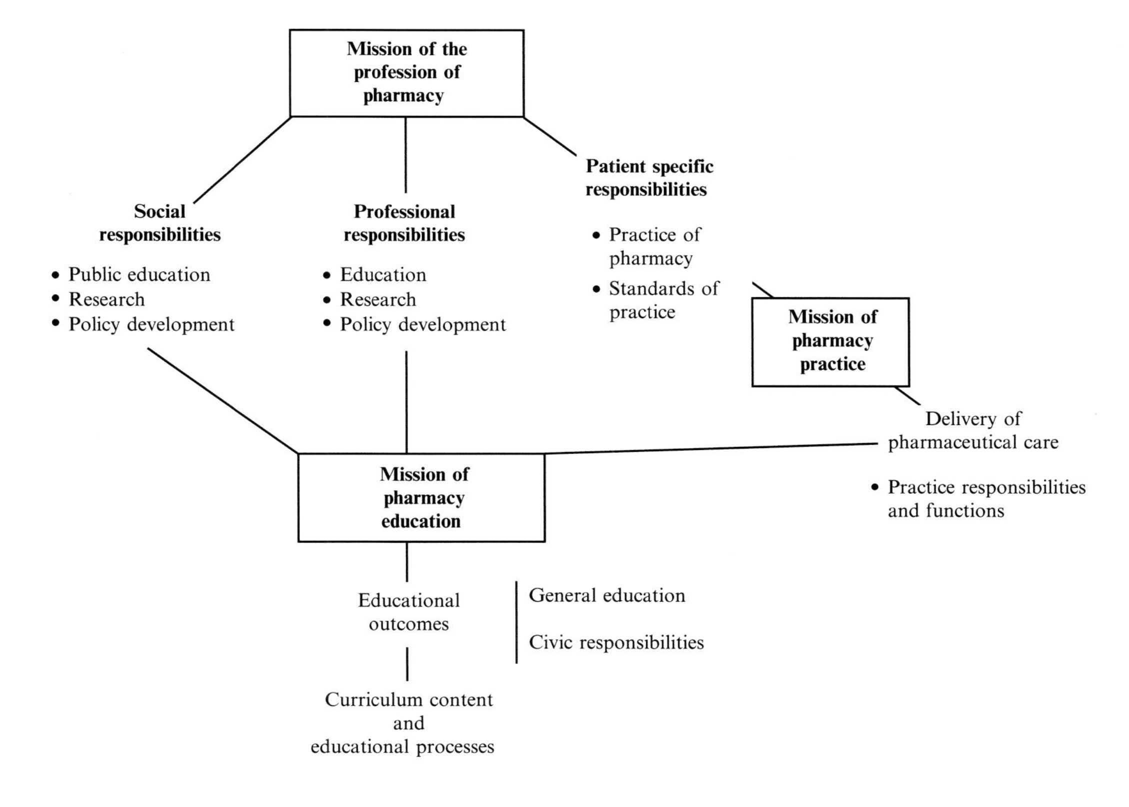

FIG. 1

Interrelationship of mission statements, responsibilities, educational outcomes, curricular content, and educational processes.

From Perrier, D. G., Winsdale, N., Pugsley, J., Lavack, L., & Strand, L. M. (1995). Designing a pharmaceutical care curriculum. American Journal of Pharmaceutical Education, 59, *113–125.*

Similarly, the EAFP Task Force for Implementing Pharmaceutical Care into the Curriculum (Tromp, 1999) proposed changes in the pharmacy undergraduate curricula in European countries. Following this, European countries including the Netherlands, Germany, Switzerland, Romania, Spain, and Portugal developed and implemented pharmaceutical care–based curricula in their undergraduate pharmacy degree programs (Fresco & Silva, 2011; Hersberger & Arnet, 2006; Martín-Calero et al., 2004; Popa, Crisan, Sandulescu, & Bojita, 2002; Van Mil et al., 2004).

Some scholars had noted early evidence of lack of clinical orientation in pregraduate pharmacy education in some European schools, where the curriculum was dominated by the traditional emphasis on molecular science that is often poorly linked to clinical application (Hudson et al., 2007).

A recent review has compared the inclusion of patient-centered care in pharmacy curricula in the United States and Europe (Nunes-da-Cunha, Arguello, Martinez, & Fernandez-Llimos, 2016). A random sample of 59 schools (23 in the United States and 36 in Europe) was selected and, based on evaluation of course descriptions from syllabi, courses were classified into one of the following: clinical sciences, other/basic sciences, sociobehavioral/administrative pharmacy sciences, or experiential training. This analysis found that colleges of pharmacy in the United States heavily focused on clinical sciences in their curricula, while their European counterparts maintained a greater focus on basic sciences and less emphasis on clinical sciences (Nunes-da-Cunha et al., 2016). Although the study was not focused specifically on pharmaceutical care education, it made several references to the term and provided some insights into the variabilities in curricula across nations. However, gradually, more schools of pharmacy in Europe are shifting toward a new combination of laboratory-based science and clinical science within the curricula (Hudson et al., 2007).

Similarly, countries of South America, such as Argentina, Brazil, Cuba, and Chile, have progressed in terms of inclusion of pharmaceutical care content in pharmacy education (Bertoldo, Huespe, Ascar, Welter, & Mainardi, 2003; Limberger, 2013; Martínez-Sánchez, 2003; Ruiz et al., 2002). Several other developing countries of Africa, the Middle East, and Asia have also progressed in implementing pharmaceutical care-based education in pharmacy curricula. As an example, pharmaceutical care education has been introduced in Malaysia, Ethiopia, Qatar, Jordan, Kuwait, and other Middle Eastern countries (Albsoul-Younes, Wazaify, & Alkofahi, 2008; Hassali, Mak, & See, 2014; Katoue, Awad, Schwinghammer, & Kombian, 2014; Kheir et al., 2008; Kheir & Fahey, 2011; Odegard et al., 2011). Indeed, pharmaceutical care education has been incorporated in the curricula of undergraduate and postgraduate pharmacy curricula in several other countries, including Australia, New Zealand, China, and Nigeria.

We do acknowledge that this review is short of exhaustive reporting for all countries and universities that have incorporated pharmaceutical care content in their pharmacy curricula worldwide. But, as indicated earlier, the intention was to highlight some examples from different parts of the world. Furthermore, a lack of published peer-reviewed literature (original investigations or reviews) does not necessarily imply a lack of pharmaceutical care content in pharmacy education in certain countries. A global review investigating pharmaceutical care education in pharmacy curricula as well as teaching methods and learning strategies is warranted.

It is increasingly recognized that initial undergraduate training cannot provide health professionals such as pharmacists with all that they need to know for a lifetime of professional practice (Anderson et al., 2008). Therefore, pharmacy students must have the preparedness and mindset of lifelong learning. In order to fully implement pharmaceutical care education and practice, postgraduate education in the form of continuing professional development (CPD) is needed (Martín-Calero et al., 2004;

Van Mil et al., 2004). Pharmacists who graduated prior to the 1990s might not have been exposed to such education and will require a knowledge and skills upgrade. It becomes obvious that those pharmacists should actively participate in CPD or similar programs to meet their professional mandates and responsibilities. Within the last two decades, numerous postgraduate courses and CPD training programs related to pharmaceutical care skills have been offered to practicing pharmacists around the world (Chiang, Lee, Lin, Yen, & Chen, 2010; de Souza, Mesquita, Antoniolli, De Lyra Júnior, & Da Silva, 2015; Koda-Kimble & Batz, 1994; Reutzel, DeFalco, Hogan, & Kazerooni, 1999). Educational outcomes and competency standards against which practice may be compared have been developed in some countries (Wiedenmayer et al., 2006). Such standards are used to assess the competency of pharmacists in licensure examinations and in CPD programs. The FIP Position Statement on CPD introduced a solid framework for pharmacists to meet this obligation (International Pharmaceutical Federation, 2002).

A systematic review of teaching methods in pharmaceutical care by de Souza and colleagues has demonstrated that simulation-based education followed by CBL and PBL was the most commonly described teaching method for pharmaceutical care in the published literature. Other reported teaching methods and technologies used include didactic lectures, experiential learning and advanced pharmacy practice experiences, discussion boards, use of an audience response system, web-based learning, and collaborative activities utilizing digital tools and service learning (de Souza et al., 2015).

The evolution of pharmaceutical care-based curricula has led to the emergence and advancement of research to assess the impact of pharmaceutical care services on patient outcomes (Berenguer et al., 2004; Martín-Calero et al., 2004; Strand, Cipolle, Morley, & Frakes, 2004). Some of the early landmark pharmaceutical care education and research projects have included the IMPROVE Project (Carter et al., 1998; Ellis et al., 2000), the Pharmaceutical Care Project in Minnesota (Tomechko, Strand, Morley, & Cipolle, 1995), the Pharmacist Implementation of Pharmaceutical Care Model (Odedina, Hepler, Segal, & Miller, 1997), and the Pharmaceutical Care Research and Education (PEP) in Canada (Kassam et al., 1999). Several of these studies on the implementation of pharmaceutical care programs enabled pharmacists to gain skills and knowledge to deliver patient-centered care and have demonstrated some evidence of benefits.

The changes outlined in the new mission for the pharmacy profession and pharmacy practice orchestrate the need to provide optimal drug therapy outcomes for patients through patient-centered care. The new mission mandates pharmacists to effectively manage all patients' drug therapy, and academic pharmacy and professional bodies have an obligation to prepare pharmacy graduates for this role (Raman-Wilms, 2012). As previously emphasized, a link between pharmacy practice and education is warranted if the educational transformation is to have a positive impact on patient care outcomes and the profession (Newton, 1991). There is a clear articulation of the guiding principles for pharmaceutical care as a new model of pharmacy practice, which in turn serves as the basis for curricular reforms (Commission to Implement Change in Pharmaceutical Education, 1993a, 1993b, 1993c, 1993d; Perrier et al., 1995). New training and educational models are in place in many countries to produce graduates that are independent and competent pharmaceutical care practitioners, who are responsible to both patients and healthcare teams. As a result of this paradigm shift in practice and training, more needs to be done in order to meet the contemporary healthcare needs of the society. Some of the milestones and educational reforms that have taken place to prepare pharmacy students and pharmacists for the expanded patient care role include introduction of new entry-to-practice degree programs such as PharmD in North America and MPharm in the UK, new educational outcomes and professional competency standards, requirements for expanded experiential education, pharmacists' specialization across a wide range of medical specialties, and clinical teaching of pharmacists (Hudson et al., 2007; Kennerly & Weber, 2013; Nash, Chalmers, Brown, Jackson, & Peterson, 2015; Raman-Wilms, 2012).

When establishing pharmaceutical care or patient-centered care services in hospitals and other healthcare settings, pharmacy leaders should take into consideration the role of academic pharmacy (Kennerly & Weber, 2013). Academia has played an important role in transforming the pharmacy practice model toward patient-centered care globally. In the United States, many stakeholders were involved in creating the Practice Model Initiative (PPMI), and academic pharmacy was a critical component of the recommendations provided. Kennerly and Weber (2013) proposed a framework such that pharmacy students can assume an integrated and accountable role in the new practice model through defined responsibilities for patient care. To achieve such a model, pharmacy students must begin their experiential training with a sound knowledge base in pharmacotherapy and a broad set of skills, such as communication, clinical reasoning, and time management, to enable them to be effective providers of direct patient care and be proactive members of an interprofessional team. This model, in turn, will produce graduates who are best suited to meet the opportunities and challenges of contemporary pharmacy practice and healthcare reforms. The pharmacy leadership in healthcare institutions should develop a specific plan for integrating trainees into the practice model and establishing strong collaborative partnerships with the pharmacy academic leadership (Kennerly & Weber, 2013; Raman-Wilms, 2012). This will ultimately lead to the attainment of the primary mission of developing patient-centered pharmacy services.

CONCLUSION AND FUTURE DIRECTIONS

Throughout the world, healthcare system and pharmacy practice have undergone enormous changes in the last few decades. Undoubtedly, pharmacists have the potential to improve therapeutic outcomes and ultimately patients' quality of life, and must position themselves appropriately within the healthcare system. With the new evolving roles and expanded scope of practice for pharmacists, the profession is faced with enormous opportunities and challenges. Pharmacy practice has undergone unprecedented changes as new roles for pharmacists, as providers of pharmaceutical care and as scientists, continue to evolve and are increasingly being recognized. While the profession articulates pharmaceutical care as its primary responsibility to the society, pharmacy education needs to develop the educational outcomes, professional competencies, curricular content, and processes that are required to prepare competent graduates to provide optimal pharmaceutical care at the time of entry into practice.

Therefore, academic pharmacy should implement curricular changes to prepare students to assume an integrated and accountable role in the healthcare system by having defined responsibilities for patient care. This will result in graduates who are best suited to meet the increasing challenges of contemporary healthcare reforms and pharmacy practice. To accomplish this, framework development is needed in order to integrate pharmacy degree programs with the new practice models and to establish relationships between leaders in pharmacy practice and those in pharmacy academia. The result will be the fulfillment of the primary mission of providing optimal patient-centered care.

Future directions for both pharmacy practice and education will include: emphasis on interprofessional education and collaborative practice; expanding the role of pharmacists in public or population health; and incorporating more intensive experiential education in teaching pharmaceutical care.

REFERENCES

Accreditation Council for Pharmacy Education. (2011). *Accreditation standards and guidelines for the professional program in pharmacy leading to the doctor of pharmacy degree*. Retrieved from https://www.acpe-accredit.org/pdf/S2007Guidelines2.0_ChangesIdentifiedInRed.pdf.

Al-Wazaify, M., Matowe, L., Albsoul-Younes, A., & Al-Omran, O. A. (2006). Pharmacy education in Jordan, Saudi Arabia, and Kuwait. *American Journal of Pharmaceutical Education*, *70*(1), 18.

Al-Worafi, Y. M. (2014). The challenges of pharmacy education in Yemen. *American Journal of Pharmaceutical Education*, *78*(8), 146. https://doi.org/10.5688/ajpe788146.

Albsoul-Younes, A., Wazaify, M., & Alkofahi, A. (2008). Pharmaceutical care education and practice in Jordan in the new millennium. *Jordan Journal of Pharmaceutical Sciences*, *1*(1), 83–90.

Allemann, S. S., Van Mil, J. W., Botermann, L., Berger, K., Griese, N., & Hersberger, K. E. (2014). Pharmaceutical care: the PCNE definition 2013. *International Journal of Clinical Pharmacy*, *36*(3), 544–555. https://doi.org/10.1007/s11096-014-9933-x.

American Association of Colleges of Pharmacy. (1998). *Educational outcomes* (p. 1998). Retrieved from http://www.aacp.org/Pages/Default.aspx.

American Association of Colleges of Pharmacy (CAPE). (2013). *Educational outcomes* (p. 2013). Retrieved from http://www.aacp.org/documents/CAPEoutcomes071213.pdf.

American College of Clinical Pharmacy. (2008). The definition of clinical pharmacy. *Pharmacotherapy*, *28*(6), 816–817.

Anderson, C., Bates, I., Beck, D. E., Brock, T., Futter, B., Mercer, H., et al. (2008). The WHO UNESCO FIP pharmacy education taskforce: enabling concerted and collective global action. *American Journal of Pharmaceutical Education*, *72*(6), 127.

Anderson, C., Blenkinsopp, A., & Armstrong, M. (2003). *The contribution of community pharmacy to improving the public's health. In Report 1, Evidence from the peer-reviewed literature 1990–2001*, ISBN 0-9538505-1-X. Retrieved from http://eprints.nottingham.ac.uk/id/eprint/1571.

Association of Faculties of Pharmacy of Canada. (2010). *Educational outcomes for first professional degree programs in pharmacy (entry-to-practice pharmacy programs) in Canada*. Retrieved from https://www.afpc.info/sites/default/files/AFPC%20Educational%20Outcomes.pdf.

Austin, Z., & Ensom, M. H. H. (2008). Education of pharmacists in Canada. *American Journal of Pharmaceutical Education*, *72*(6), 128.

Awaisu, A., & Pawluk, S. (2015). Patient assessment teaching and learning in undergraduate pharmacy curriculum: students' perspective of a pharmacist-physician instructional strategy. *Pharmacy Education*, *15*, 27–130.

Barber, N. (2001). Pharmaceutical care and medicines management—is there a difference? *Pharmacy World & Science*, *23*(6), 210–211.

Basak, S. C., & Sathyanarayana, D. (2010). Pharmacy education in India. *American Journal of Pharmaceutical Education*, *74*(4), 68.

Beney, J., Bero, L. A., & Bond, C. (2000). Expanding the roles of outpatient pharmacists: effects on health services utilisation, costs, and patient outcomes. *The Cochrane Database of Systematic Reviews*, (3). Cd000336 https://doi.org/10.1002/14651858.cd000336.

Berenguer, B., La Casa, C., de la Matta, M. J., & Martin-Calero, M. J. (2004). Pharmaceutical care: past, present and future. *Current Pharmaceutical Design*, *10*(31), 3931–3946.

Bernsten, C., Bjorkman, I., Caramona, M., Crealey, G., Frokjaer, B., Grundberger, E., et al. (2001). Improving the well-being of elderly patients via community pharmacy-based provision of pharmaceutical care: a multicentre study in seven European countries. *Drugs & Aging*, *18*(1), 63–77.

Bertoldo, P., Huespe, C., Ascar, G., Welter, A., & Mainardi, C. (2003). Pharmaceutical health care education by application of tutorial teaching. *Pharmaceutical Care España*, *5*, 170–172.

Bourdon, O., Ekeland, C., & Brion, F. (2008). Pharmacy education in France. *American Journal of Pharmaceutical Education*, *72*(6), 132.

Bradberry, J. C., Droege, M., Evans, R. L., Guglielmo, J. B., Knapp, D. A., Knapp, K. K., et al. (2007). Curricula then and now—an environmental scan and recommendations since the commission to implement change in pharmaceutical education: report of the 2006–2007 academic affairs committee. *American Journal of Pharmaceutical Education*, *71*(Suppl), S10.

Brodie, D. C. (1981). Pharmacy's societal purpose. *American Journal of Health-System Pharmacy*, *38*, 1893–1986.

Bruce, S. P., Bower, A., Hak, E., & Schwartz, A. H. (2006). Utilization of the Center for the Advancement of Pharmaceutical Education Educational Outcomes, revised Version 2004: report of the 2005 American College of Clinical Pharmacy Educational Affairs Committee. *American Journal of Pharmaceutical Education*, *70*. 4 Article 79.

Caldwell, N. A., Sexton, J. A., Green, C. F., & Farrar, K. (2001). Sowing the seeds for pharmaceutical care: developments in undergraduate clinical teaching at Liverpool School of Pharmacy. *The Pharmaceutical Journal*, *267*, 721–723.

Carter, B. L., Malone, D. C., Valuck, R. J., Barnette, D. J., Sintek, C. D., & Billups, S. J. (1998). The IMPROVE study: background and study design. Impact of managed pharmaceutical care on resource utilization and outcomes in veterans affairs medical centers. *American Journal of Health-System Pharmacy*, *55*(1), 62–67.

Chambers, S. L., Schmittgen, J., & Allen, C. R. (2000). Evaluation of peer teaching in a pharmaceutical care laboratory. *American Journal of Pharmaceutical Education*, *64*(3), 283.

Chiang, Y., Lee, C., Lin, Y., Yen, Y., & Chen, H. (2010). Impact of a continuing education program on pharmacists' knowledge and attitudes toward asthma patient care. *Medical Principles and Practice*, *19*(4), 305–311.

Cipolle, R. J., Strand, L. M., & Morley, P. C. (1998). Preparing the pharmaceutical care practitioner. In R. J. Cipolle, L. M. Strand, & P. C. Morley (Eds.), *Pharmaceutical care practice* (pp. 297–323). New York: Mc Graw-Hill.

Commission to Implement Change in Pharmaceutical Education, A. A. o. C. o. P. (1993a). Background paper I: what is the mission of pharmaceutical education? *American Journal of Pharmaceutical Education*, *57*, 374–376.

Commission to Implement Change in Pharmaceutical Education, A. A. o. C. o. P. (1993b). Background paper II: entry level, curricular outcomes, curricular content and educational process. *American Journal of Pharmaceutical Education*, *57*, 377–385.

Commission to Implement Change in Pharmaceutical Education, A. A. o. C. o. P. (1993c). Background paper III: entry-level education in pharmacy: a commitment to change. *American Journal of Pharmaceutical Education*, *57*, 366–374.

Commission to Implement Change in Pharmaceutical Education, A. A. o. C. o. P. (1993d). Background paper IV: the responsibility of pharmaceutical education for scholarship, graduate education, fellowships, and postgraduate professional education and training. *American Journal of Pharmaceutical Education*, *57*, 386–399.

de Souza, W. M., Mesquita, A. R., Antoniolli, A. R., De Lyra Júnior, D. P., & Da Silva, W. B. (2015). Teaching in pharmaceutical care: a systematic review. *African Journal of Pharmacy and Pharmacology*, *9*(10), 333–346.

Ellis, S. L., Billups, S. J., Malone, D. C., Carter, B. L., Covey, D., Mason, B., et al. (2000). Types of interventions made by clinical pharmacists in the IMPROVE study. Impact of managed pharmaceutical care on resource utilization and outcomes in veterans affairs medical centers. *Pharmacotherapy*, *20*(4), 429–435.

Fielding, D. W., Brazeau, G. A., & Wasan, K. M. (2008). Introduction to the international pharmacy education supplement. *American Journal of Pharmaceutical Education*, *72*(6), 126.

Fresco, P., & Silva, C. (2011). Pharmaceutical Care: a teaching experience. *Pharmacy Education*, *11*(1), 190–193.

Hamouda, A., Al-Rousan, R. M., & Alkhateeb, F. M. (2015). Pharmacy education in the Palestinian territories. *American Journal of Pharmaceutical Education*, *79*(1), 03. https://doi.org/10.5688/ajpe79103.

Hassali, M. A., Mak, V. S. L., & See, O. G. (2014). Pharmacy practice in Malaysia. *Journal of Pharmacy Practice and Research*, *44*(3), 125–128. https://doi.org/10.1002/jppr.1024.

Hepler, C. D. (1987). The third wave in pharmaceutical education: the clinical movement. *American Journal of Pharmaceutical Education*, *51*, 369–385.

Hepler, C. D. (2004). Clinical pharmacy, pharmaceutical care, and the quality of drug therapy. *Pharmacotherapy*, *24*(11), 1491–1498. https://doi.org/10.1592/phco.24.16.1491.50950.

Hepler, C. D., & Strand, L. M. (1990). Opportunities and responsibilities in pharmaceutical care. *American Journal of Hospital Pharmacy*, *47*(3), 533–543.

Hersberger, K. E., & Arnet, I. (2006). Pharmaceutical care—a new discipline in the curriculum: introducing pharmacy students to medication non-compliance. *International Journal for Chemistry (CHIMIA)*, *60*(1–2), 76–79. https://doi.org/10.2533/000942906777675065.

Hu, M., Yee, G., Zhou, N., Yang, N., Jiang, X., & Klepser, D. (2014). Development and current status of clinical pharmacy education in China. *American Journal of Pharmaceutical Education*, *78*(8).

Hudson, S. A., Mc Anaw, J. J., & Johnson, B. J. (2007). The changing roles of pharmacists in society. *International e-Journal of Science, Medicine & Education*, *1*(1), 22–34.

International Pharmaceutical Federation. (2000). *FIP statement of policy on good pharmacy education practice*. Retrieved from http://www.fip.org/www/uploads/database_file.php?id=188.

International Pharmaceutical Federation. (2002). *FIP statement on professional standards: continuing professional development*. Retrieved from https://www.fip.org/www/uploads/database_file.php?id=221&table_id.

International Pharmaceutical Federation. (2009). *FIP statement of policy: quality assurance of pharmacy education*. Retrieved from https://www.fip.org/www/uploads/database_file.php?id=302&table_id.

Isetts, B. J. (1999). Evaluation of pharmacy students abilities to provide pharmaceutical care. *American Journal of Pharmaceutical Education*, *63*, 11–20.

James, D., Nastasic, S., Horne, R., & Davies, G. (2001). The design and evaluation of a simulated-patient teaching programme to develop the consultation skills of undergraduate pharmacy students. *Pharmacy World & Science*, *23*(6), 212–216.

Johnson, J. A., & Bootman, J. L. (1995). Drug-related morbidity and mortality. A cost-of-illness model. *Archives of Internal Medicine*, *155*(18), 1949–1956.

Kassam, R. (2006). Evaluation of pharmaceutical care opportunities within an advanced pharmacy practice experience. *American Journal of Pharmaceutical Education*, *70*(3), 49.

Kassam, R., Farris, K. B., Cox, C. E., Volume, C. I., Cave, A., Schopflocher, D. P., et al. (1999). Tools used to help community pharmacists implement comprehensive pharmaceutical care. *Journal of the American Pharmaceutical Association*, *39*(6), 843–856.

Katoue, M. G., Awad, A. I., Schwinghammer, T. L., & Kombian, S. B. (2014). Pharmaceutical care education in Kuwait: pharmacy students' perspectives. *Pharmacy Practice*, *12*(3), 411.

Kennedy, D. T., Ruffin, D. M., Goode, J. R., & Small, R. E. (1997). The role of academia in community-based pharmaceutical care. *Pharmacotherapy*, *17*(6), 1352–1356. https://doi.org/10.1002/j.1875-9114.1997.tb03107.x.

Kennerly, J., & Weber, R. J. (2013). Role of pharmacy education in growing the pharmacy practice model. *Hospital Pharmacy*, *48*(4), 338–342. https://doi.org/10.1310/hpj4804-338.

Kennie, N. R., Schuster, B. G., & Einarson, T. R. (1998). Critical analysis of the pharmaceutical care research literature. *Annals of Pharmacotherapy*, *32*(1), 17–26. https://doi.org/10.1177/106002809803200101.

Kheir, N., & Fahey, M. (2011). Pharmacy practice in Qatar: challenges and opportunities. *Southern Med Review*, *4*(2), 45–49. https://doi.org/10.5655/smr.v4i2.1007.

Kheir, N., Zaidan, M., Younes, H., El Hajj, M., Wilbur, K., & Jewesson, P. J. (2008). Pharmacy education and practice in 13 middle eastern countries. *American Journal of Pharmaceutical Education*, *72*(6), 133.

Koda-Kimble, M. A., & Batz, F. R. (1994). Diabetes care as an active learning model of postgraduate education and training for pharmaceutical care. *American Journal of Pharmaceutical Education*, *58*, 382–385.

Limberger, J. B. (2013). Metodologias ativas de ensino-aprendizagem para educação farmacêutica: um relato de experiência. *Interface—Comunicação, Saúde, Educação*, *17*(47), 969–975.

Marriott, J. L., Nation, R. L., Roller, L., Costelloe, M., Galbraith, K., Stewart, P., et al. (2008). Pharmacy education in the context of Australian practice. *American Journal of Pharmaceutical Education, 72*(6), 131.

Martín-Calero, M. J., Machuca, M., Murillo, M. D., Cansino, J., Gastelurrutia, M. A., & Faus, M. J. (2004). Structural process and implementation programs of pharmaceutical care in different countries. *Current Pharmaceutical Design, 10*(31), 3969–3985.

Martínez-Sánchez, A. M. (2003). Pharmaceutical care: a challenge to curricula design in pharmacy careers. *Pharmaceutical Care España, 5*, 94–97.

Medina, M. S., Plaza, C. M., Stowe, C. D., Robinson, E. T., DeLander, G., Beck, D. E., et al. (2013). Center for the advancement of pharmacy education 2013 educational outcomes. *American Journal of Pharmaceutical Education, 77*(8), 162. https://doi.org/10.5688/ajpe778162.

Mikeal, R. L., Brown, T. R., Lazarus, H. L., & Vinson, C. (1975). Quality of pharmaceutical care in hospitals. *American Journal of Health-System Pharmacy, 32*(6), 567–574.

Nash, R. E., Chalmers, L., Brown, N., Jackson, S., & Peterson, G. (2015). An international review of the use of competency standards in undergraduate pharmacy education. *Pharmacy Education, 15*(1), 131–141.

Newton, G. D. (1991). Pharmaceutical education and the translation of pharmaceutical care into practice. *American Journal of Pharmaceutical Education, 55*, 339–344.

Nunes-da-Cunha, I., Arguello, B., Martinez, F. M., & Fernandez-Llimos, F. (2016). A comparison of patient-centered care in pharmacy curricula in the United States and Europe. *American Journal of Pharmaceutical Education, 80*(5), 83.

Odedina, F. T., Hepler, C. D., Segal, R., & Miller, D. (1997). The pharmacists' implementation of pharmaceutical care (PIPC) model. *Pharmaceutical Research, 14*(2), 135–144.

Odegard, P. S., Tadeg, H., Downing, D., Mekonnen, H., Negussu, M., Bartlein, R., et al. (2011). Strengthening pharmaceutical care education in Ethiopia through instructional collaboration. *American Journal of Pharmaceutical Education, 75*(7), 134. https://doi.org/10.5688/ajpe757134.

Perrier, D. G., Winsdale, N., Pugsley, J., Lavack, L., & Strand, L. M. (1995). Designing a pharmaceutical care curriculum. *American Journal of Pharmaceutical Education, 59*, 113–125.

Plumridge, R. J., & Wojnar-Horton, R. E. (1998). A review of the pharmacoeconomics of pharmaceutical care. *PharmacoEconomics, 14*(2), 175–189.

Popa, A., Crisan, O., Sandulescu, R., & Bojita, M. (2002). Pharmaceutical care and pharmacy education in Romania. *Pharmacy Education, 2*(1), 11–14.

Raman-Wilms, L. (2012). Evolution in pharmacy education: developing effective patient care practitioners. *The Canadian Journal of Hospital Pharmacy, 65*(4), 253–254.

Reutzel, T. J., DeFalco, P. G., Hogan, M., & Kazerooni, P. V. (1999). Evaluation of a pharmaceutical care education series for chain pharmacists using the focus group method. *Journal of the American Pharmaceutical Association, 39*(2), 226–234 (quiz 295-296).

Robert Gordon University. (2000). Enhancing the performance of graduates: the new pharmaceutical care centre at the Robert Gordon University, Aberdeen [editorial]. *The Pharmaceutical Journal, 264*(7090), 513–517.

Robertson, K. E. (1996). Process for preventing or identifying and resolving problems in drug therapy. *American Journal of Health-System Pharmacy, 53*(6), 639–650.

Ruiz, I., Jirón, M., Pinilla, E., Paulos, C., Pezzani, M., Rubio, B., et al. (2002). Pharmaceutical care education at the University of Chile. *American Journal of Pharmaceutical Education, 66*, 144–147.

Ryan, M., Shao, H., Yang, L., Nie, X., Zhai, S., Shi, L., et al. (2008). Clinical pharmacy education in China. *American Journal of Pharmaceutical Education, 72*(6), 129.

Sarheed, O., Al-Azzawi, A. M., & Nagavi, B. (2014). Pharmacy education in the United Arab Emirates. *American Journal of Pharmaceutical Education. 78*(2). https://doi.org/10.5688/ajpe78245.

Schumock, G. T., Butler, M. G., Meek, P. D., Vermeulen, L. C., Arondekar, B. V., & Bauman, J. L. (2003). Evidence of the economic benefit of clinical pharmacy services: 1996–2000. *Pharmacotherapy, 23*(1), 113–132.

Sosabowski, M. H., & Gard, P. R. (2008). Pharmacy education in the United Kingdom. *American Journal of Pharmaceutical Education, 72*(6), 130.

Strand, L. M., Cipolle, R. J., Morley, P. C., & Frakes, M. J. (2004). The impact of pharmaceutical care practice on the practitioner and the patient in the ambulatory practice setting: twenty-five years of experience. *Current Pharmaceutical Design*, *10*(31), 3987–4001.

Strand, L. M., Morley, P. C., Cipolle, R. J., Ramsey, R., & Lamsam, G. D. (1990). Drug-related problems: their structure and function. *Drug Intelligence and Clinical Pharmacy*, *24*(11), 1093–1097.

Tomechko, M. A., Strand, L. M., Morley, P. C., & Cipolle, R. J. (1995). Q and A from the pharmaceutical care project in Minnesota. *American Pharmacy*, *Ns35*(4), 30–39.

Touchette, D. R., Doloresco, F., Suda, K. J., Perez, A., Turner, S., Jalundhwala, Y., et al. (2014). Economic evaluations of clinical pharmacy services: 2006–2010. *Pharmacotherapy*, *34*(8), 771–793. https://doi.org/10.1002/phar.1414.

Tromp, T. F. J. (Ed.), (1999). *Report of the task force for implementing pharmaceutical care into the curriculum.* Groningen/Kampen, The Netherlands: University of Groningen Quality Institute for Pharmaceutical Care and European Association of Faculties of Pharmacy.

Van Mil, J. W., Schulz, M., & Tromp, T. F. (2004). Pharmaceutical care, European developments in concepts, implementation, teaching, and research: a review. *Pharmacy World & Science*, *26*(6), 303–311.

Wadelin, J. W. (2003). Evolving quality improvement in pharmaceutical education. *American Journal of Pharmaceutical Education*, *67*(2), 49. https://doi.org/10.5688/aj670249.

Wiedenmayer, K., Summers, R. S., Mackie, C., Gous, A., Everard, M., & Tromp, D. (2006). *Developing pharmacy practice: A focus on patient care.* Retrieved from http://apps.who.int/iris/bitstream/10665/69399/1/WHO_PSM_PAR_2006.5_eng.pdf.

Winslade, N. E., Strand, L. M., Pugsley, J. A., & Perrier, D. G. (1996). Practice functions necessary for the delivery of pharmaceutical care. *Pharmacotherapy*, *16*(5), 889–898.

CHAPTER

THE CONTRIBUTION OF PHARMACY EDUCATION TO PUBLIC HEALTH

7

Albert I. Wertheimer
College of Pharmacy, Nova Southeastern University, Ft. Lauderdale, FL, United States

INTRODUCTION

There are two general avenues to maintain and improve the health of a society. The first is the one we pharmacists are most familiar with, which is one-on-one delivery of personal health services, caring for one patient at a time. This is often referred to as episodic care, where the patient contacts the physician when an episode of illness is observed. The second avenue, called public health or population health, is just as important. Some tasks are best accomplished by one or the other of the two options, and some health challenges require a joint effort of both avenues. Public health targets a large population instead of individual patients and its emphasis is usually on disease prevention and early detection of disease. Some common examples of public health efforts are immunization campaigns and health education activities to reduce the incidence of type 2 diabetes, with promotion of healthy eating and exercise regimes to the population at risk.

To contribute to the health status of a region or country, the pharmacy student or practicing pharmacist must understand public health terminology and the history of healthcare services. Public health professionals speak about infant mortality rates, life expectancy, and the prevalence of certain diseases. They focus on patient education, screening for pathologies, and prevention activities. Public health personnel are the ones in nearly all countries who suggest the studies and policies that a Ministry of Health may adopt for the betterment of a society's health status. Let's first discuss what public health is as it is practiced today (Carter & Slack, 2010).

Public health is the discipline involved in preventing disease, promoting health, and prolonging life by organized efforts and informed choices of organizations, society, public and private groups, communities, and individuals. Health is defined by the World Health Organization (WHO) as the sense of physical, mental, and social well-being, and not just the absence of disease or infirmity. Public health differs from personal health services mainly in the targeted audience. The targeted audience is one person when a person visits their primary care provider or a specialist, while in the public health realm, the intended target audience is groups or cohorts of people. These could be seniors, high school students, or patients with specific diseases or risk factors, such as sexually active teenagers, or persons with diabetes or cancer in their family history, among many others (Krska, 2011).

Pharmacy Education in the Twenty First Century and Beyond. https://doi.org/10.1016/B978-0-12-811909-9.00007-1

Public health personnel perform what is called "needs assessment" to locate and quantify the biggest or most pressing needs for public health services. They examine vital statistics records to see whether any standards or statistics are slipping or not improving. They look at data on the burden of illness to ascertain what are the most costly pathologies within a country or region. The greatest needs may not always coincide with the health problems receiving the greatest amount of media attention. Once the public health priorities are determined, the question becomes: "What is/are the optimal strategy/strategies to provide an effective solution to the problem?" For example, we have all seen the "practice safe sex" promotional messages used by health authorities and public health personnel to combat the spread of the virus causing HIV/AIDS. Different geographic areas routinely face different public health issues. For example, in the tropics, there are public health educational efforts promoting the use of sunblocking agent to prevent skin cancers. In northern climates, there are public health messages about the steps to prevent frostbite or how to deal with it. In Africa, there are extensive efforts concerning parasitic diseases, giving information about avoiding worms and providing encouragement not to walk barefoot.

Not all public health activities are undertaken by public health workers. For example, in order to decrease deaths and injury from automobile accidents on curves and hills, the streets and roads personnel install strong metal guardrails. The restaurant inspectors from city governments check the temperature when dishes are washed, to make certain that possible microorganisms are destroyed. Similarly, restaurant inspectors check for rodents or insects and they measure the temperature of refrigerators to verify that foods requiring refrigeration or freezing are kept at the appropriate temperatures and conditions. The school street crossing guard is a type of public health worker, making certain that children can safely cross the street on their way to or from their school. School staff measure the pH of public swimming pools and add chlorine when necessary to maintain a safe antibacterial level. We receive countless messages every day from multiple sources regarding topics such as not to drive and drink alcohol, to be tested for hypertension, to get flu shots, etc. (American Society of Health-System Pharmacists, 2008).

Public health activities are not new. Beginning in the 19th century, tuberculosis patients were quarantined so as to minimize the spread of the disease to uninfected persons. Starting with smallpox, vaccinations have been used throughout the years to immunize people, to prevent diseases such as pertussis, rubella, pneumonia, diphtheria, tetanus, and many more. One could say that immunizations are individual health services and not examples of population health, but they would be only partially correct: when the immunization rate comes close to 80%, a phenomenon called *herd immunity* occurs. With about 80% of the population protected, there would likely be little transmission of the disease, since so many people would be protected and therefore unable to contract the disease and spread it to others. This is partially the reason why we immunize school children. By doing this, there is a lesser chance that children will spread a disease to their family at home.

The public health authorities also establish guidelines for individual healthcare services. Examples include recommendations for prostate gland examinations for men over 60 years, colonoscopies for persons 50 years and older every 6 years, mammography for women 40 years and older, annual seasonal flu shots, Pap smears every 3 years for women, and many others that public health expert advisory panels recommend, and that the various medical practitioner societies endorse and encourage their members to adopt (American Public Health Association, 2006).

Today, the field of public health has greatly expanded and grown, with new specialty areas and even subspecialty branches. There are people who analyze "big data" looking for trends, to give us advance warning of expected problems. These same people can compare different treatment regimens or approaches and determine what are called best practices using real-world evidence (rwe), informing policy on the optimal interventions for a large array of disease states. We see nutritionists who are prepared to help diabetic or hypertensive and other patients to have an optimal diet. Health educators teach health literacy, so that people with lesser levels of formal education can understand more about their conditions. We cannot expect patients to follow nutritional or exercise or drug-taking adherence advice if they do not understand the nature of their pathology and what steps are necessary to control symptoms or to cure the disease. Hopefully, having a better understanding of a disease state will lead to optimal patient behaviors. An example would be that it is necessary that diabetics understand that they must limit carbohydrates and not only sugars by understanding that the starch in pasta or baked goods becomes sugar in the body.

HOW IS PUBLIC HEALTH PRACTICED

Most traditional public health activities are undertaken by local county and city health departments. The federal government in the United States is also very involved through the US Public Health Service and through the National Institutes of Health (NIH) and the Centers for Disease Control and Prevention (CDC). Local county and city health departments have become the frontlines for public health activities. They inspect restaurants and food-handling establishments such as grocery stores and cold storage facilities, and organizations that use radiation, such as X-ray machines in hospitals and dentists' offices. A number of what are called "reportable diseases" are reported by physicians to the local health department, where early outbreaks might be able to be halted with the use of mass immunization campaigns. This might prevent an epidemic from occurring in that community. Local health departments also undertake work in case finding when, for example, certain sexually transmitted diseases are diagnosed, and the local public health personnel will determine the identities of previous liaison partners of the patient diagnosed so that he or she might be treated to curtail the infection of larger numbers of people. It is the local health department that erects signs and issues warnings that the water at a beach is not safe for swimming due to a high coliform bacteria count or due to an algae bloom. These same people check the quality of the air to prevent industrial pollution from local factories. They check the sewage discharge to check for prohibited substances or high levels of toxic materials. Some chemicals or substances must be incinerated at high temperature and not dumped into the water supply. They also monitor the items shipped to landfills to prevent an accumulation of harmful substances. The local health authorities have the authority to issue penalties to polluters in order to encourage them to clean up their previous practices. Repeat offenders can be fined large sums of money or even sent to jail (American Public Health Association, 2006).

At the national level, the NIH conducts research on promising drugs, vaccines, devices, and diagnostic items. Many of our most important healthcare improvements have come through NIH efforts. The CDC is probably the most important organization in the public health area. The CDC characterizes and identifies new pathogens, such as the agent (often a virus or bacteria) responsible for swine flu, bird fever, SARS, and Ebola outbreaks, among many others. They begin crafting vaccines and they determine what known drugs or biological agents might be effective against such pathogens. The CDC establishes the guidelines for the schedule of childhood vaccinations that nearly all pediatricians follow.

Recently, the US Food and Drug Administration has become more active in the public health arena. Previously, the FDA would passively receive reports from nurses and physicians and pharmacists about an unexpected adverse event, and if enough of these voluntarily submitted reports were received, the FDA might look into the matter. Today, Phase IV, postmarketing studies are required to be submitted by manufacturers to the FDA, and in addition the FDA purchases data from large hospitals and clinics to become proactive in spotting patterns of adverse events before too many patients are harmed. Clinical trials of new drugs usually involve less than 10,000 patients, so that an adverse event happening at a rate of 1 event in every 12,000 patients may not have been detected during the formal clinical trial. Now the FDA can learn about one case in Oregon, one in Missouri, one in Florida, and one in Maine, and have the clues that a problem might be developing. This would not have been possible during the previous passive era, where many more local problem cases would be needed to be observed before any patterns might be hypothesized.

All levels of health departments publish educational materials as well as videos for television and also for social media to warn, educate, and raise consciousness about various health risks. These may be quite diverse, from handling guns safely, to carefully washing fruits and vegetables, to how to cough into one's elbow, etc. Other sectors practice very specific aspects of public health. Hospitals exhaust potentially harmful gases through vents in the building roof; manufacturers require protective covering, especially of the eyes, where acids and other caustic substances are used in production; pharmaceutical companies may use masks and ventilators when workers might be harmed by some compounds if inhaled. Health department rules even limit the amount of carbon dioxide in the small booths where people collect tolls on highways. The operator of the tollbooth is responsible for adhering to those regulations. Some countries have gone well beyond the rest: The Netherlands requires that workers have access to an outside window so they can see the sun and sky to improve mental health. Even labor laws often involve public health, where a break is required for workers on the job continuously for 4 h. Walking and stretching can help prevent emboli and a bathroom break may avoid kidney or bladder problems.

TOPICS TO BE STUDIED

Law and jurisprudence are important topics. When the research or academic community report definitive findings, it is often required that the power of the law is necessary for acceptable levels of innovation. Thus the practitioner of public health must understand how something becomes a law and the processes involved. Examples abound. When it became crystal clear that the use of seatbelts in automobiles saved lives and reduced morbidity, it became necessary to introduce legislation to require the use of seatbelts while operating a vehicle. If a driver is found not wearing a seatbelt, he or she is subject to a monetary fine or penalty. We have other public health–based laws regarding required immunizations before students are permitted to enter elementary school, the use of helmets by motorcycle riders, and others. Laws are introduced by legislators, who must convince other legislators to cosponsor a "bill" and lobby other legislators to vote in favor of the bill. The public's health is the core reason that some medications require a doctor's prescription and that some other drugs, such as narcotics, have further restrictions, and it is also the reason that healthcare professionals must pass licensing examinations before being allowed to practice.

Health policy is a related area that is equally important. One must study this area to learn how to be an effective advocate. For example, if a creek overflows with foul water on a frequent basis, the public health practitioner must understand the structure and functioning of the city and county governments so as to reach the responsible agency with a minimum of referrals, to request that something be done about that creek. If these efforts are not successful, one must know who is higher in the bureaucracy to be able to apply pressure on the department that is not fulfilling its responsibilities. This advocacy may include calling in favors from local office candidates that the practitioner or their professional society supported in their election campaigns. Health policy includes knowledge of organizing coalitions of groups with common interests to apply even greater pressure on lawmakers. Since legislators need votes to be elected, they recognize the power of organized groups of voters (Fulda, Lyles, & Wertheimer, 2016).

Quality and outcomes represent another area where knowledge is necessary. We hear people saying that a certain nearby hospital is one of the best. That may be true, but civic pride is not enough to justify that statement. One must know what percentage of their surgeries or treatments are successful; what percentage of patients do not survive certain procedures; and what percentage of patients for specific conditions require subsequent interventions. Once we know this information for a hospital or clinic, or even for an individual physician or surgeon, we can compare those results with the numbers from others. Then and only then can we make a factual statement about whether the nearby hospital is excellent, average, or worse. We would like to believe that all physicians with board certification in a field provide roughly equivalent levels of care but, unfortunately, that is not true. There are always some who are more careful or skilled. Recently, a great deal of outcomes and quality data has become available from care provider websites and you should be able to help the patient navigate the information on such sites.

An understanding of **biostatistics** is important for several reasons. Perhaps the most obvious reason is to be able to read and interpret journal articles in health services research or public health journals. But the other major rationale is just as important. Sometimes it is necessary to conduct an evaluation in order to answer a question and the appropriate statistical methods must be used to optimally provide a solution to the question at hand. By mastering biostatistics or statistics, we should be able to determine a minimum sample size for a study, and make certain that we are capturing all of the relevant variables, such as age, gender, previous diseases, etc.

Environmental health is critical in maintaining high levels of public health. We must be aware of the governmental standards for water purity and particulate matter in the air, as well as for permissible levels of pollutants in the air, water, and soil. High levels of coal dust or emissions from factory smokestacks can lead to respiratory difficulties in some persons. Chronic exposure to heavy metals is a very serious problem. A federal government agency, the Environmental Protection Agency, is responsible for much in this area in the United States. Enforcement is often in the hands of local agencies.

Since 1970 the Occupational Safety and Health Administration (OSHA) has been in business establishing standards for workplace matters. Helpful websites include https://www.cdc.gov/niosh/homepage.html and https://www.epa.gov. For example, the EPA requires that no more than 0.01 mg/L of arsenic can be in drinking water. The EPA conducts risk assessment for exposure to many substances, radiation, etc.

Epidemiology is the basic or core science of public health. It is the study of disease patterns and is employed within the entire public health process. It is used to determine what factors are related to a health problem. For example, it was pioneered by Dr. John Snow in London, who determined that everyone who contracted cholera had obtained drinking water from the same Bond Street well. Armed with that information, the well was closed and no new cases of cholera were discovered. Through the use of epidemiological principles and practices, we can correlate diseases with possible causes, such as lead in old paint, radiation with cancers, sedentary lifestyles with diabetes and heart disease, etc. Two of the most commonly used tools are cohort and case-control studies. Subjects in a cohort study are enrolled without the investigator knowing whether they will come down with the disease, but he/she knows whether they were exposed to it earlier. Case-control studies also explore the strength of association exposure and development of a disease. Epidemiology measures risk by creating a risk estimate referred to as "relative risk." Another commonly used methodology is the odds ratio, which compares the likelihood that people who have a disease were exposed to people who do not have that disease. The mathematics is not complex, even if some of the terminology sounds imposing.

Development and disasters are the focus for numerous public health endeavors. While the efforts may be similar, the activities and goals are quite different. There are numerous countries around the world where the family income may not exceed US$1 per day, which clearly limits the amount of healthcare services the family can afford to consume. Missions and other generous healthcare professions visit such places and set up clinics for immunizations, dental care, cleft palate, parasitic and amoebic diseases, among many others. From preliminary studies of disease patterns, nutrition, water quality, etc. the mission members have an idea of what medical problems they will encounter. Such development activities can help the population to be healthier, to be more able to work or attend school, and hopefully to become self-sufficient and more affluent over time.

Missions are also activated for disaster relief following floods, tornados, fires, hurricanes, environmental catastrophes such as chemical spills, or famines often caused by drought or weather problems, war, or unaffordability of seeds to plant. The recent Ebola epidemic in Africa caused serious health and economic hardship as drivers, farmers, and factory and office workers became ill and many services could not function.

Demography is the study of people's characteristics. Demographic variables are essential in public health activities. We need to know about people's height, weight, gender, age, disease status, and clinical information about blood glucose levels, blood pressure, cholesterol levels, etc. It is difficult to collect all of the clinical and demographic data from a group, because it often must be obtained from multiple sources and then aggregated. But once it is available, we can search for correlations, such as increased numbers of heart attacks with specific drugs, drinking water from a certain source, eating large quantities of some food or drink. People who consume large quantities of cured meats are thought to have higher levels of colon cancers, and this is observed with smoked fish and stomach cancers, and tobacco chewing and oral cancers. When such associations are recognized, public health educators may step in with campaigns and educational programs to teach and inform the public about behaviors to avoid to improve their health status.

Value for money is a piece of economics that is used in public health. Consider the following example: A local health department has an annual budget of US$2 million. It has recommendations to hire more food and restaurant inspectors, to install more guard rails on local roads where curves occur on hills, and to hold influenza vaccine programs at local high schools. Each of these programs costs about $1 million each. Which are the priorities? The answer comes from conducting a quality of life study to determine the cost of a QALY—a Quality Adjusted Life Year. The health department would first implement the intervention that received the highest number of QALYs per $1 million, and after that, the next most cost:beneficial intervention. Of course, the pharmacist active in public health would learn about the cost–utility equation, which is used to compute the QALY numbers needed to make fund allocation decisions (Truong, Bresette, & Sellers, 2010).

CONCLUSIONS

There are many other aspects of public health that one would learn in a public health course. A recent search on "Public Health courses" located nearly 150 such courses, many of which are available online and for free. They appear to be available in numerous languages.

Masters of Public Health (MPH) courses are offered by universities all over the world, but it is also quite possible for pharmacists to study one or more of the online courses to improve their skills and knowledge in the area of public health, so that they may be optimally helpful and useful when public health efforts are needed in an area.

REFERENCES

American Public Health Association (APHA). (2006). *The role of the pharmacist in public health: Policy statement*. DC: Washington.

American Society of Health-System Pharmacists (ASHP). (2008). ASHP statement on the role of health-system pharmacists in public health. *American Journal of Health-System Pharmacy*, *65*, 462–467.

Carter, J., & Slack, M. (2010). *Pharmacy in public health: Basics and beyond*. Bethesda, MD: American Society of Health System Pharmacists.

Fulda, T., Lyles, A., & Wertheimer, A. (2016). *Pharmaceutical public policy*. Boca Raton, FL: CRC Press.

Krska, J. (2011). *Pharmacy in public health*. London: Pharmaceutical Press.

Truong, H. A., Bresette, J. L., & Sellers, J. A. (2010). *The pharmacist in public health*. Washington, DC: American Pharmacists Association.

SECTION

PHARMACY EDUCATION: FEATURES AND CONTRIBUTING FACTORS

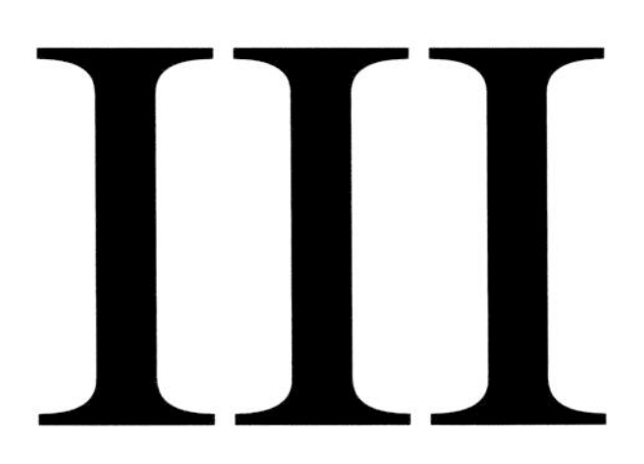

CHAPTER

CURRICULA ORIENTATIONS: CLASSICAL- VERSUS CLINICAL-ORIENTED CURRICULA

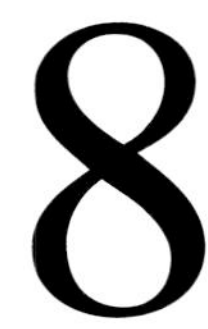

Long C. Ming*,†, Tahir M. Khan‡,§

**KPJ Healthcare University College, Nilai, Malaysia, †University of Tasmania, Hobart, TAS, Australia, ‡Monash University Malaysia, Subang Jaya, Malaysia, §University of Veterinary & Animal Sciences, Lahore, Pakistan*

INTRODUCTION

Pharmacy practice has been transformed in recent years following novel scientific discoveries, technology trends, and evolving patient needs, as well as higher competencies required of pharmacists in terms of pharmacist-provided services, active collaboration in multidisciplinary teams, and better understanding of patients' health (Gilmartin, Nguyen, Reeve, & Tan, 2016). Hence, it is imperative to ensure that the development of pharmacy education is sufficient to produce healthcare professionals who are adequately trained, especially in clinical aspects (Hadi, Long, Leng, Shaharuddin, & Adam, 2010). For the past two-and-a-half decades, the discipline of clinical pharmacy has been described as not just merely dispensing of pharmaceutical products, but the involvement of organizing, developing, and analyzing information related to pharmaceutical issues and, most importantly, counseling on drug-related information to patients and other healthcare professionals (Stohs & Muhi-Eldeen, 1990). In recent years, the pharmacy profession has evolved and been restructured in terms of focus toward patient care and development of new tools as well as approaches (Hasan et al., 2010).

Nowadays, clinical pharmacists are part of a multidisciplinary healthcare team and have a role as drug experts and pharmacotherapy consultants, meaning they have influence in decision-making on medication-related problems (Salamzadeh, 2010). Clinical pharmacists play a vital role in rational use of medicine (Salamzadeh, 2010), identifying drug-related problems, contributing to medication reviews and therapeutic recommendations, and ideally acting as a bridge to fill the gaps between patients and physicians (Francis & Abraham, 2014). It has been shown that pharmacists' active involvement in healthcare systems has a positive impact on disease management and on reducing healthcare costs. Therefore, in order to make sure pharmacy graduates are competent to meet the needs of healthcare systems, it is necessary to amplify clinical knowledge and experience of pharmacy throughout their education (Salamzadeh, 2010).

The main objectives of pharmacy education are to provide students with the competencies to function within a multidisciplinary healthcare system and to manage complex drug regimens for a myriad of medical conditions (Pearson & Hubball, 2012). Therefore various institutions are establishing and

Pharmacy Education in the Twenty First Century and Beyond. https://doi.org/10.1016/B978-0-12-811909-9.00008-3

expanding pharmacy education to meet the current requirements of the profession, as pharmacists nowadays are required to make clinical judgments and resolve therapeutic problems (Chanakit, Low, Wongpoowarak, Moolasarn, & Anderson, 2014). In order to equip the clinical pharmacist with therapeutic problem-solving capabilities and to enhance critical judgment skills, an integrated curriculum is essential, with a student-centered and problem-based rather than subject-based approach (Waterfield, 2011). The knowledge base in healthcare is continuously growing; in pharmacy education, active learning strategies like process-oriented guided inquiry learning (POGIL), computerized modules and tutorials, case studies, and team-based learning need to be incorporated, as pharmacists must analyze new information and share this new information with colleagues and patients (Stewart, Brown, Clavier, & Wyatt, 2011). Pharmacy education must equip pharmacists with knowledge of evidence-based practice and medical information, as patients are becoming increasingly knowledgeable about their diseases and current medication, along with other therapeutic options available for the management of their diseases (Marriott et al., 2008).

Classical disciplinary categories used to structure pharmacy curricula rarely place problems and situations that arise in pharmacy practice into distinct categories. Hence, it is important that the curricula of pharmacy programs integrate disciplines and theory with practice (Pearson & Hubball, 2012). Traditionally, the pharmacy profession has been considered to be a transitional discipline between chemistry and health sciences (Pearson, 2007). Classical pharmacy practice curricula focus on pharmaceutical sciences over patient-centered pharmacy practice, meaning they are limited to the traditional responsibilities of pharmacists: compounding, dispensing, administrative activities, and laboratory experience (Ryan et al., 2008). In classical curricula, students tend to spend more time listening to lectures and working individually, with cooperation discouraged. On the other hand, integrated curricula are associated with student-centered educational methods and preparing students for lifelong learning (Azzalis et al., 2012). Classical pharmacy curricula might not be sufficient, as is evidenced by the need for additional pharmacy seminar courses being introduced to impart some basic professional skills to the students, including contemporary information and issues pertaining to hospital and clinical practice. These courses typically address teaching topics or skills that do not fit into the classical curriculum but are an essential part of students' learning process (Romanelli, 2008).

The concepts of curricular integration and integrative learning are crucial in pharmacy programs where students are expected to acquire the knowledge required for competent practice (Pearson & Hubball, 2012). Integration of curricula is an essential component of contemporary approaches in pharmacy education and is designed to connect diverse disciplines and knowledge. It is vital to view the curriculum as a whole and assess students' understanding rather than just information recall (Kerr, 2000). An integrated curriculum is an educational experience designed to demonstrate to students the patterns and applications of different knowledge domains. Integration is seen as a strategy for making educational experiences engaging, relevant and coherent to assist higher-order learning among the students (Pearson & Hubball, 2012).

There are two types of integration: horizontal integration, referring to integration among the disciplines of basic science like pharmaceutics, medicinal chemistry, and pharmacology which involves crossing disciplinary boundaries; and vertical integration, referring to integration of clinical sciences and basic sciences, which involves connecting across time and between theory and practice (Pearson & Hubball, 2012). In addition, student learning can be enhanced through various approaches in sequencing an integrated curriculum, such as a spiraling curriculum (content introduced in curriculum should be proportionate to the students' intellectual development, so there is regular and episodic reutilization of the same topics with gradually greater complexity functions, like a spiral), progressive differentiation (organizing the curriculum contents into levels of detail in a way naturally learned and understood), hierarchical sequencing (following the bottom-up pattern in which the essential parts should be taught first followed by complexity at a later stage), shortest-path sequencing (teachers should first assess what the learners already know and should teach what the students have not learned), and elaboration sequencing (similar to complex sequencing) (Van Patten, Chun, & Reigeluth, 1986). Each of the sequencing approaches can be applied in different sections throughout integrated curricula.

CURRICULUM DELIVERY METHODS

Students' learning processes can be enhanced through integration of pharmacy curricula with structured experiences that allow students to apply knowledge and skills from various domains such as pharmaceutical sciences, and practice experience while in biomedical domains (life sciences, physiological science, and bioengineering) and clinical sciences (clinical therapeutics and clinical practice). Through an integrated curriculum, previously learned skills and knowledge are required to solve problems from various domains, and the abilities-based learning allows students to apply rational and logical thinking (Kerr, 2000). This approach enhances students' critical thinking and ability to recall information, which is an important skill required in real-life cases.

A carefully designed curriculum should consist of both horizontal and vertical integration, and should integrate academic and experiential learning. Courses and subjects integrated with each other at the same or successive curricular levels would assist students to view the curriculum as one whole picture (Kerr, 2000). Horizontal integration links related pharmaceutical science subjects and addresses the same concepts from various scientific domains that include similar principles or skills (Kerr, 2000). The objective of horizontal integration is to enhance students' understanding of a particular topic through interdisciplinary clerkship. For instance, students learn a disease state by learning pathophysiology, pharmacology, medicinal chemistry, and management within the same subject (Brueckner & Gould, 2011). This type of integration can be attained through eliminating departmentally oriented teaching (Elliott, 1999), and planning a coordinated course to warrant learning of a particular topic from different domains simultaneously (Kerr, 2000). Horizontal integration has been the typical curriculum standard for the past decade in medical education in the form of problem-based learning (PBL) (Barrows, 1986; Brynhildsen, Dahle, Fallsberg, Rundquist, & Hammar, 2002; Elliott, 1999).

Vertical integration, on the other hand, refers to inclusion of clinical experience into the early part of the curriculum or reintroduction of basic sciences during clinical years (Brynhildsen et al., 2002; Nierenberg, 1998; Schmidt, 1998). However, the integration of basic sciences into clinical years remains an obstacle for several schools (Rudich & Bashan, 2001). It uses a spiraling sequencing approach in which those critical elements of the curriculum are identified and recycled repeatedly throughout the curriculum. The cyclical repetitions have to be structured in such a way that the degree of complexity escalates continuously, in order to enhance critical abilities of students as they progress through the program (Kerr, 2000). For instance, management concepts can be vertically integrated throughout the 4 years of a program (Kerr, 2000).

Integration of didactic and experiential learning can be realized by including experiential learning throughout the curriculum. At each stage of the curriculum, the experiential module is a platform for students to apply and practice the knowledge and skills learned from didactic modules. At early stages of the curriculum, simple problems and cases can be used as simulation of experiential modules and the degree of complexity should be increased as the students' progress through the curriculum. Problem identification and solving complex cases may require a substantial amount of effort from students and there may be a few different but equally appropriate solutions to the cases. Integration of didactic and experiential modules allow students to develop updated and relevant knowledge and better clinical problem-solving skills (Kerr, 2000; Long, Hadi, Kassab, Yap, & Lee, 2013). The effective integration of didactic learning and experiential training approaches such as problem-based learning (PBL), enquiry-based learning (EBL), and interprofessional education (IPE) could help students to learn. Among these, PBL has been commonly executed by various healthcare professions (Long, Lim, & Hadi, 2011). This approach involves presenting students with a case-based scenario with problems that mimic real-life situations and aligns with the learning outcomes of the particular topic (Long et al., 2011; Long, Yee, Muhammad, Hussain, & Manan, 2015). It demands certain skills and abilities from the learner including critical thinking, teamwork, and self-directed learning (Wells, Warelow, & Jackson, 2009). Besides that, it has been shown in a study that self-consciousness and continual self-reflection are crucial for sustainable competency as a healthcare professional, and the PBL approach may assist students in the development of critical reflection (Waterfield, 2011; Williams, 2001).

EBL is a similar approach to PBL, but involves integration of two or more subject disciplines. This approach receives positive feedback from students, according to a questionnaire-based study (Sattenstall & Freeman, 2015).The students acknowledged that EBL provides a platform that integrates pharmaceutical chemistry into a clinical context and that it encourages self-directed learning (Waterfield, 2011). This approach has addressed other essential soft skills as a healthcare professional such as presentation skills, interpersonal skills, time management, and working in teams (Waterfield, 2011).

IPE is another type of integration focusing on two or more professions collaborating and learning from each other (Waterfield, 2011). The aim of IPE is to enhance collaboration and teamwork among different disciplines, as interdisciplinary collaboration is important in ensuring optimal patient outcomes. According to a systematic review, there is limited evidence that interprofessional learning leads to better teamwork in the workplace (Hammick, Freeth, Koppel, Reeves, & Barr, 2007). However, IPE is typically well accepted by participants and allows them to be trained in terms of skills required for collaborative working. IPE is commonly used to enhance service delivery skills and to improve the development of practice (Hammick et al., 2007).

TREND OF CLASSICAL CLINICAL-ORIENTED AND INTEGRATED CURRICULA

A study was done in the United States to determine the current status and perception of a faculty regarding integration of clinical sciences and basic sciences in the pharmacy curriculum and program (Islam, Talukder, Taheri, & Blanchard, 2016). Curriculum integration has gained a lot of importance in healthcare education and integration of basic sciences and clinical sciences has accounted for key reform in medical education. To achieve this, a survey was conducted among 132 faculty members ($n = 132$) in an accredited pharmacy program. Out of the faculty members, 112 responded, giving a response rate of 85%. Out of the 112 participating institutions (colleges and schools), 78 (70%) responded that they offered integration between clinical sciences and basic sciences, while

13 (12%) institutions had integrated a basic science course and 20 (18%) offered no integrated course (Islam et al., 2016). Among the 70 institutions with integration between basic sciences and clinical sciences, 25 institutions offered a fully integrated course of basic sciences and clinical sciences, 50 institutions offered sequential and coordinated delivery of contents, while 3 institutions offer an isolated integrated course (Islam et al., 2016). Almost 76% of the faculty members agreed/strongly agreed that integrated courses developed practice-oriented, problem-solving skills. A few barriers and challenges faced in the integrated pharmacy curriculum were a lack of coordination between the basic science faculty and practice faculty members, and a lack of consistency in course material (Islam et al., 2016). Nevertheless, the integrated science and clinical practice curricula in pharmacy education is essential to equip pharmacy graduates with the basic knowledge and skills to solve therapeutic problems. The integration helps students to understand the principles in basic sciences in an appropriate clinical context. Collaboration, appreciation and understanding of the bridging between disciplines contributes to a balanced integrated curriculum (Islam et al., 2016).

Integrated pharmacy curricula reforms have gained attention due to their relevance, their ability to engage students and diverse disciplines, and the fact that they allow high-order learning to enable pharmacy professionals to enhance their capabilities and work in large and complex healthcare systems with patient-centric activities (Pearson & Hubball, 2012). In pharmacy, the integration of science and practice in curricula enables pharmacy professionals to solve complex problems with a broad knowledge base (Husband, Todd, & Fulton, 2014). Integrated clinical and practice curricula are well designed and implemented in developed countries, but in developing countries they are not well designed and are not perceived to meet the expectations in current trends of pharmacy practice (Hussain, Malik, & Abdullah, 2017). The duration and content of a pharmacy curriculum can vary from school to school and from country to country, and the pharmaceutical care concept varies in the way it is applied in different countries, but the basic pharmaceutical courses in curricula are similar (Toklu & Hussain, 2013).

PROS AND CONS OF INTEGRATED CURRICULA

The main advantages of having integrated curricula are that it increases education efficiency and it is a beneficial learning style, especially in courses for healthcare professions. Curricula should be evaluated to identify the essentials and maintain them as core elements.

Another added benefit of interprofessional integrated courses is that they create opportunities for collaborative research between faculties (Kerr, 2000). In pharmacy education, several implementations of enhancing active learning among students have been employed, especially in pharmacotherapeutic topics such as PBL alongside case-based learning (Stewart et al., 2011). Furthermore, self-directed learning has been advocated, which motivates students to take initiative in formulating their learning process and implementing suitable learning strategies (Brady, Caldwell, Pate, & Pate, 2013).

According to a large study assessing current and ideal emphasis, the major barrier to curriculum reform in the United States is the limited availability of clinical training sites (Graber, Bellack, Lancaster, & Musham, 1999). Ideally, a ratio of student to preceptor at a clerkship site should be two to one. Up to four to one is justifiable, but it should not exceed four to one at a given time (Haase, Smythe, Orlando, Resman-Targoff, & Smith, 2008). Standardization and continuity between training sites can be ensured by giving the preceptors briefing sessions regarding outlines and concepts of the learning objectives.

SUCCESSES IN CLINICAL-ORIENTED CURRICULUM ADOPTION

In recent years, significant changes have occurred in pharmacy education and it is undeniable that attempts to implement changes in curricula have faced barriers and difficulties. There are debates and arguments regarding the necessity of changing conventional nonintegrated curricula and doubts about the benefits of newly proposed clinical-oriented curricula. It has been noted that the initial changes involved decreasing traditional lab-based working for compounding and dispensing, while putting greater emphasis on drug information and developing communication skills.

Pharmacy curricula in the United States have now evolved from science-based education into a balanced scientific background with an emphasis on a patient-oriented approach. Curricula will continue to evolve in parallel with the development of advanced areas, such as pharmacoinformatics (Neoh, Zainal, Hameed, Khan, & Ming, 2015; Zainal et al., 2016), precision medicine, oncology, and nuclear medicine (Murphy et al., 2010). Students should be taught about integrated clinical information. Besides that, pharmacy students should be taught how technology in health information could impact the delivery system of healthcare, and should also learn the scientific approach in understanding the effectiveness and safety of technologies as part of the process of medication use (Fox, Flynn, Fortier, & Clauson, 2011).

Ever since the Doctor of Pharmacy (PharmD) postbaccalaureate program was introduced in the 1970s, clinical pharmacy has been growing in importance and has become the core of this profession in developed countries. However, for developing countries the term clinical pharmacy is relatively new. The newly developed curricula with a focus on clinical pharmacy practice has given new dimensions to classical pharmacy curricula, with a strong emphasis on clinical training and evidence-based practice (Khan, 2011). The entry requirements for the PharmD degree in the United States include preprofessional undergraduate coursework, for the student to develop professional competencies, and a minimum of four academic years is required. Typically, a total of six academic years is required to meet the degree requirements. Students must complete the preprofessional fundamental curriculum with a minimum of five semesters of coursework (Gleason et al., 2013), which includes applied sciences such as chemistry, biological sciences, physical sciences, and mathematics. Furthermore, throughout the curriculum, students are exposed to behavioral sciences, social sciences, cultural and diversity awareness, humanities, moral and ethics reasoning, teamwork, critical thinking, and communication skills (Francisco, 2002; Gleason et al., 2013).

A clinical-oriented pharmacy curriculum usually includes didactic courses and practice experiences. The program is constructed with the aim of transforming students into independent learners so that, upon completion of the program, students are prepared to undergo continuous learning throughout their career (Francisco, 2002). Furthermore, the experiential elements in the curriculum help in integrating theoretical knowledge and skills so that students can excel in the provision of pharmaceutical care to patients. The practice attachments occur throughout the professional curriculum for 4 years. The attachments in the earlier part of the curriculum are usually general in nature with the aim of introducing students to the pharmacy profession and the multidisciplinary healthcare system. Attachments in the later part of the curriculum include rotation clerkship through several aspects of pharmacy practice, each rotation lasting for several weeks. Throughout the clerkship, students will spend time learning management in the practice setting, providing care to patients and carers, and interacting with other healthcare professionals. These rotations are actually the major elements in the program, as these direct practice experiences assist in the development of practice competence (Francisco, 2002).

The academic success of PharmD graduates has been evaluated and reported in the pharmacy literature, and one of the main factors is the requirement for preprofessional courses before starting pharmacy school (Gleason et al., 2013). In spite of these findings, policy administrators are still undecided on the ideal duration of the preprofessional course (Gleason et al., 2013). Nevertheless, many of these changes were not decided and implemented overnight, but happened steadily over approximately two decades, as seen from previous attempts in curricular changes (Stohs & Muhi-Eldeen, 1990). It is important to note the changes are a continuous improvement process.

CHALLENGES OF CURRICULUM REVISION

In recent years, patient-centered pharmacy practice has been gaining more attention and has focused on clinical pharmacy, which emphasizes the role of the pharmacist as a frontline healthcare provider (Rosenthal, Austin, & Tsuyuki, 2010). However, the nature of this practice change has been in discussion for some time and only a few countries have been successful in significant healthcare reform. Some common barriers are time constraints, limited remuneration models, and limited support from other healthcare colleagues (Rosenthal et al., 2010).

One of the approaches to practice change is to start with pharmacy education. However, planning a curriculum integrated with clinical components cannot be achieved just by combining existing courses into a superficial mixed course. In the decision-making process of creating a curriculum, discipline-specific content often has to be omitted, as not all of it is core information required to execute specific abilities. A curriculum should include teaching students the skills and abilities essential in problem identification, information analysis, and problem solving. Besides that, students should be given opportunities to carry out hands-on activities in order to actually learn and practice the skills and abilities needed as a pharmacist (Kerr, 2000).

Course planning and the development of integrated curriculum are time consuming for the faculty, especially during the developing stage. This is due to the complicated scheduling needed to accommodate group-based learning, self-directed learning, active learning, and participation of multiple disciplines. Notably, members from different faculties should be aware of the learning objectives of the curriculum so that the materials taught are catered specifically to pharmacy students. Besides that, new methods of examination must be designed following the curriculum change. Students' academic performances should be evaluated based on their understanding and ability to apply knowledge to solve problems instead of merely their ability to recall information (Kerr, 2000).

Taking Thailand pharmacy program development history as a case study, the first pharmacy school was formed in 1914 as a part of the Chulalongkorn University, whereby the graduates from a 3-year program received a certificate of compounding. Formal pharmacy education in Thailand began in 1923 as a part of the Faculty of Medicine at the Royal Medical School (Pongcharoensuk & Prakongpan, 2012). Over the years, the professional curriculum evolved and expanded to a 4-year program. In 1989 and 1990, the pharmacy program was further developed to include the concept of clinical pharmacy. In 2008, a 6-year pharmacy program was fully implemented by the Pharmacy Council of Thailand with the title of Doctor of Pharmacy (PharmD) (Chanakit et al., 2014; Pramyothin, Sripanidkulchai, Thirawarapan, & Khunkitti, 1999). To standardize the pharmacy profession throughout Thailand, the council has set this program as a compulsory prerequisite for application to the national pharmacist register. During the transition period, students with BPharm had to do a bridging year of coursework in order to upgrade to PharmD (Bradberry et al., 2007; Scahill, Akhlaq, & Garg, 2013). Since 2014, there have been only PharmD graduates in Thailand, as the classical BPharm has been totally phased out (Chanakit et al., 2014) (Fig. 1).

All PharmD courses in Thailand comply with the core pharmacy course structure guidelines, with at least 140 credit hours for professional content as recommended by the Pharmacy Council of Thailand. The first 4 years of the curriculum consist of core competencies for the profession and the following 2 years are designated for specialization. Students are required to do coursework in the fifth year, while the sixth year involves undergoing specialized clerkship experiences of 2000 practice hours, similar to the American pharmacy programs. Typically, the first 400 h of clerkship experiences start at the end of the fourth year. Practice experiences in hospitals and community pharmacies are compulsory, while the remaining professional practice time can be completed based on individual interests, for instance in hospitals or community settings, in research and development, in manufacturing, or in regulation and jurisdiction. The current PharmD program in Thailand has two tracks, namely pharmaceutical care and industrial pharmacy (formerly pharmaceutical sciences). The amount of time pharmacy students commit to theory, practice, and research in PharmD programs is 51.5%, 46.7% and 1.8%, respectively (Chanakit et al., 2014).

The transition from BPharm to PharmD requires significant cooperation between government, pharmacy faculties, pharmacy councils, and pharmacists in the workforce to foster a better pharmacy

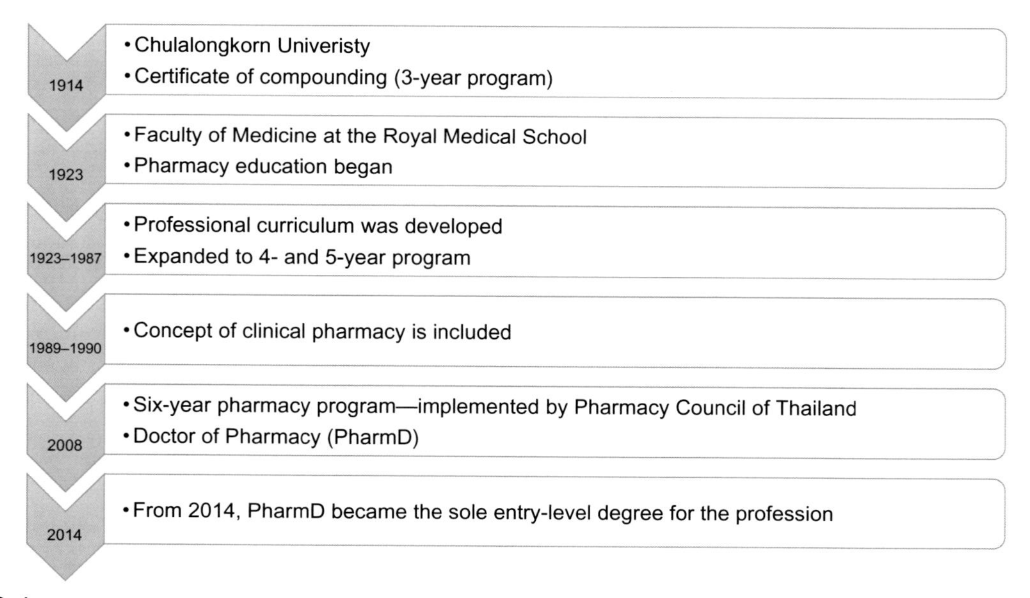

FIG. 1

Time sequence of pharmacy education evolution in Thailand.

education in different aspects, including quality of the program, curriculum validation, training-site planning, and graduates' competencies. Faculty attitudes and opinions differ depending on the degree and the type of integrated curricula being implemented.

The transition from classical and traditional curricula to clinical-oriented pharmacy practice curricula faces a huge barrier if there are negative faculty attitudes toward the change. One of the ways to overcome the perception that basic sciences are irrelevant to clinical practice can be through open line of communication between basic life science and clinical disciplines and discussion of the best way to integrate the elements (Brueckner & Gould, 2006). Besides that, faculty development programs, strong administrative leadership, and enhanced reward systems for participation are some of the other efforts imperative to transitioning to an integrated curriculum (Brueckner & Gould, 2006).

SUMMARY

Globalization and the era of technology have affected numerous sectors of society, including education. Patient-centered pharmacy practice is gaining more attention, as is clinical pharmacy, which emphasizes that the pharmacist is a frontline healthcare provider. Pharmacy curricula have evolved a lot due to the expanded role of the pharmacist in the healthcare system, from a traditional role of dispensing and compounding to clinical-oriented pharmacy practice and being a multidisciplinary healthcare team member.

The transition of pharmacy curricula and teaching methodologies could be a challenging task, but once the barriers have been overcome, it will be exciting and intellectually stimulating. Nowadays, most countries and pharmacy program accreditation councils are in the transition phase of adopting the clinical-oriented pharmacy curriculum and are in the process of modifying from the classical pharmacy curriculum. This will equip pharmacy graduates with the knowledge and skills required to meet the standards and expectations of the new healthcare system, to provide services to communities based on their strong clinical-oriented pharmacy knowledge.

REFERENCES

Azzalis, L. A., Giavarotti, L., Sato, S., Barros, N. M. T., Junqueira, V. B. C., & Fonseca, F. L. A. (2012). Integration of basic sciences in health's courses. *Biochemistry and Molecular Biology Education*, *40*(3), 204–208.

Barrows, H. S. (1986). A taxonomy of problem-based learning methods. *Medical Education*, *20*(6), 481–486.

Bradberry, J. C., Droege, M., Evans, R. L., Guglielmo, J. B., Knapp, D. A., Knapp, K. K., et al. (2007). Curricula then and now—an environmental scan and recommendations since the Commission to Implement Change in Pharmaceutical Education: Report of the 2006–2007 academic affairs committee. *American Journal of Pharmaceutical Education*, *71*, 1–11.

Brady, J. H., Caldwell, D. J., Pate, K. A., & Pate, A. N. (2013). An elective course on application of clinical pharmacy principles. *American Journal of Pharmaceutical Education*, *77*(10), 216.

Brueckner, J. K., & Gould, D. J. (2006). Health science faculty members' perceptions of curricular integration: insights and obstacles. *Journal of the International Association of Medical Science Educators*, *16*(1), 31–34.

Brueckner, J. K., & Gould, D. J. (2011). Health science faculty members' perceptions of curricular integration: Insights and obstacles. *Medical Science Educator*, *16*(1).

Brynhildsen, J., Dahle, L. O., Fallsberg, M. B., Rundquist, I., & Hammar, M. (2002). Attitudes among students and teachers on vertical integration between clinical medicine and basic science within a problem-based undergraduate medical curriculum. *Medical Teacher*, *24*(3), 286–288.

Chanakit, T., Low, B. Y., Wongpoowarak, P., Moolasarn, S., & Anderson, C. (2014). A survey of pharmacy education in Thailand. *American Journal of Pharmaceutical Education*, *78*(9), 161.

Elliott, M. K. (1999). Are we going in the right direction? A survey of the undergraduate medical education in Canada, Australia and the United Kingdom from a general practice perspective. *Medical Teacher*, *21*(1), 53–60.

Fox, B. I., Flynn, A. J., Fortier, C. R., & Clauson, K. A. (2011). Knowledge, skills, and resources for pharmacy informatics education. *American Journal of Pharmaceutical Education*, *75*(5), 1–93.

Francis, J., & Abraham, S. (2014). Clinical pharmacists: bridging the gap between patients and physicians. *Saudi Pharmaceutical Journal*, *22*(6), 600–602.

Francisco, G. E. (2002). Doctor of pharmacy. In *Encyclopedia of Clinical Pharmacy* (pp. 276–281). New York: CRC Press.

Gilmartin, J. F. M., Nguyen, T. A., Reeve, E., & Tan, E. C. (2016). Incorporating research into current pharmacy practice: the future of Australian pharmacy? *Journal of Pharmacy Practice and Research*, *46*(4), 397–398.

Gleason, B. L., Siracuse, M. V., Moniri, N. H., Birnie, C. R., Okamoto, C. T., & Crouch, M. A. (2013). Evolution of preprofessional pharmacy curricula. *American Journal of Pharmaceutical Education*, *77*(5), 95.

Graber, D. R., Bellack, J. P., Lancaster, C., & Musham, C. (1999). Curriculum topics in pharmacy education: current and ideal emphasis. *American Journal of Pharmaceutical Education*, *63*(2), 145.

Haase, K. K., Smythe, M. A., Orlando, P. L., Resman-Targoff, B. H., & Smith, L. S. (2008). Ensuring quality experiential education. *Pharmacotherapy*, *28*(12), 1548–1551.

Hadi, M. A., Long, C. M., Leng, L. W., Shaharuddin, S., & Adam, A. (2010). Developing a practice-based master in clinical pharmacy program at the Universiti Teknologi MARA, Malaysia. *American Journal of Pharmaceutical Education*, *74*(2), 32d.

Hammick, M., Freeth, D., Koppel, I., Reeves, S., & Barr, H. (2007). A best evidence systematic review of interprofessional education: BEME guide no. 9. *Medical Teacher*, *29*(8), 735–751.

Hasan, S. S., Kwai Chong, D. W., Ahmadi, K., Se, W. P., Hassali, M. A., Hata, E. M., et al. (2010). Influences on Malaysian pharmacy students' career preferences. *American Journal of Pharmaceutical Education*, *74*(9), 166.

Husband, A. K., Todd, A., & Fulton, J. (2014). Integrating science and practice in pharmacy curricula. *American Journal of Pharmaceutical Education*, *78*(3), 63.

Hussain, A., Malik, M., & Abdullah, S. (2017). Review of evolving trends in clinical pharmacy curriculum around the globe. *American Journal of Pharmacological Sciences*, *5*(1), 1–7.

Islam, M. A., Talukder, R. M., Taheri, R., & Blanchard, N. (2016). Integration of basic and clinical science courses in US PharmD programs. *American Journal of Pharmaceutical Education*, *80*(10), 166.

Kerr, R. A. (2000). Curricular integration to enhance educational outcomes. *Pharmacotherapy*, *20*(10 Pt 2), 292s–296s.

Khan, M. U. (2011). A new paradigm in clinical pharmacy teaching in Pakistan. *American Journal of Pharmaceutical Education*, *75*(8), 166.

Long, C. M., Hadi, M. A., Kassab, Y. W., Yap, Y. L., & Lee, W. L. (2013). In *Does Msc in clinical pharmacy promote a clinical pharmacy career? A qualitative study. Paper presented at The 13th Asian Conference on Clinical Pharmacy, September 13th–15th, 2013 Haiphong city, Vietnam.*

Long, C. M., Lim, Z., & Hadi, M. A. (2011). Is problem-based learning (PBL) a preferred learning method in a Malaysian context? Student and lecturer perspectives. *International Journal of Pharmacy Practice*, *19*, 49.

Long, C. M., Yee, S. M., Muhammad, A. M., Hussain, M., & Manan, M. M. (2015). In S. F. Tang & L. Logonnathan (Eds.), *Outcome base approach for a new pharmacoinformatics course for bachelor of*

pharmacy programme. Taylor's 7th Teaching and Learning Conference 2014 Proceedings—Holistic Education: Enacting Change: Springer.
Marriott, J. L., Nation, R. L., Roller, L., Costelloe, M., Galbraith, K., Stewart, P., et al. (2008). Pharmacy education in the context of Australian practice. *American Journal of Pharmaceutical Education*, *72*(6), 131.
Murphy, J. E., Green, J. S., Adams, L. A., Squire, R. B., Kuo, G. M., & McKay, A. (2010). Pharmacogenomics in the curricula of colleges and schools of pharmacy in the United States. *American Journal of Pharmaceutical Education*, *74*(1), 7.
Neoh, C. F., Zainal, I. N. A., Hameed, M. A., Khan, T. M., & Ming, L. C. (2015). Development and progress of pharmacoinformatics in pharmaceutical and health sciences. *Journal of Young Pharmacists*, *7*(3), 155–163.
Nierenberg, D. W. (1998). The use of "vertical integration groups" to help define and update course/clerkship content. *Academic Medicine*, *73*(10), 1068–1071.
Pearson, G. J. (2007). Evolution in the practice of pharmacy—not a revolution. *Canadian Medical Association Journal*, *176*(9), 1295–1296.
Pearson, M. L., & Hubball, H. T. (2012). Curricular integration in pharmacy education. *American Journal of Pharmaceutical Education*, *76*(10), 204.
Pongcharoensuk, P., & Prakongpan, S. (2012). Centennial pharmacy education in Thailand. *Journal of Asian Association of Schools of Pharmacy*, *1*(1), 8–15.
Pramyothin, P., Sripanidkulchai, B., Thirawarapan, S., & Khunkitti, W. (1999). *Strategies for managing pharmacy education in next two decades*. Thailand: Ministry of University Affairs.
Romanelli, F. (2008). Seminar series course to teach essential knowledge and skills not covered in the traditional pharmacy curriculum. *American Journal of Pharmaceutical Education*, *72*.
Rosenthal, M., Austin, Z., & Tsuyuki, R. T. (2010). Are pharmacists the ultimate barrier to pharmacy practice change? *Canadian Pharmaceutical Journal*, *143*(1), 37–42.
Rudich, A., & Bashan, N. (2001). An interdisciplinary course in the basic sciences for senior medical and PhD students. *Academic Medicine*, *76*(10), 1072–1075.
Ryan, M., Shao, H., Yang, L., Nie, X.-Y., Zhai, S.-D., Shi, L.-W., et al. (2008). Clinical pharmacy education in China. *American Journal of Pharmaceutical Education*, *72*(6), 129.
Salamzadeh, J. (2010). Clinical pharmacy in Iran: Where do we stand? *Iranian Journal of Pharmaceutical Research*, *3*(1), 1–2.
Sattenstall, M., & Freeman, S. (2015). Integrated learning: an EBL approach to pharmaceutical chemistry. *Pharmacy Education*, *9*, 1–5.
Scahill, S. L., Akhlaq, M., & Garg, S. (2013). A bibliometric review of pharmacy education literature in the context of low- to middle-income countries. *Currents in Pharmacy Teaching and Learning*, *5*(3), 218–232.
Schmidt, H. (1998). Integrating the teaching of basic sciences, clinical sciences, and biopsychosocial issues. *Academic Medicine*, *73*(9 Suppl), S24–31.
Stewart, D. W., Brown, S. D., Clavier, C. W., & Wyatt, J. (2011). Active-learning processes used in US pharmacy education. *American Journal of Pharmaceutical Education*, *75*(4), 68.
Stohs, S. J., & Muhi-Eldeen, Z. (1990). The transition to more clinically oriented pharmacy education and the clinical practice of pharmacy. *Journal of Clinical Pharmacy and Therapeutics*, *15*(6), 435–454.
Toklu, H. Z., & Hussain, A. (2013). The changing face of pharmacy practice and the need for a new model of pharmacy education. *Journal of Young Pharmacists*, *5*(2), 38–40.
Van Patten, J., Chun, I. C., & Reigeluth, C. M. (1986). A review of strategies for sequencing and synthesizing instruction. *Review of Educational Research*, *56*(4), 437–471.
Waterfield, J. (2011). Two approaches to vocational education and training. A view from pharmacy education. *Journal of Vocational Education and Training*, *63*(2), 235–246.
Wells, S. H., Warelow, P. J., & Jackson, K. L. (2009). Problem based learning (PBL): a conundrum. *Contemporary Nurse*, *33*, 191.

Williams, B. (2001). Developing critical reflection for professional practice through problem-based learning. *Journal of Advanced Nursing*, *34*(1), 27–34.

Zainal, I. N. A., Karim, N. A. A., Soh, Y. C., Suleiman, A. K., Khan, T. M., Hameed, M. A., et al. (2016). Key elements of pharmacoinformatics for the degrees of bachelor and master of pharmacy. *Therapeutic Innovation and Regulatory Science*, *51*(4), 419–425.

CHAPTER

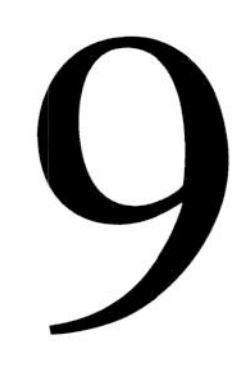

PROFESSIONAL DEGREES AND POSTGRADUATE QUALIFICATIONS IN PHARMACY: A GLOBAL OVERVIEW

Alian A. Alrasheedy*, Mohamed Azmi Hassali†

**Unaizah College of Pharmacy, Qassim University, Qassim, Saudi Arabia, †Universiti Sains Malaysia, Penang, Malaysia*

INTRODUCTION

Pharmacy education has experienced tremendous growth since the beginning of the last century. It has evolved from being a limited educational field in the 1800s and early 1900s to its current modern system of education, producing professionals considered to be an essential part of healthcare systems and capable of providing many healthcare services. In fact, in the last 150 years, pharmacy education has been in a constant state of change (DeBenedette, 2007). In the United States, the pharmacy program evolved from a graduate degree in pharmacy (PhG), to a 4-year baccalaureate degree (BSc), to a 5-year bachelor of science in pharmacy (BS Pharm), to the doctoral degree (PharmD), which has been the sole entry-level degree for the profession since 2000 (Fink III, 2012). Similarly, in Canada, it evolved from a limited education (i.e., trade and apprenticeship courses), to a 4-year science-oriented undergraduate program, to a professional pharmacy program (typically a 1+4 model), to the recently introduced entry-to-practice PharmD offered by many Canadian universities (Association of Faculties of Pharmacy of Canada (AFPC)/Association of Deans of Pharmacy of Canada (ADPC), 2010).

Similar to the West, pharmacy education in the East has also evolved rapidly over the years in many countries. For example, in Thailand it evolved from a 3-year certification in pharmacy compounding in 1913 to the current PharmD program, which has been the sole entry-to-practice professional degree since 2014, as shown in Table 1 (Chanakit, Low, Wongpoowarak, Moolasarn, & Anderson, 2015; Pongcharoensuk & Prakongpan, 2012).

In fact, not only have the qualifications offered in pharmacy and their durations changed, but also the number of pharmacy programs has tremendously increased in recent years in many countries. For example, in the United States, the number of accredited pharmacy colleges/schools progressively increased from a total of 87 in 2005 to 129 in early 2014 (a 48% increase) (University of California, 2014). In Malaysia, the first professional program in pharmacy (Bachelor of Pharmacy) was established by the School of Pharmaceutical Science, Universiti Sains Malaysia (USM) in 1972. More than 20 years later, in 1996, two other universities started offering pharmacy degrees (AB Fatah &

Pharmacy Education in the Twenty First Century and Beyond. https://doi.org/10.1016/B978-0-12-811909-9.00009-5

Table 1 Development of Pharmacy Education in Thailand

Period	Offered degree	Duration (years)
1913–1934	Certification in Pharmacy Compounding	3
1935–1936	Certification in Pharmacy	3
1937–1940	Associate Degree in Pharmacy	3
1940–1956	BSc in Pharmacy	4
1957–2010	BSc in Pharmacy	5
1999–2010	BSc in Pharmacy and Doctor of Pharmacy (PharmD)	5 and 6
2014	All PharmD	6

From Chanakit, T., Low, B. Y., Wongpoowarak, P., Moolasarn, S., & Anderson, C. (2015). Does a transition in education equate to a transition in practice? Thai stakeholder's perceptions of the introduction of the doctor of pharmacy programme. BMC Medical Education, 15*(1), 205; Pongcharoensuk, P., & Prakongpan, S. (2012). Centennial pharmacy education in Thailand.* Journal of Asian Association of Schools of Pharmacy, 1*(1), 8–15.*

Bahari, 2004). Currently, there are 21 pharmacy schools offering pharmacy programs in Malaysia (Pharmacy Board Malaysia, 2017). Similarly, in Saudi Arabia the pharmacy programs have increased tremendously. The first pharmacy program was established in 1959 at King Saudi University (Asiri, 2011). More than 40 years later, in 2001, another university—King Abdulaziz University—started offering a pharmacy degree (Faculty of Pharmacy-King Abdulaziz University, 2017). Currently, there are 28 pharmacy schools offering pharmacy programs in Saudi Arabia (Al-Jedai, Qaisi, & Al-Meman, 2016).

This chapter provides a comprehensive overview of qualifications and degrees offered in pharmacy. In particular, the chapter covers the following topics:

- *First professional pharmacy degrees*: An overview and discussion of the "entry-level degree for the profession." The chapter provides details about the requirements for the degrees according to regulatory or registration bodies to practice the pharmacy profession, with comparisons between some countries/continents and regions (i.e., the United States, Canada, Australia, Europe, Middle East, Asia). These include Bachelor of Science in Pharmacy (BScPharm, BSPharm), Bachelor of Pharmacy (BPharm), Master of Pharmacy (MPharm), and PharmD. Also, accelerated pharmacy degrees such as accelerated PharmD and other similar pathways (e.g., entry-level graduate MPharm degree for nonpharmacy graduates) are discussed.
- *Postgraduate qualifications in pharmacy*: An overview of postgraduate qualifications in pharmacy, with a focus on the professional postgraduate qualifications and the countries in which these degrees are offered, is provided. These include master of clinical Pharmacy (MClinPharm), MPharm (Postgraduate level), PharmD (postgraduate level), and professional doctorates in pharmacy, such as Doctor of Clinical Pharmacy (DClinPharm), and Doctor of Pharmacy (DPharm).
- *Residency and specialty certificates in pharmacy*: An overview and discussion of postgraduate structured trainings such as residencies, fellowships, and specialty certificates is provided.
- *Certifications in pharmacy*: The certifications in pharmacy such as Board Specialty certifications (e.g., Board Certified Pharmacotherapy Specialist (BCPS), Board Certified Oncology Pharmacist (BCOP)) and other certifications such as Certified Diabetes Educator (CDE) are introduced in the chapter.

- A brief overview of academic graduate degrees in pharmacy and pharmaceutical sciences is presented.
- *Equivalency and qualification frameworks*: A comparison between qualifications across countries will be provided and whether qualifications with the same title/name in different countries are actually equivalent is discussed in the chapter.

ENTRY-LEVEL DEGREES FOR THE PROFESSION

The first pharmacy degree required by the regulatory bodies in order to be registered or licensed as a pharmacist varies widely between countries. Moreover, within some countries, more than one degree can lead to the profession of pharmacy. In this chapter, many countries are reviewed, including the United States, the United Kingdom, France, Australia, Canada, Malaysia, Saudi Arabia, India, Singapore, and Thailand. Also, the additional education/training required for registration as a pharmacist is discussed.

REVIEWED COUNTRIES

The United States

In 2000, the sole entry-level degree for the profession in the United States became the PharmD degree. The PharmD degree requires at least 2 years of prepharmacy (preprofessional) undergraduate coursework, followed by four academic years in a professional program (2+4 program). Some colleges of pharmacy accept students directly from high school into a 6-year pharmacy program (0+6 program) that combines the prerequisite undergraduate coursework with the professional program. Some colleges offer an accelerated PharmD program (conducted over three calendar years) for individuals with a bachelor's degree in a related health or science field (American Association of Colleges of Pharmacy (AACP), 2016a; Knoer, Eck, & Lucas, 2016). Structured practical training is incorporated into the curriculum. In fact, the Accreditation Council for Pharmacy Education (ACPE) requires all pharmacy programs to include interprofessional education (IPE), introductory pharmacy practice experiences (IPPEs), and advanced pharmacy practice experiences (APPEs) in the curriculum. The IPPEs should not be less than 300 h and should be purposely integrated into the didactic curriculum. The IPPEs need to be conducted equally between community pharmacy and institutional pharmacy practice (at least 150 h in each section). APPEs are conducted during the fourth year of the professional program after completion of the didactic curriculum and all IPPEs. They consist of core and elective rotations covering both inpatient and outpatient services, acute and chronic conditions, and diverse patient populations. As per the ACPE requirements, the duration of APPEs should not be less than 36 weeks (1440 h) with a minimum of 4 weeks for each rotation (160 h) (ACPE, 2015). In all states, candidates for pharmacy licensure must pass the North American Pharmacist Licensure Examination (NAPLEX) and a law examination is also required (Knoer et al., 2016).

The United Kingdom

The entry-level degree to the practice in the United Kingdom is the MPharm program. This is a 4-year professional program (General Pharmaceutical Council (GPhC), 2011, 2012). This is considered an "undergraduate" master's degree because a bachelor's degree is not required before registration into this program (Global Knowledge Exchange Network on Healthcare (GKEN), 2009). Beyond the coursework, clinical placements and practicum are relatively limited in the program, compared to the US pharmacy programs. However, all MPharm graduates are required to complete a 52-week preregistration training (GPhC, 2011, 2012). Recently, some UK schools of pharmacy started a 5-year MPharm degree, which integrates academic study with the preregistration year. The GPhC expect this integrated degree to be predominant in the near future (GPhC, 2011). The 5-year integrated MPharm degree is currently offered at some universities, such as the University of Nottingham (University of Nottingham, 2017). Besides the MPharm degree and the preregistration training, the applicant must pass a registration assessment by GPhC to be registered as a UK pharmacist.

Australia

The entry-level degrees for practice in Australia are BPharm and a graduate-entry MPharm. The BPharm program is a 4-year undergraduate degree while the MPharm is a 3-year full-time (or equivalent) degree. Therefore, the MPharm program could be conducted over either six semesters over 3 years or six trimesters over 2 years (Australian Pharmacy Council, 2012). The experiential education and clinical training incorporated into the curriculum varies among pharmacy schools in Australia (Marriott et al., 2008). As an example, at the University of Queensland, over 350 h of clinical placements and internships are incorporated into the curriculum and are conducted in different clinical settings (i.e., community and hospital settings) (University of Queensland, 2017). Before registration, candidates are required to complete 1824 h of Board-approved supervised practice, including an accredited intern training program (Pharmacy Board of Australia, 2017). In addition, the pharmacists must pass written and oral exams conducted by the Australian Board (Pharmacy Board of Australia, 2017). Recently in Australia the School of Pharmacy and Pharmaceutical Sciences at the University of Monash introduced a new combined BPharm(Hons)/MPharm program. This degree is 5 years in duration and was introduced to prepare future pharmacists to meet the current complex healthcare system demands beyond the bachelor's degree. In this combined degree, the required internship and intern training programs are incorporated into the final fifth year (University of Monash, 2017). Hence, after graduation the students will be ready for registration as pharmacists upon completion of other requirements of the Board.

Malaysia

The entry-level degrees for practice in Malaysia are BPharm(Hons) and an undergraduate MPharm. The duration of these programs is 4 years (Pharmacy Board Malaysia, 2017). The BPharm is offered by public universities while the MPharm is offered at private colleges or campuses of international universities (usually as a twinning program). For example, MPharm at the University of Nottingham Malaysia is a full-time, 4-year program in which the first 2 years are conducted in Malaysia and the last 2 years in the United Kingdom (i.e., 2 + 2 MPharm) (University of Nottingham Malaysia, 2017). After graduation, the graduates need to register with the Board of Pharmacy Malaysia as a provisional registered pharmacist (PRP). The Registration of Pharmacists Act, 1951 requires PRPs to gain at least 1 year of experience/training satisfactory to the Board before being granted full registration as a pharmacist (Hassali, Shafie, Guat See, & Wong, 2016; Registration of Pharmacists Act, 1951). In addition to the academic degree and the preregistration experience, the PRPs must pass the Pharmacy Jurisprudence Examination conducted by the Pharmacy Board Malaysia (Hassali et al., 2016).

India

The Pharmacy Council of India Education Regulations 1991 in Chapter 1 stipulated that Diploma in Pharmacy is the minimum qualification for registration as a pharmacist (Pharmacy Council of India, 1991). Other registerable degrees include BPharm and PharmD (Basak & Sathyanarayana, 2010). The Diploma in Pharmacy consists of two academic years and practical training (500h conducted over a period not less than 3months) (Pharmacy Council of India, 1991). The duration of the BPharm and PharmD are 4 and 6years, respectively. In terms of practical training, BPharm programs require at least 150h (over 4weeks) of training in a pharmaceutical industry or hospital, while in the PharmD program the sixth year is devoted to clinical training as internship/residency training. The internship consists of four rotations (6months in general medicine and 6months in three other different specialties—2months for each) (Pharmacy Council of India, 2008, 2016). Therefore, the competencies of these three registerable degrees are not the same. The Diploma in Pharmacy is mainly meant to prepare students to serve in community and hospital settings (i.e., compounding and dispensing); the BPharm is industry and product oriented; while PharmD is a clinically oriented curriculum (Basak & Sathyanarayana, 2010; Karim & Adnan, 2016).

Canada

The entry-level degrees for practice in Canada are currently Baccalaureate in Pharmacy (BScPharm) and Doctor of Pharmacy (PharmD). In fact, many Canadian universities are now replacing the BSc degree with the PharmD as the first professional degree. These include the University of British Colombia, University of Toronto, University of Waterloo, University of Saskatchewan, Université de Montréal, Memorial University of Newfoundland, and Université Laval (Canadian Council for Accreditation of Pharmacy Programs (CCAPP), 2017). In fact, CCAPP stated that "Canada moves inexorably closer to the goal of graduating all pharmacists with a First Professional Degree Doctorate of Pharmacy." (CCAPP, 2016, page 2) The professional program requires at least four academic years, or an equivalent. The BScPharm is required to have at least 16weeks (640h) of practical training with a focus on direct patient care experiences. However, the PharmD program is required to have at least 40weeks (1600h) of practical training with a focus on direct patient care experiences. Before admission to these programs, applicants need to undertake preprofessional postsecondary coursework in general education, biomedical, and basic sciences (CCAPP, 2016). For example, currently the Faculty of Pharmacy and Pharmaceutical Sciences at University of Alberta requires completion of at least 30 credit hours before admission into the BScPharm and 60 credit hours for PharmD (University of Alberta, 2017). The University of British Columbia Faculty of Pharmaceutical Sciences requires for admission to the PharmD at least 60 credits completed within the last 10years (University of British Columbia, 2017). Therefore, the pharmacy degree in Canada is 4years in length (whether it is a BScPharm or a PharmD). Prior to starting the pharmacy degree, individuals must complete a minimum of 1 or 2years of an appropriate course of undergraduate study, so the total time is 5 or 6years. Before registration, pharmacists are required to successfully pass the Pharmacy Examining Board of Canada Qualifying Exam Parts I & II. Also, the jurisprudence exam is required (the jurisprudence exam is a provincial requirement) (National Association of Pharmacy Regulatory Authorities (NAPRA), 2017).

France

In France, the entry level to practice is the Doctor of Pharmacy degree "diplome d'Etat de docteur en pharmacie." This is a 6-year program and consists of coursework, training, and internship. Since 2010 the first year has been a common curriculum with other fields (i.e., medical studies, midwifery, and dentistry). After completion of this year, students are required to pass a competitive exam to advance into the pharmacy program. In the fifth year, students complete a 12-month internship half-time at a university hospital. In the sixth year, depending on the student's interest, a 6-month full-time internship in community pharmacy or industrial pharmacy needs to be completed. Also, in the fifth year, students may choose a 9-year option by applying for the *Internat* (this is a 4-year paid internship/residency program). Therefore, depending on the option the students selected, at the end of the 6-year option, students will be awarded Doctor of Pharmacy (PharmD), whereas those who choose the 9-year option will be awarded a special degree called the "Diplome d'Etudes Spécialisées" (DES, Specialized Studies Diplomas), as well as a PharmD. Pharmacists must register with the French College of Pharmacists before they enter the practice. The DES is required for those who wish to specialize in hospital pharmacy, medical biology, biomedical industrial pharmacy, research, and teaching. However, those who choose to work in other sectors/industries where there is not a need for pharmaceutical liability are not required to register with the College (Bourdon, Ekeland, & Brion, 2008; Campus France Agency, 2016; GKEN, 2009).

Thailand

Since 2014, the entry-level degree for practice has been a 6-year PharmD program as required by the Pharmacy Council of Thailand (PCT). The BPharm program was stopped in 2010 and now has been completely replaced by the new 6-year PharmD. Currently, there are two types/tracks of PharmD programs in Thailand. These are a Pharmaceutical Care-PharmD (PC-PD) program and an Industrial Pharmacy-PharmD (IP-PD) program (Chanakit et al., 2015). In the sixth year of the program, the students are required to obtain at least 2000 h of training and practice in the relevant track of the program (i.e., patient-oriented rotations or industry-oriented rotations) (Chaiyakunapruk, Jones, Dhippayom, & Sumpradit, 2016; Pongcharoensuk & Prakongpan, 2012). The pharmacist licensure is granted by the PCT after all the requirements are met, including a pharmacist licensure exam (Pongcharoensuk & Prakongpan, 2012).

Saudi Arabia

The entry-level degrees to the practice are currently the BPharm and PharmD. However, most Saudi universities are now offering the PharmD program. The duration of the BPharm program is at least 5 years, while the PharmD is at least 6 years. The BPharm usually includes one semester of practical training (i.e., 15 weeks) or the equivalent, while the PharmD program includes a 1-year internship program with a focus on patient care experiences. Pharmacists in Saudi Arabia are required to register with the Saudi Commission of Health Specialties (SCHS) (Al-Jedai et al., 2016).

ANALYSIS AND COMPARISONS

As shown in Table 2, the entry-level degree for the pharmacy profession varies widely between countries. For example, in the United States, France and Thailand, the minimum qualification is PharmD, while in other countries the minimum qualifications are MPharm in the United Kingdom, BPharm in

Table 2 Entry-Level Degrees for the Profession

	United States	United Kingdom	Australia	Malaysia	Canada	France	India	Thailand	Saudi Arabia
The Degree(s)	PharmD	MPharm	BPharm, MPharm (graduate entry)	BPharm, MPharm	BSc (Pharm), PharmD	PharmD	Diploma in Pharmacy, BPharm, PharmD	PharmD	BPharm, PharmD
Training/ practice/ experiential education required before full registration as a pharmacist. (Integrated in the degree versus a separate preregistration)	• Integrated • IPPE: at least 300h • APPEs: at least 36 weeks (1440h)	• For the 4-year MPharm: a 52-week preregistration training. • For the 5-year integrated MPharm: incorporated in the 5th year	• Preregistration 1 year of supervised practice including an accredited intern training program (1824h) • Combined BPharm(Hons)/ MPharm program: incorporated in the 5th year	• 1 year of experience/ training before registration	• Integrated: • BScPharm: at least 16 weeks (640h) • PharmD: at least 40 weeks (1600h) • Some provinces require additional preregistration training	• Integrated: • 12-month internship half-time at a university hospital • And a 6-month full-time internship in community pharmacy or industrial pharmacy	• Pre-registration: • Diploma in Pharmacy: (500h over a period not less than 3 months) • Integrated: • BPharm: at least 150h (over 4 weeks) • PharmD: One year of as internship/ residency training	• Integrated: • At least 2000h of training and practice in the relevant track of the program	• BPharm: one semester of practical training (i.e., 15 weeks) or equivalent PharmD: one year internship program
The route for registration (minimum duration in years)[a]	6	5	5	5	5	6	2 and 3 months for Pharmacy diploma 4 for BPharm 6 for PharmD	6	5
The orientation of the degree (pharmacy practice versus industry)	Practice oriented	Practice oriented	Practice oriented	Practice oriented	Practice oriented	Three tracks: community pharmacy, hospital pharmacy, and industrial pharmacy	BPharm: industry oriented PharmD: practice oriented	Two tracks: Pharmaceutical Care-PharmD (PC-PD) and Industrial Pharmacy-PharmD (IP-PD) programs	BPharm: pharmaceutical sciences oriented PharmD: practice oriented

[a] *In countries with more than one degree qualifying for registration as a pharmacist, the minimum duration is calculated based on the degree with the shortest duration.*

Australia and Malaysia, and Diploma in Pharmacy in India. Moreover, in some countries such as the United States, United Kingdom, France and Thailand, there is only one degree as the entry-level degree, while in other countries such as Malaysia, Saudi Arabia, India, and Australia there is more than one degree that is considered an entry-level degree for the profession.

In countries where there is more than one first professional degree, the general competencies/orientation of these programs are the same in some countries (e.g., BPharm and MPharm degrees in Australia). However, in some other countries, the general competencies and orientation of these degrees are different. For example, in India, the BPharm is an industry-oriented program while the PharmD is designed to be a practice-oriented qualification. A similar situation occurs in Saudi Arabia, where the BPharm focuses on pharmaceutical sciences while the PharmD mainly focuses on practice and patient care services. It should also be noted that even in some countries that have a sole degree for entrance into the profession, there are tracks/professional pathways into the final stage of the program that allow for specialization (e.g., in Thailand, there are two tracks: Pharmaceutical Care PharmD or Industrial Pharmacy PharmD).

As summarized in Table 2, the route to full registration as a pharmacist takes at least 5 years in countries such as Malaysia, Australia, and the United Kingdom, while it takes longer (i.e., 6 years) in other countries (e.g., the United States, France and Thailand). However, in India, the situation is exceptional, with only a 2-year diploma program, and with an additional 3 months of training, the individual can register as a pharmacist.

Countries also differ in terms of the practice/experiential training of pharmacists. In some countries, such as the United States, France and Saudi Arabia, the training is incorporated and integrated within the professional degree. In this case, after meeting other requirements, the graduates will be ready for registration as a pharmacist. However, in some countries, such as the United Kingdom, Malaysia, and Australia, the major components of practice/experiences are completed after graduation as a separate year (i.e., 1 year of preregistration training or supervised practice). However, there is a move to integrate this preregistration training into the professional degree. For example, in the United Kingdom some universities recently introduced the integrated Mpharm, as discussed earlier.

In summary, the first pharmacy professional degrees vary widely between countries and also within some countries in terms of duration, orientation, and structure.

POSTGRADUATE QUALIFICATIONS IN PHARMACY

An overview of postgraduate qualifications in pharmacy is presented with a focus on the professional postgraduate qualifications, such as MClinPharm, DClinPharm, PharmD (postgraduate level), MPharm (postgraduate level), and DPharm, and the countries in which these degrees are offered, including Singapore, Malta, India, Nepal, Australia, the UK, and Malaysia.

SELECTED PROGRAMS AND THE COUNTRIES IN WHICH THEY ARE OFFERED

Postgraduate PharmD in Singapore

PharmD at the National University of Singapore was introduced to meet the needs of providing specialization in pharmacy in Singapore. The aim of the program is to produce advanced generalist and specialist pharmacists to provide direct patient care services. It is a 2-year full-time postgraduate program (or equivalent part-time). The first year is didactic coursework (44 modular credits) including advanced pharmacotherapy courses and other related courses for pharmacy and clinical practice. The second year is devoted to clinical clerkships (40 modular credits). These include eight rotations (five core rotations and three are electives) and each rotation is 5 weeks in duration. The core rotations include ambulatory care, adult acute care medicine, adult general medicine, critical care medicine, and drug information. This PharmD program is the benchmark for entry into the Specialist Pharmacist Register of the Ministry of Health, Singapore (National University of Singapore, 2017).

Doctorate in pharmacy (PharmD) in Malta

PharmD at the University of Malta is a specialized degree in clinical pharmacy. This is the highest professional level (level eight doctorate, i.e., equivalent in status to a PhD). This program aims to prepare pharmacists to specialize and take leadership roles in clinical pharmacy practice. This is a 3-year full-time program and combines both advanced clinical pharmacy knowledge and skills with research training. The program consists of three components. The first component includes courses in pharmacotherapeutics, drug information and statistics, principles of pharmacoeconomics, and health systems in the United States and Europe. The other components include experiential education, clinical rotations, and a doctoral research dissertation (University of Malta, 2016).

Postbaccalaureate PharmD in India and Nepal

Besides the entry-level PharmD degree, a postbaccalaureate PharmD is offered in India. This program aims to bridge the gap between BPharm holders and the entry-level PharmD holders. This is a 3-year program and has almost the same curriculum of the last 3 years of the entry-level PharmD. The program consists of two phases. The first phase is mainly a didactic phase and includes courses in pharmacotherapy, clinical pharmacokinetics and therapeutic drug monitoring, pharmacoepidemiology, pharmacoeconomics, among others. The second phase is the internship year and it is similar to the entry-level PharmD internship (Basak & Sathyanarayana, 2010; Manipal University, 2017; Pharmacy Council of India, 2008). The PharmD curriculum in India is standardized throughout the country.

Similarly, a postbaccalaureate PharmD is offered in Nepal. It is a 3-year program where the last year is fully devoted to a clinical internship. An example of this is the PharmD at Kathmandu University (Kathmandu University, 2016).

UK DPharm

The professional doctorate in pharmacy (DPharm) is currently offered at several UK universities. This is a postgraduate degree combining both taught modules/program and a research component (commonly one-third of the program is modules and the other two-thirds is devoted to research). It is equivalent to the traditional PhD. This program targets employed, registered pharmacists who have gained significant professional experience and are currently actively engaged in a relevant area of practice. It is usually part-time and requires 4–7 years to be completed. The overall aim of the DPharm is to equip registered pharmacists with advanced knowledge in their area of practice and research skills (Keele University, 2017; University of Birmingham, 2017; University of Bradford, 2017; University of Strathclyde, 2017). It is considered an alternative route to the PhD for practicing pharmacists for whom a PhD might not be the most appropriate qualification (University of Strathclyde, 2017). In DPharm, the pharmacists can engage in a research project relevant to their practice area while they continue their work (Keele University, 2017; University of Birmingham, 2017; University of Bradford, 2017; University of Strathclyde, 2017). The program can be a leading qualification to a consultant pharmacist position (University of Bradford, 2017).

DClinPharm in Australia

DClinPharm is offered at some Australian universities. It is a 3-year full-time (or equivalent) professional doctorate program. At the University of Queensland and University of South Australia, the program aims to provide the students with advanced knowledge, skills and abilities necessary for the clinical pharmacy practitioner (i.e., to provide specialist clinical pharmacy services). The program consists of taught courses (e.g., pharmacotherapy, advanced skills for clinical pharmacy practice), clinical placements, and a doctoral research project (University of Queensland, 2013; University of South Australia, 2014).

The DClinPharm at the University of Western Australia is designed as a research-oriented degree in clinical pharmacy for practicing clinical pharmacists. The program consists of 144 credit points of which 24 points are dedicated for coursework and 120 points are dedicated for a doctoral thesis in a specialty area of clinical pharmacy practice (University of Western Australia, 2017).

Postgraduate masters in clinical pharmacy (many countries)

A master's degree in clinical pharmacy is an academic postgraduate degree aimed to provide pharmacists with specialized knowledge, skills and abilities to practice as a clinical pharmacist and to provide specialist pharmaceutical services in different clinical environments. This is taught in many countries such as the United Kingdom, Australia, New Zealand, Malaysia, Hong Kong, and Saudi Arabia. The name of the degree varies among countries. It is a MSc (Clinical Pharmacy) in the United Kingdom and Saudi Arabia, MClinPharm in Australia, New Zealand, and Hong Kong, and MPharm (Clinical Pharmacy) in Malaysia. Other forms of nomenclature also exist for this degree. The degree curriculum consists of coursework (e.g., pharmacotherapy, clinical pharmacy practice, evidence-based practice), clinical training/rotations, and a research project or dissertation. However, there is a major difference in terms of the experiential clinical training, as it can be limited or not included in some programs and it can be extensive in other programs (i.e., a major component of the program). Also, these programs vary in terms of study duration and type (full-time only, part-time only, or both, distance-learning, face-to-face, etc.).

The MPharm(ClinPharm) established in 1992 at the School of Pharmaceutical Sciences, Universiti Sains Malaysia is an example of a clinically oriented postgraduate MPharm program. The curriculum of this program is presented in Table 3.

ANALYSIS AND COMPARISON

As shown in Table 4, the postgraduate professional training in pharmacy differs widely among countries. Moreover, the postgraduate qualifications differ widely in terms of the main orientation/aim (i.e., patient care, research, or both), duration, and structure (clinical rotations, research component, coursework). For example, in Singapore, the 2-year postgraduate PharmD aims mainly to produce advanced generalist and specialist level pharmacists capable of providing direct patient care services, while in Malta the 3-year professional PharmD aims to prepare pharmacists to have leadership in both clinical pharmacy practice and research. In Australia, clinical pharmacy programs such as MClinPharm and

Table 3 MPharm(ClinPharm) at Universiti Sains Malaysia

Didactic coursework

- Pharmacotherapeutics I
- Pharmacotherapeutics II
- Pharmacotherapeutics III
- Pharmacotherapeutics IV
- Pharmacotherapeutics V
- Clinical Pharmacy Practice
- Biostatistics and Research Methodology
- Clinical Pharmacokinetics

Clinical rotations/clerkships

- Internal Medicine I & II
- Intensive Care Medicine
- Infectious Diseases
- Surgery
- Pediatrics

Research Project and Dissertation

From Universiti Sains Malaysia. (2017). Master of Pharmacy (Clinical Pharmacy). *Retrieved 24 September 2017, from http://www.pha.usm.my/index.php/en/programmes/postgraduate/about-research-programmes/master-of-pharmacy*

DClinPharm prepare clinical pharmacists with advanced training. The DClinPharm can be either a practice-oriented degree or a mainly research-oriented degree. In the United Kingdom, several opportunities for advanced education in clinical pharmacy and professional practice exist, including the MSc in clinical pharmacy and professional DPharm. The UK DPharm—with its major research component—is an alternative route to the PhD for practicing pharmacists to gain advanced knowledge and research skills. In Malaysia, MPharm in clinical pharmacy is offered by several universities to provide advanced training in clinical pharmacy. In some countries, such as the United States, the postgraduate professional training is completed via residency and fellowship programs. This is discussed in the following section.

RESIDENCY AND SPECIALTY CERTIFICATES IN PHARMACY

In Pharmacy, postgraduate structured training includes residencies, fellowships, and specialty training. This is available in several countries such as the United States, France, Saudi Arabia, and Singapore.

RESIDENCY AND FELLOWSHIP IN THE UNITED STATES

In the United States, the history of pharmacy residency dates back to the early 1930s. Originally, these were called internships and were focused mainly on training pharmacists for the management of pharmacy services in hospitals. The postgraduate research-oriented programs (i.e., fellowships) in pharmacy started to develop in 1972 (American Society of Health-System Pharmacists (ASHP), 1987). ASHP defined the residency as "an organized, directed, postgraduate training program in a defined area of

Table 4 Postgraduate Academic Qualifications in Pharmacy

The Degree	Country	Duration	Level of Degree	Orientation/Description
Doctor of Pharmacy (PharmD)	Singapore	2 years full-time or equivalent part-time	Postgraduate level (advanced generalist and specialist level)	- The aim of the program is to produce advanced generalist and specialist pharmacists to provide direct patient care - The program consists of didactic coursework (1st year) and to clinical clerkships (2nd year)
Doctorate in Pharmacy (PharmD)	Malta	3 years full-time	The highest professional level (equivalent in status to a PhD)	- This is a specialized degree in clinical pharmacy - The program consists of three components: coursework, experiential education and clinical rotations, and a doctoral research dissertation
PB Doctor of Pharmacy (PB PharmD)	India	3 years full-time	Postbaccalaureate professional level	- The aim of the program is to bridge the gap between the BPharm holders and the entry-level PharmD holders - The program consists of coursework (2 years) and internship (1 year)
PB Doctor of Pharmacy (PB PharmD)	Nepal	3 years full-time	Postbaccalaureate professional level	- The aim of the program is to bridge the gap between the BPharm holders and the entry-level PharmD holders - The program consists of coursework (2 years) and internship (1 year)
Doctorate in Pharmacy (DPharm)	The UK	3 years full-time (typically 4–7 years part-time)	The highest professional level (equivalent in status to a PhD)	- The aim of the program is to equip registered pharmacists with advanced knowledge in their area of practice and research skills - The program consists of taught modules/program and research component (commonly, one-third of the program is taught and the other two-thirds is devoted to research)
Doctor of Clinical Pharmacy (DClinPharm)	Australia	3 years full-time or equivalent	The highest professional level (equivalent in status to a PhD)	- The aim of the program is to provide registered pharmacists with advanced knowledge, skills and abilities necessary for a clinical pharmacy practitioner - The program consists of coursework clinical placements and a doctoral research project - The DClinPharm at the University of Western Australia is designed mainly as a research-oriented degree

pharmacy practice" while the fellowship is defined as "a directed, highly individualized, postgraduate program designed to prepare the participant to become an independent researcher" (ASHP, 1987).

In the United States, residency training is divided into two postgraduate years known as postgraduate year one (PGY-1) and postgraduate year two (PGY-2). PGY-1 provides more generalized training in a broad range of disease states, building on the knowledge, skills, and experiences gained from the entry-level professional pharmacy degree. PGY-2 provides a more specialized training in a specific area of interest, building on the knowledge, skills and experiences gained from PGY-1 (American College of Clinical Pharmacy (ACCP), n.d.). Therefore, after completing PGY-1, the pharmacy residents can specialize in PGY-2. The current PGY-2 specialties include (ACCP):

- Ambulatory Care
- Cardiology
- Critical Care
- Drug Information
- Emergency Medicine
- Geriatrics
- Infectious Diseases
- Informatics
- Internal Medicine
- Managed Care Pharmacy Systems
- Medication-Use Safety
- Nuclear Pharmacy
- Nutrition Support
- Oncology
- Pediatrics
- Pharmacotherapy
- Health-System Pharmacy Administration
- Psychiatrics
- Solid Organ Transplantation

CERTIFICATE OF CLINICAL PHARMACY SPECIALTY IN SAUDI ARABIA

In Saudi Arabia, the first pharmacy residency program was introduced at a tertiary hospital in Riyadh in 1997 (Al-Jedai et al., 2016). In 2001, the national residency program was established by the Saudi Commission for health specialties. This general clinical training aimed to equip the residents with the knowledge, skills, and abilities to provide pharmaceutical care services. In 2013, a specialty residency program was introduced and the residency program was restructured into two residency programs. One program is 2 years in duration and is called a general clinical pharmacy diploma program. The first year focuses on hospital pharmacy practice and administration (in-patient care, ambulatory care, administration, medication safety, sterile preparations, drug information, etc.). The second year includes nine clinical rotations (e.g., internal medicine, cardiology, critical care, etc.) (Saudi Scientific Council of Pharmacy, 2017).

The second residency program is called the Saudi Certificate in Clinical Pharmacy. This is a 3-year program. The first 2 years of the program are identical to the clinical pharmacy diploma program. The third year is devoted to specialty training (e.g., internal medicine, oncology, pediatrics, etc.).

The 3-year specialty certificate is considered equivalent to a professional doctorate and qualifies the resident for registration as a consultant in clinical pharmacy after meeting other requirements set forth by the Saudi Commission for Health Specialties (Saudi Scientific Council of Pharmacy, 2017).

PHARMACY RESIDENCY IN SINGAPORE

In Singapore, the national pharmacy residency programs were officially launched in 2016. Similar to the US residency programs, the residency training consists of PGY-1 and PGY-2. The PGY-1 provides the residents with general clinical competencies to deliver direct patient care services in a broad range of disease states. Hence, the PGY-1 includes a broad range of clinical rotations (i.e., infectious diseases, general medicine, critical care, ambulatory care, medication safety and informatics, practice management and leadership, and research, etc.). PGY-2 is designed to provide advanced training in a particular specialty. The current PGY-2 specialties include cardiology, geriatrics, infectious diseases, oncology, and psychiatry (Department of Pharmacy-NUS, 2016; Ministry of Health Singapore, 2016). Besides these national residency programs, in conjunction with Tan Tock Seng hospital, Department of Pharmacy at NUS runs the (PGY2) Ambulatory Care Pharmacy Residency (Department of Pharmacy-NUS, 2017).

PHARMACY RESIDENCY IN FRANCE

In France in the early 1980s a 4-year specialized residency training was established (Bourdon et al., 2008; Slimano, Gervais, Masse, & Langree, 2014). The pharmacy residency program "Internat en Pharmacie" is conducted at university hospitals affiliated with colleges of pharmacy. Currently, there are 23 university hospitals (or groups of hospitals in the largest cities) in France that have pharmacy residency programs and there are three residency specialties for pharmacists, including medical biology, hospital pharmacy, and pharmaceutical innovation and research. To be eligible for admission into the residency program, the pharmacist students need to pass a national written ranking exam. By national ranking order, they then choose their specialties. The number of positions for each specialty and for each university hospital is determined jointly by the ministries of health and universities. Hence, this results in a national quota by specialty (Fardel, 2017).

In France, medical biology is equivalent to clinical pathology in the United States. Similar to physicians, pharmacists can specialize in this field in France (Fardel, 2017). In fact, pharmacists play a major role in medical biology activities, including being a director of ambulatory laboratories (Bourdon et al., 2008). Pharmaceutical Innovation and Research includes areas such as cell therapy and biotechnology. This specialty can also be accessed through other routes such as research degrees (e.g., master's and doctoral) and by other scientists/professionals not holding a PharmD (Fardel, 2017). After successful completion of one's residency, the resident is awarded the "Diplôme d'études spécialisées" (DES, Specialized Studies Diploma) as well as the PharmD degree (Bourdon et al., 2008; Fardel, 2017).

ANALYSIS AND COMPARISON

As shown in Fig. 1, pharmacy residency in the United States consists of two postgraduate years (PGY-1 followed by PGY-2). As discussed earlier, there are many specialties available for pharmacists in the United States. Similarly, the pharmacy residency in Singapore is similar to the US model, having both PGY-1 and PGY-2. However, currently there are six specialties, as mentioned earlier. In Saudi Arabia, the pharmacy residency consists of three postgraduate years (the 2-year diploma followed by a 1-year

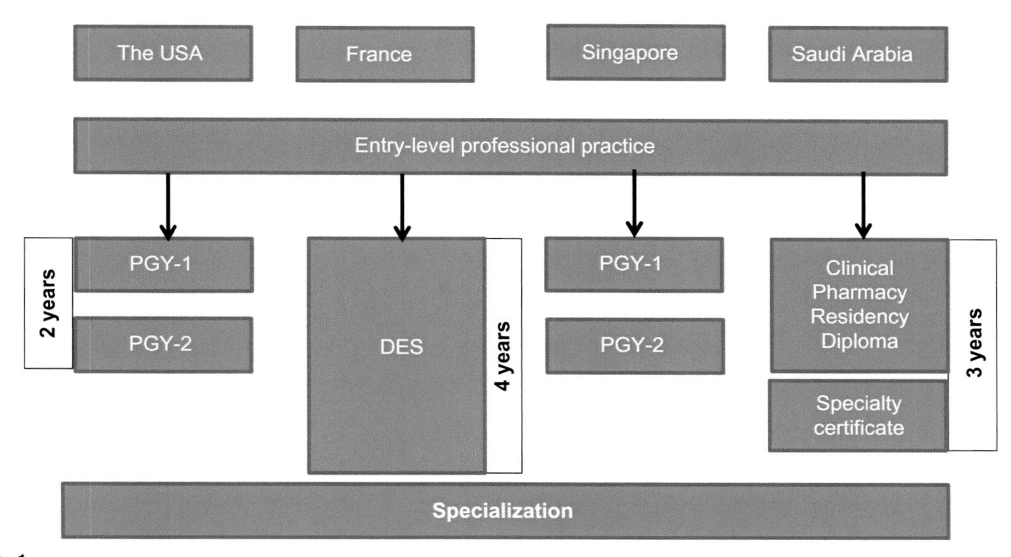

FIG. 1

The route to specialization via residency programs in the United States, France, Singapore, and Saudi Arabia.

specialty). There are many specialties available for pharmacists in Saudi Arabia. In France, the residency program consists of 4 years and currently there are three specialization areas for pharmacists in this program.

CERTIFICATIONS IN PHARMACY

In addition to academic qualifications, licensure, and postgraduate education/training, many pharmacists seek certification to have additional evidence that they have the skills and expertise to provide care services directly to patients (US Council on Credentialing in Pharmacy (CCP), 2014). The US CCP (2014, page 1829) provided the following definitions to explain the terminology:

> *A certificate is a document issued to an individual after the successful achievement of a predetermined level of performance in an education and/or training program* (e.g., *an immunization training program, a pharmacy residency, a fellowship).*
>
> *Certification is a voluntary process by which a nongovernmental agency or an association grants recognition to an individual who has met certain predetermined qualifications specified by that organization. This formal recognition is granted to designate to the public that the individual has attained the requisite level of knowledge, skill, and/or experience in a well-defined, often specialized, area of the total discipline.*

Certification can be pharmacist-only certification (i.e., Pharmacy Board specialty certification) or multidisciplinary certification. In pharmacist-only certification, only pharmacists are eligible to apply for this certification (US CCP, 2012). In the United States, the Board of Pharmacy Specialties, established

Table 5 US Board of Pharmacy Specialties

Specialty	Name of the Credential/Certification
Ambulatory Care Pharmacy	Board Certified Ambulatory Care Pharmacist (BCACP)
Critical Care Pharmacy	Board Certified Critical Care Pharmacist (BCCCP)
Geriatric Pharmacy	Board Certified Geriatric Pharmacist (BCGP)
Nuclear Pharmacy	Board Certified Nuclear Pharmacist (BCNP)
Nutrition Support Pharmacy	Board Certified Nutrition Support Pharmacist (BCNSP)
Oncology Pharmacy	Board Certified Oncology Pharmacist (BCOP)
Pediatric Pharmacy	Board Certified Pediatric Pharmacy Specialist (BCPPS)
Pharmacotherapy[a]	Board Certified Pharmacotherapy Specialist (BCPS)
Psychiatric Pharmacy	Board Certified Psychiatric Pharmacist (BCPP)

[a]*Two added qualifications within the pharmacotherapy specialty: cardiology and infectious diseases.*

in 1976, is a postlicensure certification agency that provides specialty certification for pharmacists in the United States and worldwide (Board of Pharmacy Specialties, n.d.). Currently, the board provides certification in nine pharmacy specialties (Table 5).

In addition, pharmacists can obtain multidisciplinary certification. In addition to pharmacists, this certification is open to other healthcare providers such as physicians, nurses, and assistant physicians (US CCP, 2012). Examples of these certifications are presented in Table 6.

Table 6 Examples of Multidisciplinary Certifications Available to Pharmacists in the United States

Area of Certification	Name of the Credential/ Certification	Organization Responsible for the Certification
Anticoagulation care	Certified Anticoagulation Care Provider (CACP)	National Certification Board for Anticoagulation Providers (NCBAP)
Asthma education	Certified Asthma Educator (AE-C)	National Asthma Educator Certification Board (NAECB)
Clinical pharmacology	Accredited in Applied Pharmacology (AP)	American Board of Clinical Pharmacology (ABCP)
Diabetes education	Certified Diabetes Educator (CDE)	National Certification Board for Diabetes Educators (NCBDE)
Diabetes management-advanced	Board Certified-Advanced Diabetes Management (BC-ADM)	The American Association of Diabetes Educators (AADE)
Pain education	Credentialed Pain Educator (CPE)	American Society of Pain Educators (ASPE)
Pain management	Credentialed Pain Practitioner (CPP)	American Academy of Pain Management (AAPM)
Lipids	Clinical Lipid Specialist	Accreditation Council for Clinical Lipidology (ACCL)

Data from Council on Credentialing in Pharmacy (CCP). (2012). Certification programs for pharmacists. *Retrieved 24 September 2017, from http://www.pharmacycredentialing.org/files/certificationprograms.pdf.*

ACADEMIC GRADUATE DEGREES IN PHARMACY AND PHARMACEUTICAL SCIENCES

Pharmacists have the opportunity to advance their knowledge and skills by completing further academic studies including a master's degree and PhD in many fields. These include pharmaceutical sciences and related disciplines (medicinal chemistry, pharmaceutics, pharmacology, toxicology, pharmacokinetics, etc.), clinical pharmaceutical sciences, and clinical and experimental therapeutics. In addition to these traditional fields, pharmacists can specialize in pharmacy practice, social and administrative pharmacy, and other related disciplines, including regulatory affairs, regulatory sciences, pharmaceutical outcomes and policy, pharmacoepidemiology and medication safety, and pharmacoeconomics (AACP, 2016b).

OTHER TRAINING PROGRAMS

In 2003, pharmacists in the United Kingdom were given prescribing rights (i.e., supplementary prescribing). This prescribing privilege can be obtained following a successful completion of a supplementary prescribing course at a UK school of pharmacy and subsequent registration with the regulatory body (Baqir, Miller, & Richardson, 2012). In 2006, the prescribing rights were extended to independent prescribing. A pharmacist independent prescriber can prescribe autonomously for any condition within their clinical competence (with the exception of three controlled medicines for addiction). To be an independent prescriber (IP), the pharmacists must successfully complete a GPhC accredited independent prescribing program. These accredited programs are offered by many UK universities. The program is typically part-time and is conducted over 6 months. It consists of at least 26 days of teaching and learning activity (component taught at the university) followed by at least 12 days of practice/training under the guidance of a medical practitioner. There are also GPhC accredited conversion programs at several universities to allow supplementary prescribers to become qualified independent prescribers (GPhC, 2017). The prescribing rights are considered an important milestone in pharmacy practice in the United Kingdom.

EQUIVALENCY AND QUALIFICATION FRAMEWORKS

This provides general guidance and discussion of equivalency and the qualification framework of pharmacy degrees across some countries. In fact, qualifications of the same title/name are not necessarily equivalent. They can differ in terms of level of education (entry-level, postgraduate, highest professional level, etc.). For example, PharmD in the United States, France, Thailand, and Saudi Arabia is considered an entry-to-the-practice professional degree, while in Singapore it is a postgraduate (specialist) degree and it is a postgraduate highest professional doctorate (PhD level) in Malta. In India, PharmD is an entry-level degree (6-year program) and a postbaccalaureate program (3-year program for BPharm holders). The DPharm is the highest professional qualification in pharmacy in the UK (PhD level).

Similarly, MPharm differs in terms of level of education across countries. In the United Kingdom, MPharm is an undergraduate program and the only entry-level degree for the profession. In Australia, the MPharm is a graduate-entry master of pharmacy degree and an accelerated route (usually 2-year full-time program) for nonpharmacy graduates from related disciplines (it is also an entry-level degree). In some countries such as Malaysia, MPharm is a postgraduate degree for specialization in clinical pharmacy and pharmacy practice. To differentiate it from undergraduate masters, the specialization usually follows the title of the degree (i.e., MPharm (Clinical Pharmacy)). On the other hand, in India the MPharm degree is offered as a postgraduate degree in any pharmacy-related disciplines (e.g., pharmacognosy, pharmaceutics, pharmacology, pharmacy practice, and pharmaceutical chemistry, etc.).

Lastly, in some countries, degrees offered in pharmaceutical sciences are not considered a pharmacy degree (i.e., not a registerable degree—it does not qualify for registration or licensure as a pharmacist). These programs are offered by some universities in several countries such as the United States, United Kingdom, and Australia. These include, for example, the Bachelor of Science in Pharmaceutical Sciences (BSPS) in the United States, Bachelor of Pharmaceutical Science(s) in Australia, and BSc in Pharmaceutical Science in the UK. These programs aim to prepare graduates in pharmaceutical and other healthcare industries, drug development, research, and further postgraduate studies.

CONCLUSION

Pharmacy education has evolved from a limited educational field in the 1800s and early 1900s to the current modern pharmacy education system. In fact, in the last 150 years pharmacy education has been changing in terms of the type of entry-level pharmacy degree programs, program duration, and program orientation (patient care versus product oriented). Moreover, the number of pharmacy programs has also increased tremendously in recent years in many countries. Currently, the entry-level degree for the pharmacy profession varies widely between countries and sometimes within the same country. These include PharmD, MPharm, BPharm, and BScPharm. Moreover, in some countries there is more than one degree that is considered an entry-level degree for the profession, with different competencies in some countries as well. The postgraduate professional training in pharmacy also differs widely among countries, including the main orientation/aim (i.e., patient care, research, both), duration, and structure (clinical rotations, research component, coursework, etc.). The current postgraduate opportunities include the master's degree in clinical pharmacy, professional doctorate in pharmacy (e.g., PharmD, DClinPharm, DPharm), fellowships, residencies, and MScs and PhDs in pharmaceutical sciences, pharmacy practice, and related disciplines.

ACKNOWLEDGMENT

The authors of this chapter would like to thank the following experts for their review of the parts related to their countries. The authors greatly appreciate their help to ensure that the information provided is up-to-date and correct.

The United States
Professor Donald E. Letendre
Dean,
The University of Iowa College of Pharmacy,
Iowa, United States.

The United Kingdom
Professor Derek Stewart
School of Pharmacy and Life Sciences,
Robert Gordon University,
Aberdeen, Scotland,
United Kingdom.

France
Dr. Florian Slimano
Department of Pharmacy,
Reims University Hospital,
45 Avenue du Général Koenig, 51100, Reims,
France.

Thailand
Professor Nathorn Chaiyakunapruk
School of Pharmacy,
Monash University Malaysia,
Malaysia.

Nepal
Dr. Bhuvan KC
School of Pharmacy,
Monash University Malaysia,
Malaysia.

Canada
Professor Zubin Austin
Leslie Dan Faculty of Pharmacy,
University of Toronto,
Toronto, Ontario
Canada.

Singapore
Associate Professor Alexandre Chan
Department of Pharmacy,
National University of Singapore,
Singapore.

Malta
Professor Lilian M Azzopardi
Pharmacy,
Faculty of Medicine & Surgery,
University of Malta,
Msida, Malta.

India
Dr. Suhaj Abdulsalim
Unaizah College of Pharmacy,
Qassim University,
Saudi Arabia.

REFERENCES

AB Fatah, A. R., & Bahari, M. B. (2004). Master's program in clinical pharmacy at a Malaysian pharmacy school. *American Journal of Health-System Pharmacy*, *61*, 2687–2689.

Accreditation Council for Pharmacy Education (ACPE). (2015). *Accreditation standards and key elements for the professional program in pharmacy leading to the doctor of pharmacy degree "Standards 2016."* Retrieved 24 September 2017, from https://www.acpe-accredit.org/pdf/Standards2016FINAL.pdf.

Al-Jedai, A., Qaisi, S., & Al-Meman, A. (2016). Pharmacy practice and the health care system in Saudi Arabia. *The Canadian Journal of Hospital Pharmacy*, *69*(3), 231–237.

American Association of Colleges of Pharmacy (AACP). (2016a). *Doctor of Pharmacy (PharmD) Degree*. Retrieved 24 September 2017, from http://www.aacp.org/resources/student/pharmacyforyou/Documents/PharmD.pdf.

American Association of Colleges of Pharmacy (AACP). (2016b). *Graduate degrees defined*. Retrieved 24 September 2017, from http://www.aacp.org/resources/student/graduateresearchstudents/Pages/GraduateDegreesDefined.aspx.

American College of Clinical Pharmacy (ACCP) (n.d.). What is a residency and how do I get one? Retrieved 24 September 2017, from https://www.accp.com/stunet/compass/residency.aspx

American Society of Health-System Pharmacists (ASHP). (1987). Definitions of pharmacy residencies and fellowships. *American Journal of Hospital Pharmacy*, *44*, 1142–1144.

Asiri, Y. A. (2011). Emerging frontiers of pharmacy education in Saudi Arabia: the metamorphosis in the last fifty years. *Saudi Pharmaceutical Journal*, *19*(1), 1–8.

Association of Faculties of Pharmacy of Canada (AFPC)/Association of Deans of Pharmacy of Canada (ADPC). (2010). *Position Statement and Joint Resolution on the Doctor of Pharmacy (PharmD) for the First Professional Degree at Universities in Canada*. Retrieved 24 September 2017, from http://www.afpc.info/sites/default/files/AFPC_ADPC_PharmD_Position_Statement_Resolution_Sept_2010.pdf.

Australian Pharmacy Council Ltd. (2012). *Accreditation Standards for Pharmacy Programs in Australia and New Zealand*. Retrieved 24 September 2017, from https://www.pharmacycouncil.org.au/media/1032/accreditation-standards-pharmacy-programs-aunz-2014.pdf.

Baqir, W., Miller, D., & Richardson, G. (2012). A brief history of pharmacist prescribing in the UK. *European Journal of Hospital Pharmacy: Science and Practice*, *19*(5), 487–488.

Basak, S. C., & Sathyanarayana, D. (2010). Pharmacy education in India. *American Journal of Pharmaceutical Education*, *74*(4). article no. 68.

Board of Pharmacy Specialties. *About BPS: What we do*. Retrieved 24 September 2017, from https://www.bpsweb.org/about-bps/.

Bourdon, O., Ekeland, C., & Brion, F. (2008). Pharmacy education in France. *American Journal of Pharmaceutical Education*, *72*(6). article no. 132.

Campus France Agency. (2016). *Pharmacy*. Retrieved 24 September 2017, from http://ressources.campusfrance.org/catalogues_recherche/domaines/noindex/es/pharmacie_en.pdf.

Canadian Council for Accreditation of Pharmacy Programs (CCAPP). (2017). *Canadian University Degree Programs*. Retrieved 24 September 2017, from http://ccapp-accredit.ca/find-an-accredited-program/#deg.

Canadian Council for Accreditation of Pharmacy Programs (CCAPP). (2016). *Accreditation standards for Canadian first professional degree in pharmacy programs-2018*. Retrieved 24 September 2017, from http://ccapp-accredit.ca/wp-content/uploads/2016/01/Accreditation-Standards-for-Canadian-First-Professional-Degree-in-Pharmacy-Programs.pdf.

Chaiyakunapruk, N., Jones, S. M., Dhippayom, T., & Sumpradit, N. (2016). Pharmacy practice in Thailand. In A. I. Fathelrahman, M. I. Mohamed Ibrahim, & A. I. Wertheimer (Eds.), *Pharmacy practice in developing countries* (pp. 3–22). Academic Press.

Chanakit, T., Low, B. Y., Wongpoowarak, P., Moolasarn, S., & Anderson, C. (2015). Does a transition in education equate to a transition in practice? Thai stakeholder's perceptions of the introduction of the doctor of pharmacy programme. *BMC Medical Education*, *15*(1), 205.

Council on Credentialing in Pharmacy (CCP). (2012). *Certification programs for pharmacists*. Retrieved 24 September 2017, from http://www.pharmacycredentialing.org/files/certificationprograms.pdf.

Council on Credentialing in Pharmacy (CCP). (2014). Credentialing and privileging of pharmacists: A resource paper from the council on credentialing in pharmacy. *American Journal of Health-System Pharmacy*, *71*(21), 1891–1900.

DeBenedette, V. (2007). *Pharmacy education: Change is the only constant*. Retrieved 24 September 2017, from http://drugtopics.modernmedicine.com/drug-topics/content/pharmacy-education-change-only-constant.

Department of Pharmacy (NUS). (2016). *National Pharmacy Residency Programmes. Retrieved 24 September 2017, from* http://pharmacy.nus.edu.sg/national-pharmacy-residency-programmes/.

Department of Pharmacy (NUS). (2017). *Specialty Residency in Ambulatory Care Pharmacy Practice (PGY 2)*. Retrieved 30 October 2017, from https://pharmacy.nus.edu.sg/specialty-residency-in-ambulatory-care-pharmacy-practice-pgy-2/.

Faculty of Pharmacy-King Abdulaziz University. (2017). *About us*. Retrieved 24 September 2017, from http://pharmacy.kau.edu.sa/Pages-01200-faculty-en.aspx.

Fardel, O. (2017). Relationship between pharmacy residency examination rank and specialty choice for French pharmacy residency-admitted students. *Pharmacy Practice*, *15*(1), 912.

Fink, J. L., III (2012). *Pharmacy: A brief history of the profession*. Retrieved 24 September, 2017, from https://www.studentdoctor.net/2012/01/pharmacy-a-brief-history-of-the-profession/.

General Pharmaceutical Council (GPhC). (2011). *Future pharmacists Standards for the initial education and training of pharmacists*. Retrieved 24 September 2017, from https://www.pharmacyregulation.org/sites/default/files/GPhC_Future_Pharmacists.pdf.

General Pharmaceutical Council (GPhC). (2012). *Criteria for registration as a pharmacist*. Retrieved 24 September 2017, from https://www.pharmacyregulation.org/sites/default/files/Registration%20criteria%20for%20pharmacists%20September%202012_0.pdf.

General Pharmaceutical Council. (2017). *Pharmacist independent prescriber*. Retrieved 24 September 2017, from https://www.pharmacyregulation.org/education/pharmacist-independent-prescriber.

Global Knowledge Exchange Network on Healthcare (GKEN). (2009). *An Overview of Education and Training Requirements for Global Healthcare Professionals-Pharmacists*. Retrieved 24 September 2017, from http://gken.org/Docs/Workforce/Pharmacy%20Education%20FINAL%20102609.pdf.

Hassali, M. A., Shafie, A. A., Guat See, O., & Wong, Z. Y. (2016). Pharmacy practice in Malaysia. In A. I. Fathelrahman, M. I. Mohamed Ibrahim, & A. I. Wertheimer (Eds.), *Pharmacy Practice in Developing Countries* (pp. 23–40). California: Academic Press.

Karim, S., & Adnan, M. (2016). Pharmacy practice in India. In A. I. Fathelrahman, M. I. Mohamed Ibrahim, & A. I. Wertheimer (Eds.), *Pharmacy practice in developing countries* (pp. 117–146). California: Academic Press.

Kathmandu University. (2016). *PharmD (Post Baccalaureate)*. Retrieved 24 September 2017, from http://www.ku.edu.np/pharmacy/index.php?go=PharmDcourses.

Keele University. (2017). *Professional Doctorate in Pharmacy (DPharm)*. Retrieved 24 September 2017, from https://www.keele.ac.uk/pgresearch/professionaldoctorates/dpharm/.

Knoer, S. J., Eck, A. R., & Lucas, A. J. (2016). A review of American pharmacy: education, training, technology, and practice. *Journal of Pharmaceutical Health Care and Sciences*, *2*(1). article no. 32.

Manipal University. (2017). *PharmD (Post Baccalaureate)*. Retrieved 24 September 2017, from https://manipal.edu/mcops-manipal/programs/program-list/pharmd-post-baccalaureatel.html.

Marriott, J. L., Nation, R. L., Roller, L., Costelloe, M., Galbraith, K., Stewart, P., et al. (2008). Pharmacy education in the context of Australian practice. *American Journal of Pharmaceutical Education*, *72*(6). article no. 131.

Ministry of Health Singapore. (2016). *National pharmacy residency programmes*. Retrieved 24 September 2017, from https://www.moh.gov.sg/content/moh_web/healthprofessionalsportal/pharmacists/programmes/pharma_residency_programme.html.

National Association of Pharmacy Regulatory Authorities (NAPRA). (2017). *Initial licensure-pharmacists. Retrieved 24 September 2017, from* http://napra.ca/pages/Licensing_Registration/initial_licensure.aspx.

National University of Singapore. (2017). *Doctor of pharmacy (PharmD)*. Retrieved 24 September 2017, from http://pharmacy.nus.edu.sg/doctor-of-pharmacy-pharm-d/.

Pharmacy Board Malaysia. (2017). *List of authorized local universities offering pharmacy course*. Retrieved 24 September 2017, from http://www.pharmacy.gov.my/v2/en/content/list-authorized-local-universities-offering-pharmacy-course.html.

Pharmacy Board of Australia. (2017). *Registration: internships*. Retrieved 24 September 2017, from http://www.pharmacyboard.gov.au/Registration/Internships.aspx#internships.

Pharmacy Council of India. (1991). *Education regulations (1991) for the diploma course in Pharmacy*. Retrieved 24 September 2017, from http://www.pci.nic.in/RulesRegulations/EducationRegulations1991/Chapter1.aspx.

Pharmacy Council of India. (2008). *PharmD. Regulations 2008*. Retrieved 24 September 2017, from http://www.pci.nic.in/PDF-Files/PharmD-Revised-A.pdf.

Pharmacy Council of India. (2016). *Rules & Syllabus for the Bachelor of Pharmacy (B. Pharm) Course*. Retrieved 24 September 2017, from http://www.pci.nic.in/GeneralInformation/AboutPCI/Syllabus_B_Pharm.pdf.

Pongcharoensuk, P., & Prakongpan, S. (2012). Centennial pharmacy education in Thailand. *Journal of Asian Association of Schools of Pharmacy*, *1*(1), 8–15.

Registration of Pharmacists Act, 1951 (Revised—1989). Retrieved 24 September 2017, from http://www.pharmacy.gov.my/v2/sites/default/files/document-upload/registration-pharmacists-act-1951-act-371.pdf.

Saudi Scientific Council of Pharmacy., & Saudi Commission for Health Specialties (SCHS). (2017). *Candidate information for clinical pharmacy residency programs* (2nd ed.). Retrieved 24 September 2017, from http://www.scfhs.org.sa/en/MESPS/TrainingProgs/TrainingProgsStatement/ClinicalPharmacy/Documents/Program%20Booklit.pdf.

Slimano, F., Gervais, F., Masse, C., & Langree, B. (2014). Hospital pharmacy residency in France in 2014: to a recognition of the specialization? *Annales Pharmaceutiques Francaises*, *72*(5), 317–324.

University of Alberta. (2017). *Admission requirements for Faculty of Pharmacy and Pharmaceutical Sciences*. Retrieved 24 September 2017, from http://calendar.ualberta.ca/content.php?catoid=20&navoid=5079#doctor-of-pharmacy-pharmd.

University of Birmingham. (2017). *Professional Doctorate in Pharmacy (DPharm). Retrieved 24 September 2017, from* http://www.birmingham.ac.uk/postgraduate/courses/combined/med/dpharm.aspx#CourseOverviewTab.

University of Bradford. (2017). *Pharmacy DPharm*. Retrieved 24 September 2017, from http://www.bradford.ac.uk/study/courses/info/pharmacy-dpharm-part-time.

University of British Colombia. (2017). *Admission requirements for Faculty of Pharmaceutical Sciences*. Retrieved 24 September 2017, from https://pharmsci.ubc.ca/programs/entry-practice-pharmd-degree/admissions-and-finances/admission-requirements.

University of California. (2014). *An era of growth and change: A closer look at pharmacy education and practice*. Retrieved 09 October 2017, from http://www.ucop.edu/uc-health/_files/pharmacy-an-era-of-growth-and-change.pdf.

University of Malta. (2016). *Doctorate in Pharmacy: Overview description*. Retrieved 24 September 2017, from http://www.um.edu.mt/ms/overview/PPPHDPHRFTT4-2016-7-O.

University of Monash. (2017). *Undergraduate Pharmacy*. Retrieved 24 September 2017, from https://www.monash.edu/pharm/future/courses/pharmacy.

University of Nottingham. (2017). *Pharmacy (with Integrated Pre-registration Scheme) MPharm*. Retrieved 24 September 2017, from https://nottingham.ac.uk/ugstudy/courses/pharmacy/mpharm-pharmacy-with-integrated-pre-registration-scheme.aspx.

University of Nottingham Malaysia. (2017). *Pharmacy MPharm (Hons)*. Retrieved 24 September 2017, from http://www.nottingham.edu.my/Study/Undergraduate-courses/Pharmacy/Pharmacy-MPharm-Hons.aspx.

University of Queensland. (2013). *Doctor of Clinical Pharmacy (DClinPharm)*. Retrieved 24 September 2017, from https://www.uq.edu.au/study/program.html?acad_prog=5005.

University of Queensland. (2017). *Bachelor of Pharmacy (Honours): program details*. Retrieved 24 September 2017, from https://future-students.uq.edu.au/study/program/Bachelor-of-Pharmacy-Honours-2373.

University of South Australia. (2014). *Doctor of Clinical Pharmacy*. Retrieved 24 September 2017, from http://study.unisa.edu.au/degrees/2014/267-862.

University of Strathclyde. (2017). *DPharm Pharmacy*. Retrieved 24 September 2017, from https://www.strath.ac.uk/courses/research/biomedicalsciences/dpharmpharmacy/.

University of Western Australia. (2017). *Doctor of Clinical Pharmacy*. Retrieved 24 September 2017, from http://handbooks.uwa.edu.au/courses/coursedetails?id=c146.

FURTHER READING

Universiti Sains Malaysia. (2017). *Master of Pharmacy (Clinical Pharmacy)*. Retrieved 24 September 2017, from http://www.pha.usm.my/index.php/en/programmes/postgraduate/about-research-programmes/master-of-pharmacy.

CHAPTER

TEACHING STRATEGIES USED IN PHARMACY

10

Ahmad A. Almeman, Saleh A. Alrebish
Qassim University, Buraidah, Saudi Arabia

ABBREVIATIONS

ACPE	Accreditation Council for Pharmacy Education
DRPs	drug-related problems
GPhC	General Pharmaceutical Council
GPA	grade point average
gRAT	Group Readiness Assurance Test
HPS	human patient simulation
iRAT	Individual Readiness Assurance Test
KPIs	key performance indicators
PBL	problem-based learning
PharmD	Doctor of Pharmacy
RAP	readiness assurance process
SDL	self-directed learning
TBL	team-based learning
UK	United Kingdom
US	United States

INTRODUCTION

The Conference of Teaching Colleges of Pharmacy (1870–84) in the United States was one of the first organized conferences in the field of pharmacy education (Kremers & Sonnedecker, 1986). During the mid-1990s, there was a rapid expansion in pharmacy education, and many colleges and associations were established. In 2000, the number of pharmacy colleges increased significantly, with huge variety in their curricula among different countries. In the years since, the number of pharmacy colleges has continued to grow (Grabenstein, 2016). One important reason for the relatively rapid increase in pharmacy colleges is the fact that the world has a shortage of skilled pharmacists. Consequently, governments are keen to train more of these professionals and develop a healthcare system capable of serving the population.

Most pharmacy programs include the following departments or subsections: pharmacognosy, pharmacology, pharmaceutical chemistry, pharmacy practice, clinical pharmacy, and pharmaceutics. They also adhere to common methods of evaluation, with a particular focus on laboratory testing, written examinations, and short essays. When students approach graduation, their final-year projects feature

Pharmacy Education in the Twenty First Century and Beyond. https://doi.org/10.1016/B978-0-12-811909-9.00010-1

detailed reports and an oral examination. Many programs give students the chance to enroll in internships after their courses have ended. A typical internship lasts approximately 12 months and, if the learner does well, it may lead to a paid position. The fact that most pharmacy colleges use similar methods, content, and learning objectives means that there is no significant variation among the degree programs. As a result, some of the recent pharmacy colleges have tried to apply different approaches. In the years to come, many other teaching colleges are expected to follow accordingly.

Some of the significant issues include syllabi that are too dense and complex, courses heavily skewed toward particular subjects, a separation between theory and practical application, poor quality training in social and communication skills, and an academic divide between the core scientific disciplines and the pharmaceutical subjects. For instance, many researchers suggest that clinical degrees and programs are not shaped to fit the practical needs of the real-life practice. For a long time, the decisions associated with course content and teaching methods were primarily based on tradition and what was already familiar. In many countries, pharmacy colleges are responsible for structuring their own programs and content. Therefore, decisions about course subjects, marking schemes, learning objectives, and testing techniques are all handled by internal staff. It is up to the academic leaders to decide how to pass pharmacy knowledge on to their students. In contrast, some well-known bodies have clear competencies, such as the Accreditation Council for Pharmacy Education (ACPE) in the United States, the General Pharmaceutical Council (GPhC) in the United Kingdom, and the Australian Pharmacy Council. Moreover, accreditation bodies may play an important role toward reforming curriculums, course designs, learning outcomes, and assessment methods (Alrebish, Jolly, & Molloy, 2017). Regardless of the educational style, programs must be designed in such a way to train the students based on the described skills and competencies.

AN OVERVIEW: WHAT DOES "TEACHING AND LEARNING STRATEGY" MEAN IN THE HIGHER EDUCATION CONTEXT?

There are countless theories and ideas designed to explain how human beings acquire knowledge. The term learning, in its most general form, refers to the process of obtaining information and skills, usually through academic study, teaching, or practical encounters. Learning is closely linked to experience, and it results in fundamental changes in principles, values, behaviors, and beliefs. For instance, activity theory suggests that learning methods and results are a product of direct involvement in valuable actions. However, this is only one academic interpretation of what constitutes learning. In regard to different methods of learning, there is a similar degree of variation. The problem with this is that it is a primarily subjective judgment. The learner is the one who determines the learning method, which means that it is influenced by all kinds of complex internal and external factors (Cassidy, 2004). According to Newble and Entwistle (1986), the term learning style suggests "mostly consistent attributes of an individual personality which highlight a desired approach to the pursuit of knowledge." As Schatteman, Carette, Couder, and Eisendrath (1997) explain, it is possible for learning methods to change, emerge, or disappear according to the current needs of the learner.

The evaluation of personal learning styles is useful for teachers because it gives them an opportunity to shape courses and educational programs to fit the needs of students. The work of Baker and Marks (1981) suggests that students who share similar learning styles actually perform better when constructive contact is allowed. Moreover, when teachers and their students have similar learning preferences, they have healthier interactions and course content is more likely to be understood. However, it is important to note that distinctions between the various learning styles are important too. Within schools, there is a huge variety of learning styles, and, if applied correctly, they can all be valuable. For this reason, teachers should be aware of the fact that students learn in different ways and respect their individual needs.

According to academic experts, combining compatible teaching and learning methods is the right way to increase student contributions and encourage better performance (Highfield, 1988; Rezler & Rezmovic, 1981). There is much evidence showing that, when presented with learning and teaching styles that are well suited, students achieve at a greater rate, produce higher scores, and go on to have better careers (Dunn & Griggs, 2000). However, there are some experts who believe that the opposite is also true and that deliberately pairing incompatible teaching and learning styles actually forces students to improve skills that would otherwise be left unrefined (Baker et al., 1988; Cavanagh & Coffin, 1994; Grasha, 1981; Kosower & Berman, 1996; Partridge, 1983). It is likely that, if the same teaching method is used again and again, students will lose interest at some point.

A broad variety of learning styles and teaching methods exists. The question of what is more important, commitment or performance, continues to be an issue for pharmacy colleges. In fact, the number of approaches can make the educational process quite bewildering for both students and their teachers, especially because they are all designed for the same objective: helping students to graduate or complete courses. Even so, some methods emphasize the right attitudes to education, while others seem to focus more heavily on grades and scores.

To successfully improve student performance and the ways in which students acquire knowledge, there first needs to be a full understanding of the different learning styles. This is no easy feat, because there are no clear and immutable definitions or characterizations. Even when different approaches to learning are identified, they can vary depending on the personality and preferences of the user. Nevertheless, it is widely agreed that students select a suitable approach to learning and consistently improve it in accordance with three types of triggers: conscious triggers derived from the individual desires, ambitions, and needs of the learners themselves; unconscious triggers relating to the same areas; and triggers originating from outside sources (Riding & Cheema, 1991). The key concepts relating to learning methods first emerged during the 1970s. They were thought to provide a valuable framework because learning styles have a real-world, practical application as well as a theoretical one. According to Riding and Cheema (1991), the term learning style was, for a time, used as an alternative to cognitive style and described variations within intellectual perspectives. However, it is now agreed that cognitive style is just one element of the broader approach to learning. Hence, the term learning style demonstrates an attempt to emphasize the whole learning process and not just its constituent parts.

In pharmacy education, students are required to gain an understanding of the methods that are being used to teach them. For example, if a person is in training to be a teacher himself, he needs to know how to instruct and impart knowledge. It is important for him to become comfortable and confident with the various learning styles. It is a complex process, but it plays a vital role in preparing trainee teachers for their future positions (Kurtz, Silverman, & Draper, 1998). Within pharmacy education, there is a greater need for small group learning, which enables mentors to monitor levels of student progress and ensures that all students can interpret and apply the key concepts (Bokey, Chapuis, & Dent, 2014). The science-based subjects seem to produce a higher failure rate than others, so it is imperative that pharmacy colleges implement the right forms of evaluation and testing (Astin, 2012).

There are important links between small and large group learning, just as there are crucial connections between the individual pursuit of knowledge and formalized teaching. The issue is made yet more complex by the introduction of digital technologies. For the most part, they offer students some obvious benefits. For instance, they make it much easier to access content, they allow students to interact with their teachers, and ensure that teachers respond to queries and requests for help in a timely fashion, and they open up space for a much more diverse variety of learning styles and methods. Crucially, the way in which these technologies are used depends on the learning environment. They can be rigidly structured or shaped to fit individual needs. For example, the smaller the class, the more likely it is that different approaches to the use of technology will be evident in the same environment. In all cases, successful teaching requires a great deal of preparation and access to high-quality materials. One such resource is support staff, who can help classroom leaders prepare for learning sessions.

It is important to understand that there is no optimal learning or teaching style, because it all depends on the needs of the students and their environment. Nevertheless, this chapter discusses some of the most common approaches and explains why they are suitable for pharmacy education.

DIDACTIC LECTURES

The best place to begin is with the traditional lecture. The traditional lecture, which is often referred to as "large group instruction," has been the most common teaching style for centuries. It is only in the last decade that academic experts have been highlighting the weaknesses of this method. In contrast, interactive methods, which are usually referred to as "small group learning," encourage two-way discussions, as well as making time for teachers to listen to their students (Felicia, 2011). The students are permitted to voice their opinions, make suggestions, and collaborate on tasks. Learning is successful when students can recall information when promoted (Jones, 2007).

Didactic lectures are considered unidirectional. The teacher speaks, and the students listen, which leaves no room for interaction. This can lead to a frustrating experience as students tend to get bored if they cannot contribute. However, there must be a reason lecturing has been such a popular teaching style for so long. Ultimately, lectures can be hugely beneficial. They have the potential to be motivating and exciting, but their quality depends upon the skills of the presenter. The introduction of modern technologies means that lecturers can keep their students interested by adding video content, online activities, image galleries, music, and more (Tavangar, 2014). Today, lectures are largely seen as supplementary tools that are most valuable when combined with interactive approaches such as seminars and group work.

The didactic lecture is a method of teaching that is based on direct instruction. It places considerable focus on the movement of knowledge from teacher to student and less on interactions between the two. The most important materials are textbooks and lecture notes. Students advance by being gradually introduced to more difficult topics and challenges. They are assessed with the use of one-on-one evaluations, performance scores, and personalized feedback.

Didactic instruction is the oldest form of teaching. It has been in existence for centuries, and most colleges still adhere to it. In fact, even the learning centers that embrace a variety of teaching approaches tend to prioritize one-directional instruction or at least consider it an essential part of every course. It is often described as "surface learning," because it does not always move beyond the provision and receipt of facts. The driving force behind surface learning is usually extrinsic. In other words, the products of surface learning are largely limited to an ability to receive and recall facts at convenient times (for example, for the purposes of a test). It certainly has many weaknesses, but it also offers some important benefits and it remains a vital part of modern education (Hannafin & Hannafin, 2010).

In basic terms, didactic methods involve the movement of information from teacher to student. The broader aim is for the student to be able to apply this information in environments that are different from the classroom. The role of the teacher is lead assessor and knowledge provider. Didactic learning promotes a culture that is individualistic and competitive.

DEEP LEARNING

Opposite to surface learning is so-called deep learning. Deep learning offers many advantages to the practitioners of didactic teaching. It provides a way to explore a more fundamental definition of knowledge. Consequently, it focuses on a full and comprehensive interpretation of key concepts, ideas, and applications. The driving force behind this type of learning is intrinsic. It relates to the personal fulfillment that one feels after mastering a new subject or piece of information. For this reason, deep learning incorporates more than just instruction (Johnson, 2013). It should demonstrate different ways of implementing knowledge and make room for exciting and dynamic methods of presenting facts.

Deep learning has many key features and obstacles. Optimizing the features and avoiding the obstacles will successfully achieve a reasonable educational system. However, some obstacles are unavoidable or at least are difficult to avoid in this educational system.

Key Features:

1. Intrinsic (personal) incentives
2. Individualized progression
3. Proactive learning/understanding
4. Cooperation and teamwork
5. Willingness to question oneself
6. Compatible content and course structures
7. Carefully paired learning goals and testing techniques

Obstacles:

1. Extrinsic (outside) incentives
2. Recalling facts for the purposes of testing
3. Passive learning (one-way instruction)
4. Lack of collaboration
5. Lack of cohesion between subjects/topics

TEAM-BASED LEARNING

During the 1970s, the concept of team-based learning (TBL) was created by Dr. Larry Michaelsen, of the University of Oklahoma (Michaelsen, Watson, Cragin, & Fink, 1982). Michaelsen and Sweet (2008) state that "the key learning goal of TBL is to move past the simple offering of knowledge and create different ways for students to apply it to practical obstacles." Dr. Michaelsen encouraged his students to function as small groups of learners. When in teams, they collaborated and focused on using knowledge to solve basic and intricate challenges, with the professor as their guide. Dr. Michaelsen was interested in finding ways to help students transition from a unidirectional didactic learning style to an active pursuit of information. Since this approach was developed in the United States, it is most commonly used there and in some other countries.

WHY DO WE USE TBL?

There are many reasons TBL is a successful method of teaching, particularly in comparison with conventional forms of instruction. For one thing, it is equally beneficial for both students and teachers. It supports collaboration, structured group activities, the application of skills, and the importance of two-directional interaction. These attributes are all crucial to the healthcare field (Allen et al., 2013; Al-Meman, Al-Worafi, & Saleh, 2014; Hincapie, Cutler, & Fingado, 2016). TBL is characterized by a greater emphasis on practical implementations, as opposed to basic concepts. This is a great way to get students using their imaginations and connecting with information from multiple perspectives.

In recent years, TBL has grown in prominence among pharmacy colleges (Allen et al., 2013). At least one of the reasons for this relates to larger classrooms and expanding student populations. The traditional learning environment is still characterized by a select group of students who work from the same space. However, if the groups keep growing in size, the teachers will have to come up with increasingly creative methods of engagement and assessment. In many countries, PharmD courses make use of TBL teaching methods (Nation, Tweddell, & Rutter, 2016). They are also evident in a number of digital pharmacy courses (Franklin, Markowsky, De Leo, Normann, & Black, 2016).

TBL makes room for direct instruction, but it tries to avoid making teachers present to overly large groups (Schatteman et al., 1997). Instead, students are split into small teams. This is an effective way to streamline and simplify learning in larger colleges, with the largest student populations. The overarching goal of TBL is to create chances for students to actually apply knowledge, rather than be expected only to receive and recall it. They are encouraged to use new information to solve challenges and not just answer questions correctly (Bleske et al., 2016). Crucially, TBL moves the role of the teacher from a basic provider of insights to a supportive guide for efficient, valuable learning application.

It is clear then that TBL supports a much more active form of teaching than conventional "I speak, you listen" approaches to learning (Dunn & Griggs, 2000). It first began to grow in popularity during the 1990s, after a number of prestigious business colleges espoused its benefits. Just a decade later, the TBL techniques were being utilized in a huge variety of fields and industries. They are now considered to be an essential part of everything from veterinary to pharmacology, dentistry, nursing studies, and more. According to researchers, they lead to a greater understanding of educational resources, improved critical thinking skills, and higher levels of intellectual dexterity. Moreover, TBL helps students realize the value of listening to and accepting the views of their peers (Grasha, 1981). This technique fosters a greater degree of professionalism and teaches students how to collaborate effectively (Schmeck, 2013).

The goal of TBL is to encourage students to contribute more readily to classroom activities and to help them see the benefit of becoming more skilled, active learners. This is very different from traditional forms of instruction, which focus only on the receipt of information and, at later points, its efficient recall. The reason for this is that it refines and improves teaching results, helps students to become responsible for their own learning, supports autonomous development, facilitates collaboration, motivates the desire to achieve, and guides students throughout the application of new skills. For all of these reasons, TBL must continue to be an important part of pharmacy education.

TBL is the superior option for students because it increases the overall amount of knowledge gained. It also develops the understanding of most topics, expands critical thinking skills, helps learners progress through intellectual challenges, and encourages more respect for peers. It should be noted that, although approval rates for TBL are very high, it is natural to assume that teachers and learners who have always used this approach (as opposed to transitioning from a unidirectional style) will have more positive opinions of it (Frame et al., 2015, 2016; Gallegos & Peeters, 2011; Nation et al., 2016).

TBL DESIGN

TBL consists of several steps. These steps may be adjusted in several ways based on the needs of the class (Parmelee, Michaelsen, Cook, & Hudes, 2012; Sibley & Ostafichuk, 2015).

- **iRAT (Individual Readiness Assurance Test).** The iRAT must begin promptly, at the same time as the class is due to commence (for example, 8 or 9 am). All papers are submitted after 15 min. Students who arrive after the test has started may still be permitted to enter, but only up to around 5 min late. Within the next 5 min, the students are organized into groups (5–7 each).

The TBL teams should not be altered, as this is likely to damage the construction of a group spirit and a cohesive atmosphere. Students need to be given sufficient opportunity to get acquainted, and this cannot occur if the groups are constantly being reshuffled. Ultimately, late-stage changes mean that students have to begin building a team from scratch. Therefore, the groups established at the start are the ones that will be used throughout the entire semester. It is important that teams are formed according to GPAs. Each one should include members of varying abilities.

- **gRAT (Group or Team Readiness Assurance Test).** The allocated time for a gRAT is 30 min. Standard IF-AT forms are used to operate gRAT. All teams receive the same iRAT questions for exploration, discussion, debate, solution, and explanation. If the groups cannot agree on one unified response, they are encouraged to vote for the best answer. This is a good way to start healthy, productive debate among peers.

The following 20-min period is used for group presenting. The teams, after picking the best answer, are invited to share it with the class. Every member of the group should contribute to this process and there should be a clear attempt to explain and defend the response.

a. The following 20 min are spent on an open discussion
b. The following 20 min are spent on peer assessments.
c. After this point, there is a mandatory break (following G(T)RAT).
d. Following the mandatory break, 2 h are spent on application tasks. They are centered on practical case scenarios.

For students who are more familiar with older forms of instruction and teaching, the introduction of TBL needs to be controlled and consistent. If TBL is pushed onto unwilling learners too quickly, it will not be effective and the learners may choose to reject it. The recommended strategy is to commit to a forward TBL for the inaugural semester and then transition to a backward TBL (the optimal style) if the trial period is satisfactory. Forward and backward refer simply to the rearrangement of the iRAT and gRAT to be the first or last. The study program, reading tasks, and overall learning aims should be handed out to the students before teaching begins. It may help, particularly for those unfamiliar with TBL, to carry out a number of introductory sessions. These are genuine lessons, with real resources, but they do not impact grades or scores. In regard to the teachers themselves, those who are new to TBL should be provided with the necessary training in the form of structured lessons. They will also receive a supplementary guide book for additional support. It is best to arrange a TBL "catch up" session for teachers at least once every month so that they can share their experiences and voice any relevant concerns (Parmelee et al., 2012; Sibley & Ostafichuk, 2015).

When using forward TBL, the Group Readiness Assurance Test (gRAT) and the Individual Readiness Assurance Test (iRAT) are conducted after the practice session or presentation. It is structured this way to help the students feel ready for a complete move to TBL strategies. It is important to remember that the transitional period is not supposed to be permanent. It was designed to support those students and teachers who are not immediately familiar with TBL and need to be guided through a slower replacement process. New students (who have never used any other teaching systems) are exposed to the TBL strategies right away. They are likely to listen more closely than they would during a conventional presentation, because they are aware that they will be tested shortly afterwards. However, it is just as essential for students to ready themselves before the start of the class too. The amount of time allocated to the presentation is intentionally insufficient and they need to put their own time and effort in if they want to score well on the examination. Each teacher must provide the required information without giving away any answers to either test, because all the insights needed to excel are included in the presentation materials. Therefore, it is more than possible for the students to take control of their own learning and make sure that they receive a good grade. The teachers may think about transitioning to backward TBL, if forward TBL strategies produce satisfactory results during the inaugural semester. This means that the gRAT and iRAT tests are conducted at the start of each class instead of at the end. The materials, equipment, resources, and topics remain the same in both cases. More importantly, the structure of the tests is not altered. The only difference is that the teacher must configure the content of the exams in a "backwards" manner and highlight any concepts or ideas which they think might end up needing more explanation.

The 20-min period after gRAT is used for team and parallel presentations of the correct answers. Every team needs to appoint a member who can explain their choices and opinions on the subject matter. It is a good idea to rotate the order of the teams in each new class so that the same group does not end up presenting first on every occasion. The parallel debate is carried out among the teams (simultaneously), and the members vote to add a level of collaboration and interactivity to the process. They must then defend and explain the answers that they have selected. The next part of the class is spent answering any leftover queries and making sure that all the concepts covered have been fully understood. There is a mandatory rest period, because the students perform better at the next task if they are given a short interval for chat and cognitive respite. The application tasks are based on genuine case stories from the hospital. There is an abundance of case ideas for pharmacokinetics, pharmacy practice, therapeutics, and patient assessment. They are all introduced and described with the use of a PowerPoint slide show. The case stories are selected by the education leaders as part of a collective effort that is updated on a regular basis. Often, former students make contributions to this collection of concepts and application ideas, and this helps to keep the classroom tasks fresh and exciting. Every class uses two or three case stories, depending on the number of students and how quickly they progress.

ASSESSMENT

The method of assessment is quite distinct, and it has little in common with the older forms of evaluation. In fact, it can be a little dense and difficult to follow at times. If students do not fully understand the way in which they are being assessed, they will receive a lower grade, so it is not likely to please all of them. In contrast to conventional strategies, assessments are cumulative and consistent. Therefore, they can put considerable extra pressure on students.

There have been many variations among researchers. However, each college may design their own appropriate model. For instance, marks may be distributed as follows:

a. IRAT (15 marks for each session to be divided by the total)
b. GRAT (25 marks for each session to be divided by the total)
c. Peer evaluation (10 marks for each evaluation to be divided by the total).
d. 2 bonus marks are given as a reward for students or groups who have the critical thinking needed to solve and identify drug-related problems (DRPs) and other questions during the case discussion.
e. The final exam will be 50 marks.

TWELVE TIPS FOR DOING EFFECTIVE TBL (ADAPTED FROM PARMELEE & MICHAELSEN, 2010)

1. Tell the students why TBL is beneficial
2. Begin with a well-structured course
3. Utilize "backwards TBL" when designing the course content
4. Put KPIs in place to identify when and how students have fulfilled key learning objectives
5. Conduct application tasks to encourage deep thinking and debate
6. Fully exploit the value of the RAP (readiness assurance process)
7. Identify responsibility and personal accountability as key assets
8. Include an efficient appeals system
9. Stick with peer assessment techniques even if they are difficult
10. Give clear, straightforward instructions about what to prepare and why
11. Arrange the groups so that they contain varying levels of ability
12. Consider the use of small "props" to help students complete application tasks

THE FOUR ESSENTIAL PRINCIPLES OF TEAM-BASED LEARNING (ADAPTED FROM HTTP://WWW.TEAMBASEDLEARNING.ORG & CONFERENCE OF TEAM-BASED LEARNING, 2013)

Principle 1—Groups Must Be Properly Formed.

1. At the start, make sure that old/existing teams are deconstructed.
2. The students should not form their own teams.
3. Teams should include a variety of abilities.
4. Teams should contain between five and eight.
5. Teams must remain the same for the entire semester.

Principle 2—Students Must Be Made Accountable.

1. Preparing well for the class
2. Readiness Assurance Tests (gRAT and iRAT)
3. Peer evaluations
4. Application tasks and clinical case

Principle 3—Team Assignments Must Promote Both Learning and Team Development.
All suitable TBL tasks will include the following features:

1. Team collaboration and communication
2. Clear, straightforward choices and brief accounts
3. Demonstrable value for the students
4. Tasks should be the same for every team
5. Parallel voting

Principle 4—Students Must Receive Frequent and Immediate Feedback.

PROBLEM-BASED LEARNING

According to Boud and Feletti (1997), problem-based learning (PBL) is oriented around "a challenge, question, or riddle which the student needs to solve." The researchers' work furthers this explanation by arguing that PBL is a type of teaching that forms the context of the class out of an interesting challenge. The desire to unravel the conundrum is the motivating force to learn. To be precise, PBL teaching starts when the challenge emerges or presents itself. This is an important point to remember, because it is the same way challenges develop for pharmacists (Bokey et al., 2014). Looking at colleges in the United Kingdom and United States, it may seem that PBL is considerably more common in the United Kingdom and European countries than in the United States, in comparison to TBL. This trend can be seen throughout the published data, based on our research. However, the actual data may vary as some are using either system without any publication.

WHY PBL?

From a general perspective, PBL first originated during the early 1970s. It was designed to support and assist medical students. In the decades since, it has been consistently improved and applied to a broad range of teaching contexts. PBL, as a teaching strategy, was created by Tamblyn and Barrows (1980) at McMaster University in Ontario. It features case stories or "challenges," which are used to encourage students to explore different solutions. The system is highly regarded and, even though it continues to be tweaked and changed, the core principles remain the same. Currently, PBL is used in pharmacy colleges in China, Brazil, Iran, the United Kingdom, the United States, Qatar, and many other countries (Cisneros, Salisbury-Glennon, & Anderson-Harper, 2002; Galvao, Silva, Neiva, Ribeiro, & Pereira, 2014; Love & Shumway, 1983; Shaw, Lacey, Leighton, & Warner, 2006; Vatanpour, 2012; Yamaki et al., 2016). Although it is a widely applied system, it could be argued that TBL has overtaken PBL as far as prominence and range of applications (Cisneros et al., 2002). PBL classes include carefully designed and allocated "conundrums" that motivate students to seek critical information, find solutions to key challenges, take responsibility for their education, and collaborate with their peers. This is significant, because it extends beyond the time in class. The problem-solving process can be applied to a huge number of challenges that the students will go on to face outside of the classroom, in their personal lives and careers. For scientific mediums, PBL has signaled a move away from unidirectional presentations (in which the teacher talks and the students listen) to a more open and cooperative environment. It is believed that combining aspects of pharmacy with PBL strategies is a good way to enhance critical reasoning skills (Cheng, Alafris, Kirschenbaum, Kalis, & Brown, 2003; Cisneros et al., 2002; Novak, Shah, Wilson, Lawson, & Salzman, 2006; Shaw et al., 2006).

Some pharmacy colleges have implemented PBL as a supplement or a substitute for a conventional didactic approach. The system incorporates a number of key features. For one thing, the teaching is entirely focused on the needs of the student. They are encouraged to start and lead discussions, rather than take cues from the teacher. Like TBL, discussions occur among small groups. They are presented with a problem or scenario and they must find a suitable solution, so they learn how to structure information and respond to professional contexts in a structured, safe environment. The point is that there are multiple solutions to every challenge. It is the job of the students to target just one solution and explain why it is the best choice. According to Wood (2003), the aim of healthcare teaching should be "to use clinical information as a trigger for learning and help students recognize the value of fundamental scientific principles, ideas, and concepts."

The PBL system is characterized by its focus on real-world scenarios and faux "crises" or challenges. The scenario is the trigger for deep thinking and intellectual exploration. The students transition from a point of little understanding to a point of probable solution and success. The system allows them to take control of and direct their own modes of thought so that they can test the limits of their ability. As with introducing TBL, implementing PBL in a classroom of learners who are not familiar with it can be a daunting process (Haworth, Eriksen, Chmait, & Matsuda, 1998). It can take time for students to become comfortable with the move from a passive to an active stance. It is possible to streamline the process by taking a closer look at their individual approaches to learning. According to several different medical researchers (Kaufman & Mann, 1996), students express a preference for PBL, in relation to traditional didactic strategies, but only if the new system is introduced in the right way.

PBL DESIGN

The PBL element of the syllabus focuses on the formation of small teams (between 8 and 10 members) and uses a learner-oriented approach to teaching. The team discussions are observed and guided by teachers who have had extensive training as part of a teacher-focused session. In a pharmacy context, the guide is a qualified pharmacist or clinical practitioner. As course guides, the teachers congregate every fortnight to talk about issues relating to the course content and whether their team systems are proving successful. Normally, a PBL "challenge" or scenario is solved over the course of 2 weeks, with one session per week. The students are presented with the problem, and they must come to an agreement about the probable solution. It is important that the given scenario is not too familiar to the teams or they will not need to think too deeply to solve it. The best place to start is with an initial brainstorm session, as this is a good way to bring the existing knowledge of all the team members together. They should talk about what they do not understand or do not know about the scenario and identify the points that must be clarified to complete the task. The teacher may provide a list of learning objectives or "triggers" on the whiteboard as a prompt. However, it is up to the teams to decide which objectives are the most important and how the challenges should be approached. If the teacher decides that certain topics or subjects are very important and must be covered by all students, they have the choice to directly assign them (Armstrong, 1997; Wood, 2003).

After the first PBL class and before the second, the students are encouraged to conduct their own research into the assigned learning triggers. This is achieved by engaging with information from academic papers, websites, textbooks, and academic papers. It is customary to ask each learner to create a written summary of what they have learned and hand it to the teacher at the start of the second class. They can then talk about their findings with the rest of the team and evaluate the new information. It is important that students feel comfortable speaking about their research, because converting written information into a personal account is a very effective way to grasp intellectual concepts. The job of the teacher, throughout this process, is to interject with relevant, open-ended queries designed to determine the range, depth, quality, and accuracy of the information being offered and discussed. At the end of the second class, the teacher provides feedback to every learner, telling them how well they have functioned as a group and whether they have found an adequate solution to the given dilemma. Lastly, each team is instructed to write a collective paper on their classroom experiences. They have about 7 days to complete the task. If the PBL session was a success, the teams should have no problem summarizing the key points and formulating an account of how they solved the challenge. The seven stages of PBL are as follows:

1. Presenting the key terms/issues
2. Explaining the problem/challenge
3. Brainstorming/team discussion
4. Structuring and theorizing
5. Learning goals/targets
6. Looking for additional insights
7. Synthesizing (bringing all knowledge together)

ROLE OF TUTOR

The contribution of the teachers is very important for PBL learning. It is their job to direct, observe, guide, and supervise the students as they figure out the best ways to learn and understand. The best PBL guides know exactly when they should interject and offer support and when they should step back to let students control their own deep-thinking processes (Chan, 2008; Walsh, 2005).

When the class starts, the teacher spends time making sure that all learners understand the purpose of PBL. They explain the core principles and the rules of the system so that students know what they stand to gain from it if they engage fully.

Throughout the class, the students may need assistance in regard to exploring different challenges and bringing their collective knowledge together. If necessary, the teacher can offer prompts and learning triggers to help teams grasp complex ideas. In some cases, they might have a general understanding of what is required to solve a problem without fully understanding the concepts, so close supervision is recommended.

Consequently, the job of the teacher is quite different from the role that a traditional teacher, in a didactic context, is expected to provide. They are a source of support and guidance, but they are not in control of how students learn and where they find their insights. The PBL system places considerably more accountability in the hands of the learner, but this does not mean that the teacher has no active contribution. Teachers must remain alert and engaged throughout the class and ensure that every student maintains an appropriate level of motivation.

The teacher must determine whether individual learners are managing to grasp the key concepts and whether teams are successfully integrating their ideas and functioning as an intellectual unit. This is achieved by asking testing questions, providing learning triggers, making suggestions, and evaluating progress.

The most skilled teachers are those with a varied knowledge base, a dynamic, versatile skillset, and an open-minded attitude to learning.

ROLE OF STUDENTS

The PBL system requires learners to engage more actively in their own educational journey. It is common for students to direct and lead classes (with the supervision of a teacher). The transition from conventional learner, with the basic instruction to receive and interpret information, to fully active team member is a major change. It can be intimidating at first, but most students end up having a real appreciation for the interactive nature of PBL.

There are many benefits to allowing students to operate in teams. It supports the rapid procurement of knowledge, and it enhances a broad range of skills, from personal awareness to peer evaluation, peer support, perceptiveness, communication, accountability, and more. Perhaps most importantly, working among friends and peers is a great way to teach students the value of respect for those around them. As they, essentially, start to teach themselves, they accept more responsibility, become more reliable, and take more pride in their achievements.

Ultimately, PBL is about independence. The students are expected to engage with the critical analysis of data sources, literature, and practical scenarios. They must hold themselves accountable for their achievements (or lack thereof) and learn how to identify the fastest routes to intellectual success.

There is one issue that educational systems are still trying to solve. How do you motivate a student to learn for the sake of learning, as opposed to seeing learning only as a way to pass tests and make it through college? It is a major question for teachers and course creators. PBL is a response to the need for more practical, applicable skills in colleges. Therefore, every case study or scenario presented in class must be directly relevant or useful to the students. Even if it is not certain that they will encounter a specific dilemma or situation in their future lives, its core principles must contribute to their growth as human beings and academic professionals.

STUDENT ROLE-PLAYING AND SIMULATED PATIENT ROLE-PLAYING

The value of simulation-based training is most often recognized in high-risk industries. For instance, healthcare professionals recommend the use of simulation when training students. Many experts agree that it is an effective way to enhance learning results, prepare students for future work, and increase levels of patient safety. Moreover, it is a vital part of helping learners identify and manage hazards (Knowles, 1984; Kosower & Berman, 1996). For many years, its use has been explored and discussed by the pharmaceutical sector.

The most common form of simulation is role-playing. It is an experiential technique that encourages learners to engage with scenarios in the same way they would if the situation were real and were actually being played out in front of them. Normally, actors are brought into the class to formulate and direct the scenario, but they take steps to involve the learners, particularly when key decisions are needed. The beauty of role-playing is that it allows students to explore high-risk situations without the fear of dangerous consequences if they make a mistake.

Within the pharmaceutical sector, simulation is a popular and commonplace style of teaching. It can incorporate an almost endless variety of situations and challenges. For instance, actors may pretend to be patients who need urgent attention from a healthcare professional. It is the job of the learner to figure out what needs to be done and how to help the "patient." In fact, this is a technique that is utilized by paramedics and first-aid providers all the time. They feign an emergency or accident, and the class is expected to respond quickly and correctly. For a pharmacist, the objective is to help the patient and avoid death or injury.

However, it is worth pointing out that not everybody agrees with the efficacy of simulation, particularly within the healthcare sector. There are some experts who believe that clinical problems and challenges (particularly pharmaceutical issues) are far too complex to be feigned in suitable detail. However, digital technologies are gradually lessening the impact of this concern (Smithson, Bellingan, Glass, & Mills, 2015). For instance, virtual reality technology is already transforming medical simulations and allowing learners to experience extremely life-like scenarios without actually being there.

There is considerable evidence to suggest that simulation produces more skilled, confident, and prepared emergency responders. However, there are countless ways to create a clinical simulation, and each one offers varying degrees of value. The two most common forms involve human patient simulations and standardized patient simulations.

The work of Hofmann (2009) explores the efficacy of medical simulations for the training of students in high-level, high-risk professions. It states that "simulations are an effective way to improve responses to high stake scenarios and facilitate engaged, dynamic learning." Kunkler (2006) expresses similar views and explains that "medical simulations are valuable resources, particularly in regard to assessing the degree of learner awareness and their ability to select appropriate responses, practices, methods, and tools." The advantages of using simulation can be split into four groups: affordability, patient security, educational experience, and consistent learning opportunities (Kunkler, 2006). From a wider perspective, simulations are useful because they give learners the chance to experience high-risk, high-stakes situations without needing an actual emergency to occur first. In other words, learners are able to carry out consistent, cohesive learning at all times and not just when hands-on responses are required. At a deeper level, pharmacological simulations provide detailed access to data and tools, which can enhance learner skillsets and improve the provision of key services (Kunkler, 2006).

The two most common forms of patient simulation are standardized patient simulation and human patient simulation (HPS). The former is carried out by local actors, volunteers, or the students and teachers themselves. Together, they role-play a given situation or scenario. The latter involves high-fidelity digital mannequins and task-oriented trainers (Smithson et al., 2015). Alternatively, in some cases, it may include low-level, low-fidelity simulations, such as preserved animal tissues.

According to existing literature on the efficacy of simulation for healthcare training, students gain a broad variety of high-level, professional skills when they engage with standardized patient simulation. This is a view supported by experts such as Jones, Passos-Neto, and Braghiroli (2015) and

Gallimore, George, and Brown (2008), who argue that students feel more confident in tests and exam situations after experiencing standardized patient simulation. It helps them to perform substantially better on skill-based tests (Hofmann, 2009; Michaelsen, 1992), especially throughout the foundational stages of the course (Gallimore et al., 2008; Smithson et al., 2015).

The notion that healthcare professionals must be exposed to real patients during their training is broadly endorsed. However, it is also recognized that the educational need has to be combined with a commitment to patient security and safety (Young, Rohwer, Volmink, & Clarke, 2014). This is one of the reasons simulation is such a popular tool. It provides this hands-on experience without putting real patients in danger (Smithson et al., 2015). Therefore, simulation minimizes the ethical issues associated with practicing on real patients. For pharmacist trainees, it is fast becoming an invaluable part of learning and practical application.

INDEPENDENT STUDY/SELF-DIRECTED LEARNING

The system of independent study is most commonly found in universities. It is often called "self-directed" learning (SDL). The purpose of the system is to encourage students to take full control of their pursuit of knowledge. There is very minimal guidance from teachers, and, in some cases, there is no guide at all. Usually, teachers help learners choose a suitable topic and define the study goals, and then they leave them to figure out the rest alone.

The value of self-directed learning has been a subject of debate for many years. In fact, academics and educational leaders have been exploring its value since the early 1990s. It can be tricky to follow these arguments sometimes, because so many different ways exist to refer to this style of learning (Titmus, 2014). It may be called self-education, independent learning, autonomous study, andragogy, self-planned study, lifelong study, or autodidacticism. However, one of the clearest descriptions of SDL is offered by Knowles (1975), who states that "from a broad viewpoint, SDL is a learning style whereby the student controls the course of their understanding and acknowledgement. This may be achieved either with or without any assistance. They are responsible for identifying key learning objectives, finding the right data sources, selecting and applying suitable learning methods, and analyzing the results of these methods."

The primary aim of SDL is to develop the capacity to learn, which is why the focus is on giving students room to explore alternative methods and strategies, rather than giving them a path to follow. With the use of SDL, students can acquire sophisticated metacognitive abilities and become evaluators of their own pursuit of knowledge (Kasworm, 2011). This should not be underestimated, because the importance of autonomous learning is enormous. We live in a world that is constantly changing and shifting. Once we leave formal education, there are fewer support systems in place to guide our experiences, and we must be comfortable directing the course of our own lives and intellectual journeys. Ultimately, it is not possible for those training to perform high-pressure, high-risk jobs to have constant access to a personal guide. It is essential that they learn to take responsibility for their own progress.

In addition, it is necessary to note that the concept of "self" is always in danger of thwarting learning efforts. Educational progress is inevitably and unavoidably influenced by cultural biases. Consequently, the notion of self is inaccurate to some degree, because there is no identity that is free of the pressures exerted by external factors. As Flannery and Abraham (1993) explain, we cannot disregard the fact that learning (SDL included) must occur within its own cultural boundaries. It is simply impossible for teachers and mentors, no matter how skilled they are or how perceptive their methods may be, to isolate the provision of knowledge from the influences of their own character and experiences. The important thing is that we remain able to utilize strategies of autoassessment and self-reflection to acknowledge why our perceptions of value are so closely tied to cultural attributes. The right way to become autonomous learners (and to employ SDL effectively) is to first understand ourselves. There must be a high level of awareness in regard to personal biases, unconscious preferences, and social preconceptions. This can be achieved by scrutinizing our personal motivators and determining what it is that inspires the desire to learn.

The work of Candy (1991) introduces some interesting points. It argues that overvaluing SDL can result in the construction of faux democracies. In other words, teachers and course creators feel like they lose out on the right to champion the content that they, personally, believe is essential for learners. Candy (1991) notes that teachers should not feel like they're intruding on students' freedoms just because they have more knowledge and want it to be utilized. When autonomous study is employed in the wrong way, it has the potential to reduce the role of the teacher and complicate matters for the student. However, it is difficult to agree with the notion that encouraging independent learning is akin to forcing teachers to give up their power as leaders and academic guides. Although some individuals may lament the chance to take a hands-on approach with students, it is quite a stretch to view SDL as an attempt at pedagogic rebellion or an antielitist statement. In fact, independent learning is an important academic convention that asserts that there should be room for personal selection of what is important and relevant to the individual. Aversion to SDL is then, in large part, associated with a fear of losing control and a reluctance to accept that the job of teachers is to supervise learning and not necessarily to construct it (Brookfield, 1993).

If one thing is clear, particularly for healthcare students and their teachers, it is that context must be used to dictate and determine the optimal learning style. For instance, the best learning methods for practice at a patient's bedside are not necessarily going to be the same as those for the emergency department or the pharmacy. Every situation comes with its own educational possibilities and consequences.

To summarize, TBL and PBL are teaching styles that emphasize the role of the student and encourage students to explore concepts and ideas in an independent manner. This is in contrast to more traditional teaching methods that prioritize didactic "I talk, you listen" approaches. In contrast, SDL is a type of autonomous teaching style that places the responsibility for progress and achievement with the student. It involves minimal (sometimes no) supervision, and the learners must monitor the course of their own intellectual investigations.

WORKSHOPS AND SEMINARS

The "workshop" is another common learning and teaching method. Normally, it involves small teams. They are carefully arranged to form a mixture of abilities and ensure that each member of the group feels confident making contributions. The seminar is a similar strategy, because it also involves small teams and encourages intergroup discussion. The difference is that seminars usually start with a brief presentation or lecture from the teacher. It introduces the key topics and learning objectives for the session. Workshops are slightly less structured than seminars, because the latter make use of both informal debate and unidirectional "teacher to student" exchanges.

Seminars and workshops are under the umbrella of "small group teaching" strategies. The teacher is required to put in a reasonable amount of preparation before the class and make sure that the right topics are covered. Normally, a facilitator role is essential to keep students on track and give them the best possible chance of success. The teacher or facilitator must also monitor group and individual progress. The advantage of working in small teams is that students can work together to explore possible solutions to intellectual and practical challenges. It enhances communication skills, heightens interpersonal awareness, and emphasizes the value of respect for peers (Davis, 2009). According to most educational experts, the value of small group learning is evident across almost all disciplines and academic fields. Students tend to retain information more easily if they are allowed to discuss it out loud with others (Allen et al., 2013; Baird & Munir, 2015; Davis, 2009; Galvao et al., 2014).

Researchers such as Choi (2004), Arthur (2001), and Rideout et al. (2002) discovered that seminar-based strategies can improve knowledge and enhance general perspectives on the value of education. Ultimately, students seem to be very happy with the teaching style. This statement is supported by Morales-Mann and Kaitell (2001) and White, Amos, and Kouzekanani (1999), who argue that seminars boost learning independence, critical thinking skills, communications skills, and overall achievement.

One of the possible solutions is a move toward seminar-based strategies. Healthcare teachers and clinicians are particularly fond of this approach because it combines direct instruction with autonomous, independent discussion (Gunn, 2007). In fact, seminars and workshops are now a common feature in universities across the world. It is widely agreed that seminars support active learning via assisted contributions from students, both as individuals and as part of teams (Fry, Ketteridge, & Marshall, 2009). They produce a more comprehensive awareness of the consequences of key theories and the practical applications of core concepts. According to Forbes, Duke, and Prosser (2001), the seminar strategy is a good way to improve the capacity to assimilate ideas and their real-world uses. In addition, they let students explore alternative opinions, help them to communicate more effectively, increase their overall level of interest, and improve their handling of abstract concepts (Brookfield & Preskill, 2005).

It should be noted that, even though the depth and scope of modern education continue to expand, the core strategies used to teach students have remained mostly constant and unaltered (Kavanagh & Drennan, 2008). Nevertheless, the rebellion against unidirectional learning styles is becoming more prominent (Hrepic, Zollman, & Sanjay Rebello, 2007). There is a growing feeling, particularly among healthcare mentors, that lecture formats do not encourage the development of certain key skills.

CONCLUSION

This chapter has discussed the most common teaching and learning strategies in pharmacy education. There are countless theories and ideas designed to explain how human beings acquire knowledge. According to academic experts, combining compatible teaching and learning methods is the right way to increase student contributions and encourage better performance.

It is important to understand that there is no optimal learning or teaching style because it all depends on the needs of the student and their environment. Nevertheless, this chapter has outlined some of the most common approaches and explained why they are suitable for pharmacy education.

In pharmacy education, students are required to gain an understanding of the methods that are being used to teach them. It is important for them to become comfortable and confident with the various learning styles. It is a complex process, but it plays a vital role in preparing trainee teachers for their future positions.

If one thing is clear, particularly for healthcare students and their teachers, it is that context must be used to dictate and determine the optimal learning style. Every situation comes with its own educational possibilities and consequences.

REFERENCES

Al-Meman, A., Al-Worafi, Y. M., & Saleh, M. (2014). Team based learning (TBL) as a new learning strategy in pharmacy college, Saudi Arabia: Student perceptions. *Universal Journal of Pharmacy*, *3*, 57–65.

Allen, R. E., Copeland, J., Franks, A. S., Karimi, R., McCollum, M., Riese, D. J., et al. (2013). Team-based learning in US colleges and schools of pharmacy. *American Journal of Pharmaceutical Education*, *77*(6), 115. https://doi.org/10.5688/ajpe776115.

Alrebish, S. A., Jolly, B. C., & Molloy, E. K. (2017). Accreditation of medical schools in Saudi Arabia: a qualitative study. *Medical Teacher*, *39*(Suppl. 1), S1–S7. https://doi.org/10.1080/0142159X.2016.1254746.

Armstrong, E. G. (1997). A hybrid model of problem based learning. In D. Boud & G. Feletti (Eds.), *The challenge of problem-based learning* (2nd ed., pp. 137–150). London: Kogan Page.

Arthur, D. (2001). The effects of the problem-based alcohol early-intervention education package on the knowledge and attitudes of students of nursing. *Journal of Nursing Education*, *40*(2), 63–72.

Astin, A. W. (2012). *Assessment for excellence: The philosophy and practice of assessment and evaluation in higher education*. Lanham, Maryland: Rowman & Littlefield Publishers.

Baird, K., & Munir, R. (2015). The effectiveness of workshop (cooperative learning) based seminars. *Asian Review of Accounting*, *23*(3), 293–312. https://doi.org/10.1108/ara-03-2014-0038.

Baker, J. D., Cooke, J. E., Conroy, J. M., Bromley, H. R., Hollon, M. F., & Alpert, C. C. (1988). Beyond career choice: the role of learning style analysis in residency training. *Medical Education*, *22*(6), 527–532. https://doi.org/10.1111/j.1365-2923.1988.tb00798.x.

Baker, J. D., & Marks, W. E. (1981). Learning style analysis in anesthesiology education. *Anesthesiology Review*, *8*(7), 31–34.

Bleske, B. E., Remington, T. L., Wells, T. D., Klein, K. C., Guthrie, S. K., Tingen, J. M., et al. (2016). A randomized crossover comparison of team-based learning and lecture format on learning outcomes. *American Journal of Pharmaceutical Education*, *80*(7), 120. https://doi.org/10.5688/ajpe807120.

Bokey, L., Chapuis, P. H., & Dent, O. F. (2014). Problem-based learning in medical education: One of many learning paradigms. *The Medical Journal of Australia*, *201*(3), 134–136. https://doi.org/10.5694/mja13.00060.

Boud, D., & Feletti, G. (1997). *The challenge of problem-based learning*. London: Routledge.

Brookfield, S. (1993). Self-directed learning, political clarity, and the critical practice of adult education. *Adult Education Quarterly*, *43*(4), 227–242. https://doi.org/10.1177/0741713693043004002.

Brookfield, S. D., & Preskill, S. (2005). *Discussion as a way of teaching*. San Francisco, CA: Jossey-Bass.

Candy, P. C. (1991). *Self-direction for lifelong learning: A comprehensive guide to theory and practice*. San Francisco, CA: Jossey-Bass.

Cassidy, S. (2004). Learning styles: an overview of theories, models, and measures. *Educational Psychology*, *24*(4), 419–444. https://doi.org/10.1080/0144341042000228834.

Cavanagh, S. J., & Coffin, D. A. (1994). Matching instructional preference and teaching styles: a review of the literature. *Nurse Education Today*, *14*(2), 106–110. https://doi.org/10.1016/0260-6917(94)90112-0.

Chan, L. C. (2008). The role of a PBL tutor: A personal perspective. *The Kaohsiung Journal of Medical Sciences*, *24*(Suppl. 3), S34–S38. https://doi.org/10.1016/S1607-551X(08)70092-5.

Cheng, J. W. M., Alafris, A., Kirschenbaum, H. L., Kalis, M. M., & Brown, M. E. (2003). Problem-based learning versus traditional lecturing in pharmacy students' short-term examination performance. *Pharmacy Education*, *3*(2), 117–125. https://doi.org/10.1080/1560221031000151282.

Choi, H. (2004). The effects of PBL (problem-based learning) on the metacognition, critical thinking, and problem solving process of nursing students. *Journal of Korean Academy of Nursing*, *34*(5), 712–721. https://doi.org/10.4040/jkan.2004.34.5.712.

Cisneros, R. M., Salisbury-Glennon, J. D., & Anderson-Harper, H. M. (2002). Status of problem-based learning research in pharmacy education: a call for future research. *American Journal of Pharmaceutical Education*, *66*(1), 19–26.

Davis, B. G. (2009). *Tools for teaching*. Hoboken, NJ: John Wiley & Sons.

Dunn, R. S., & Griggs, S. A. (2000). *Practical approaches to using learning styles in higher education*. Connecticut: Bergin & Garvey.

Felicia, P. (2011). *Handbook of research on improving learning and motivation through educational games: Multidisciplinary approaches*. Huddersfield: IGI Global.

Flannery, J., & Abraham, I. (1993). Psychometric properties of a cognitive functioning scale for patients with traumatic brain injury. *Western Journal of Nursing Research*, *15*(4), 465–482. https://doi.org/10.1177/019394599301500406.

Forbes, H., Duke, M., & Prosser, M. (2001). Students' perceptions of learning outcomes from group-based, problem-based teaching and learning activities. *Advances in Health Sciences Education*, *6*(3), 205–217. https://doi.org/10.1023/a:1012610824885.

Frame, T. R., Cailor, S. M., Gryka, R. J., Chen, A. M., Kiersma, M. E., & Sheppard, L. (2015). Student perceptions of team-based learning vs traditional lecture-based learning. *American Journal of Pharmaceutical Education*, *79*(4), 51. https://doi.org/10.5688/ajpe79451.

Frame, T. R., Gryka, R., Kiersma, M. E., Todt, A. L., Cailor, S. M., & Chen, A. M. H. (2016). Student perceptions of and confidence in self-care course concepts using team-based learning. *American Journal of Pharmaceutical Education*, *80*(3), 46. https://doi.org/10.5688/ajpe80346.

Franklin, A. S., Markowsky, S., De Leo, J., Normann, S., & Black, E. (2016). Using team-based learning to teach a hybrid pharmacokinetics course online and in class. *American Journal of Pharmaceutical Education*, *80*(10), 171.

Fry, H., Ketteridge, S., & Marshall, S. (2009). *A handbook for teaching and learning in higher education*. Oxon: Routledge.

Gallegos, P. J., & Peeters, J. M. (2011). A measure of teamwork perceptions for team-based learning. *Currents in Pharmacy Teaching and Learning*, *3*(1), 30–35. https://doi.org/10.1016/j.cptl.2010.10.004.

Gallimore, C., George, A. K., & Brown, M. C. (2008). Pharmacy students' preferences for various types of simulated patients. *American Journal of Pharmaceutical Education*, *72*(1), 04.

Galvao, T. F., Silva, M. T., Neiva, C. S., Ribeiro, L. M., & Pereira, M. G. (2014). Problem-based learning in pharmaceutical education: a systematic review and meta-analysis. *The Scientific World Journal*, *2014*. https://doi.org/10.1155/2014/578382.

Grabenstein, J. D. (2016). Trends in the numbers of US colleges of pharmacy and their graduates, 1900 to 2014. *American Journal of Pharmaceutical Education*, *80*(2), 25.

Grasha, A. (1981). In *Learning style: The journey from Greenwich Observatory (1796) to Dalhousie University (1981). Paper presented at the Dalhousie conference on learning style in continuing medical education*. Nova Scotia: Halifax.

Gunn, V. (2007). *Approaches to small group learning and teaching*. Glasgow: University of Glasgow Learning and Teaching Centre.

Hannafin, M. J., & Hannafin, K. M. (2010). Cognition and student-centered, web-based learning: Issues and implications for research and theory. In J. M. Spector, D. Ifenthaler, P. Isaias, Kinshuk, & D. Sampson (Eds.), *Learning and instruction in the digital age* (pp. 11–23). Boston, MA: Springer.

Haworth, I. S., Eriksen, S. P., Chmait, S. H., & Matsuda, L. S. (1998). A problem based learning, case study approach to pharmaceutics: faculty and student perspectives. *American Journal of Pharmaceutical Education, 62*(4), 398.

Highfield, M. E. (1988). Learning styles. *Nurse Educator, 13*(6), 30–32.

Hincapie, A. L., Cutler, T. W., & Fingado, A. R. (2016). Incorporating health information technology and pharmacy informatics in a pharmacy professional didactic curriculum-with a team-based learning approach. *American Journal of Pharmaceutical Education, 80*(6), 107.

Hofmann, B. (2009). Why simulation can be efficient: on the preconditions of efficient learning in complex technology based practices. *BMC Medical Education, 9*, 48. https://doi.org/10.1186/1472-6920-9-48.

Hrepic, Z., Zollman, D. A., & Sanjay Rebello, N. (2007). Comparing students' and experts' understanding of the content of a lecture. *Journal of Science Education and Technology, 16*(3), 213–224. https://doi.org/10.1007/s10956-007-9048-4.

Johnson, E. (2013). *The student centered classroom. Social studies and history: Vol. 1*. London: Routledge.

Jones, L. (2007). *The student-centered classroom.* Cambridge: Cambridge University Press.

Jones, F., Passos-Neto, C. E., & Braghiroli, O. F. M. (2015). Simulation in medical education: Brief history and methodology. *Principles and Practice of Clinical Research, 1*(2), 56–63.

Kasworm, C. (2011). New perspectives on post-formal cognitive development and self-directed learning. *International Journal of Self-Directed Learning, 8*(1), 18–28.

Kaufman, D. M., & Mann, K. V. (1996). Comparing students' attitudes in problem-based and conventional curricula. *Academic Medicine, 71*(10), 1096–1099.

Kavanagh, M. H., & Drennan, L. (2008). What skills and attributes does an accounting graduate need? Evidence from student perceptions and employer expectations. *Accounting & Finance, 48*(2), 279–300. https://doi.org/10.1111/j.1467-629X.2007.00245.x.

Knowles, M. S. (1975). *Self-directed learning: A guide for learners and teachers.* New York, NY: Association Press.

Knowles, M. S. (1984). Introduction: The art and science of helping adults learn. In M. S. Knowles (Ed.), *Andragogy in action: Applying modern principles of adult learning* (pp. 1–21). San Francisco, CA: Jossey-Bass.

Kosower, E., & Berman, N. (1996). Comparison of pediatric resident and faculty learning styles: Implications for medical education. *American Journal of the Medical Sciences, 312*(5), 214–218. https://doi.org/10.1016/S0002-9629(15)41818-X.

Kremers, E., & Sonnedecker, G. (1986). *Kremers and Urdang's history of pharmacy.* Madison, WI: American Institute of the History of Pharmacy.

Kunkler, K. (2006). The role of medical simulation: an overview. *The International Journal of Medical Robotics and Computer Assisted Surgery, 2*(3), 203–210. https://doi.org/10.1002/rcs.101.

Kurtz, S. M., Silverman, J., & Draper, J. (1998). *Teaching and learning communication skills in medicine.* Oxford: Radcliffe Medical Press.

Parmelee, D., Michaelsen, L. K., Cook, S., & Hudes, P. D. (2012). Team-based learning: A practical guide: AMEE guide no. 65. *Medical Teacher, 34*(5), e275–287. https://doi.org/10.3109/0142159x.2012.651179.

Love, D. W., & Shumway, J. M. (1983). Patient-oriented problem-solving instruction in pharmacotherapeutics. *American Journal of Pharmaceutical Education, 47*(3), 228–231.

Michaelsen, L. K. (1992). Team learning: A comprehensive approach for harnessing the power of small groups in higher education. In D. H. Wulff & J. D. Nyquist (Eds.), *Vol. 11. To improve the academy: Resources for faculty, instructional, and organizational development* (pp. 107–122). Stillwater, OK: The Professional and Organizational Development Network in Higher Education. New Forums Press.

Michaelsen, L. K., & Sweet, M. (2008). The essential elements of team-based learning. *New Directions for Teaching and Learning, 2008*(116), 7–27. https://doi.org/10.1002/tl.330.

Michaelsen, L. K., Watson, W. E., Cragin, J. P., & Fink, L. D. (1982). Team-based learning: A potential solution to the problems of large classes. *Exchange: The Organizational Behavior Teaching Journal, 7*(1), 18–33.

Morales-Mann, E. T., & Kaitell, C. A. (2001). Problem-based learning in a new Canadian curriculum. *Journal of Advanced Nursing*, *33*(1), 13–19. https://doi.org/10.1046/j.1365-2648.2001.01633.x.

Nation, L. M., Tweddell, S., & Rutter, P. (2016). The applicability of a validated team-based learning student assessment instrument to assess United Kingdom pharmacy students' attitude toward team-based learning. *Journal of Educational Evaluation for Health Professions*, *13*, 30. https://doi.org/10.3352/jeehp.2016.13.30.

Newble, D. I., & Entwistle, N. J. (1986). Learning styles and approaches: implications for medical education. *Medical Education*, *20*(3), 162–175. https://doi.org/10.1111/j.1365-2923.1986.tb01163.x.

Novak, S., Shah, S., Wilson, J. P., Lawson, K. A., & Salzman, R. D. (2006). Pharmacy students' learning styles before and after a problem-based learning experience. *American Journal of Pharmaceutical Education*, *70*(4), 74. https://doi.org/10.5688/aj700474.

Parmelee, D. X., & Michaelsen, L. K. (2010). Twelve tips for doing effective team-based learning (TBL). *Medical Education*, *32*(2), 118–122. https://doi.org/10.3109/01421590903548562.

Partridge, R. (1983). Learning styles: a review of selected models. *Journal of Nursing Education*, *22*(6), 243–248.

Rezler, A. G., & Rezmovic, V. (1981). The learning preference inventory. *Journal of Allied Health*, *10*(1), 28–34.

Rideout, E., England-Oxford, V., Brown, B., Fothergill-Bourbonnais, F., Ingram, C., Benson, G., et al. (2002). A comparison of problem-based and conventional curricula in nursing education. *Advances in Health Sciences Education*, *7*(1), 3–17. https://doi.org/10.1023/a:1014534712178.

Riding, R., & Cheema, I. (1991). Cognitive styles—an overview and integration. *Educational Psychology*, *11*(3–4), 193–215. https://doi.org/10.1080/0144341910110301.

Schatteman, A., Carette, E., Couder, J., & Eisendrath, H. (1997). Understanding the effects of a process-orientated instruction in the first year of university by investigating learning style characteristics. *Educational Psychology*, *17*(1–2), 111–125. https://doi.org/10.1080/0144341970170108.

Schmeck, R. R. (2013). *Learning strategies and learning styles.* New York, NY: Springer Science & Business Media.

Shaw, S., Lacey, J., Leighton, B., & Warner, B. (2006). How problem-based learning supports continuing professional development. *The Pharmaceutical Journal*, *277*(7415), 254.

Sibley, J., & Ostafichuk, P. (2015). *Getting started with team-based learning.* Sterling, Virginia, LLC: Stylus Publishing.

Smithson, J., Bellingan, M., Glass, B., & Mills, J. (2015). Standardized patients in pharmacy education: an integrative literature review. *Currents in Pharmacy Teaching and Learning*, *7*(6), 851–863. https://doi.org/10.1016/j.cptl.2015.08.002.

Tamblyn, R. M., & Barrows, H. S. (1980). *Problem-based learning: An approach to medical education.* New York, NY: Springer Publishing Company.

Tavangar, H. (2014). *The out of Eden walk: An experiential learning journey from the virtual to the real.* Retrieved 16 March 2016, from https://www.edutopia.org/blog/out-of-eden-experiential-learning-homa-tavangar.

Titmus, C. J. (Ed.), (2014). *Lifelong education for adults: An international handbook.* Leeds, UK: Elsevier.

Vatanpour, H. (2012). To what extent would PBL be best incorporated into a pharmacy curriculum? *Iranian Journal of Pharmaceutical Research*, *11*(4), 999–1000.

Walsh, A. (2005). *The tutor in problem-based learning: A novice's guide.* Hamilton: McMaster University.

White, M. J., Amos, E., & Kouzekanani, K. (1999). Problem-based learning: an outcomes study. *Nurse Educator*, *24*(2), 33–36. https://doi.org/10.1097/00006223-199903000-00011.

Wood, D. F. (2003). ABC of learning and teaching in medicine: problem based learning. *British Medical Journal*, *326*(7384), 328–330. https://doi.org/10.1136/bmj.326.7384.328.

Yamaki, K., Ueda, M., Ueda, K., Emoto, N., Mizutani, N., Ikeda, K., et al. (2016). Interdisciplinary subject "Yakugaku Nyumon" for first-year students constructed with lectures and problem-based learning. *Journal of the Pharmaceutical Society of Japan*, *136*(7), 1051–1064. https://doi.org/10.1248/yakushi.15-00255.

Young, T., Rohwer, A., Volmink, J., & Clarke, M. (2014). What are the effects of teaching evidence-based health care (EBHC)? Overview of systematic reviews. *PLoS ONE*, *9*(1):e86706 https://doi.org/10.1371/journal.pone.0086706.

CHAPTER

ASSESSMENT METHODS AND TOOLS FOR PHARMACY EDUCATION

11

Abubakr A. Alfadl

Unaizah College of Pharmacy, Qassim University, Qassim, Saudi Arabia

OVERVIEW

INTRODUCTION

As an approach to this chapter, and before providing an overview, it is necessary to provide an unambiguous definition of assessment. Unfortunately, the word "assessment" has taken on a variety of meanings within higher education. On some occasions, it is used to refer to the process of grading student course assignments. On other occasions, when an institution seeks external accreditation, assessment refers to standardized testing imposed to demonstrate the degree of compliance. On many occasions, assessment refers to any activity designed to collect information on the success of a curriculum, program, or course. Maybe that is why most people have a simple understanding of assessment as a collection of data for measuring student learning that gives them a grade at the end of a course or program. However, whatever the disagreement upon the exact meaning, there is a general agreement that assessment is a very important component of the curriculum. It is even mentioned in the literature that assessment is not just a method of grading, but moreover it significantly influences the learning process (Editorial, 1976). Some researchers have gone further to claim that the most profound impact on what the students eventually learn is due to the evaluation system rather than the educational objectives or curriculum or teaching techniques (Lorin & David, 2001; Miller, 1973). Hence, defining the term "assessment" is a crucial start of this chapter.

The most profound impact on what the students eventually learn is due to the evaluation system rather than the educational objectives or curriculum or teaching techniques.

A number of definitions of assessment could be retrieved through reviewing the scientific literature on medical education. It is defined by some researchers as the continuous collection of information regarding student learning activities (Walvoord, 2010). University of Northern Iowa (2006) anticipates assessment in higher education as a process of five steps, and consequently defines it as follows:

Pharmacy Education in the Twenty First Century and Beyond. https://doi.org/10.1016/B978-0-12-811909-9.00011-3

"Assessment of student learning is a participatory, iterative process that:

- Provides data/information you need on your students' learning
- Engages you and others in analyzing and using this data/information to confirm and improve teaching and learning
- Produces evidence that students are learning the outcomes you intended
- Guides you in making educational and institutional improvements
- Evaluates whether changes made improve/impact student learning, and documents the learning and your efforts."

It is noticed in this definition that the term "evaluation" is used as part of the assessment process. Other researchers differentiate between the two terms as follows:

"Assessment" is used to refer to the process of gathering, interpreting, and using evidence to make judgments about students' achievement in education. The term "evaluation" is reserved for this process of using evidence in relation to programs, procedures, materials, or systems (Harlen, 2007).

Regardless of the differences in the definition, the process of assessment always starts with identification of learning objectives to specify where the institution intends to go. This is followed by the collection and analysis of data as a prerequisite for identifying weaknesses and gaps and suggestion and implementation of necessary changes and improvements. The last step is to obtain feedback about the changes and start again with the first step to close the circle, which is considered essential for continuous development in higher education (Buzzetto-More & Alade, 2006). Another assessment process, which is specific for clinical competence, was proposed in the form of a hierarchical model with the cognition assessment placed at the bottom of the model and behavior in practice at the apex (Miller, 1990). Different assessment tools were assigned for the different levels of the hierarchy as appropriate. As one of the main objectives of this chapter is to help the reader identify the most appropriate assessment method to use for collection of assessment data, our focus will be mainly on these tools and which tool is better for any specific assessment situation.

THE ROLE OF ASSESSMENT IN HIGHER EDUCATION

The central role of assessment in higher education is gathering of information with the purpose of improvement of institutional practice. However, although it looks simple, the design of efficient assessment to achieve full educational benefits remains challenging. This is because, as noticed by the Centre for the Study of Higher Education (CSHE), the two main stakeholders, i.e., students and teaching staff, are thinking about the assessment process in opposite ways.

That is, while the teaching staff considers assessment after other curriculum decisions are made, students focus most on getting marks and consequently work "backwards" through the curriculum through focusing first on how they will be assessed and then what is required to demonstrate what they have learned (CSHE, 2002).

Teaching staff considers assessment after other curriculum decisions being made.

Students work "backwards" through the curriculum, through focusing first on how they will be assessed and then what is required to demonstrate what they have learned.

Regardless of these challenges, teaching staff can design efficient assessment that plays several important roles, such as:

- Provision of information about knowledge and skills that students have when they enter a program, which facilitates better designing of learning objectives students should master when they finish the program.
- Provision of rich, reliable data about faculty members, the curriculum, teaching methods, and instructional techniques, which facilitates making better decisions about change and improvements, and also facilitates identification of chances for future instructional development.
- Provision of evidence about success and progression of students' learning, which increases the satisfaction and motivation of teaching staff.

STRATEGIES OF ASSESSMENT

There are three forms of assessment: summative, formative, and diagnostic, which are differentiated according to the purpose of use (Crisp, 2009).

Summative assessment is used as a part of the grading process to summarize the learning progress of students at a particular time. It is thus a periodic evaluation of students. In addition to its importance for the grading process, the information collected in summative assessment can also be used for diagnostic purposes. Also, it has proved useful in detecting possible shortcomings of courses and evaluating the configuration of the goals and objectives of a curriculum or a program. However, in spite of the benefits, the main weakness of summative assessment is that it can offer information only after a period of time of teaching, so corrective action cannot be taken during the learning process. This goal is only possible to be achieved using formative assessment (Garrison & Ehringhaus, 2007).

Summative Assessment:

Used to summarize the learning progress of students at a particular time.
A periodical evaluation of students.
Can be used for diagnostic purposes.
Useful in detecting possible shortcomings of courses and evaluating the configuration of the goals and objectives of a curriculum or a program.
The main weakness is that corrective action cannot be taken during the learning process.

Formative Assessment:

Used to offer feedback for both teachers and learners to help the former decide how teaching should be adjusted and improved, and to help the latter learn better.

Diagnostic Assessment:

Used to give information about students' prior knowledge.
Helps in designing the most suitable educational program for each student.

Formative assessment is used to offer feedback for both teachers and learners, to help the former decide how teaching should be adjusted and improved and to help the latter learn better. Hence, using formative assessment enables teachers to evaluate and adjust their teaching methods and techniques during the teaching period for positive influence on students and better achievement of teaching outcomes; it also enables students to revise and adjust their learning to achieve better results at the end (Boston, 2002).

Diagnostic assessment is used to give information about students' prior knowledge. This information about strengths and weaknesses of each student could help in designing a more suitable educational program for each student. Therefore, this type of assessment saves time and money that could otherwise be wasted in teaching a student an unsuitable program (Miller, Imrie, & Cox, 1998).

In summary, any specific assessment strategy should be implemented with the purpose of determining whether or not intended outcomes are being achieved and whether students have acquired the knowledge, skills, and competencies of the program, as well as how the program could be improved.

ASSESSMENT METHODS AND TOOLS

It is very difficult for one assessment measure to satisfy the need for assessment within a pharmacy curriculum. Therefore, use of a variety of assessment measures is inevitable. Use of those different measures should reflect the diversity of the learning outcome in the pharmacy curriculum. That is, use of a measure should align with the designed learning outcome of the curriculum, taking into consideration the taxonomy level of the verbs used in preparing the outcomes. When it is possible, a single assessment method is used to measure simple foundational knowledge, but sometimes more than one method needs to be used to assess high-order outcomes.

This section is not intended to be exhaustive in covering all assessment methods. Only some common assessment tools are described here, along with their construction guidelines.

WRITTEN TESTS

When thinking about written tests, many question formats are available, each with its own advantages and disadvantages. As mentioned earlier, it is difficult for one type of question to achieve the purpose of measuring all specified outcomes of a topic. Therefore, multiple formats are used to counteract the anticipated bias associated with the use of a single format.

Multiple choice questions

Multiple choice questions (MCQs) were defined by Vinu and Kumar (2015) as a 3-tuple (S, K, D), where S (stem) is a statement that introduces the problem, K (keys) is a nonempty set of correct solutions to S, and D (distractors) is a nonempty set of incorrect solutions to S. The MCQ is one of the most commonly used type of questions. It is used extensively in almost all kinds of examinations. Most MCQs are context-free, involving a simple thought process, hence testing exclusively factual knowledge (Schuwirth, Verheggen, Van der Vleuten, Boshuizen, & Dinant, 2001). However, although the main usage of MCQs in medical education is the assessment of knowledge in undergraduate and postgraduate students (Hamdorf & Hall, 2001; Liyanage, Ariyaratne, Dankanda, & Deen, 2009), well-constructed MCQs can be used to test problem-solving skills as well. This can be achieved by including clinical or laboratory scenarios in the question. In addition to conveying authenticity and validity, this strategy can also facilitate focusing on important information. The thought process involved is not as simple as when using a context-free question, but is rather complex, with students evaluating different pieces of information against each other before a decision can be made (Schuwirth et al., 2001).

Construction guidelines

Construction of MCQs is relatively easy, in addition to these questions having high reliability per hour of testing, since they can be used to sample a broad content domain. Construction requires preparation of an opening question or stem and a list of options from which the learner must recognize and choose the most correct answer. Usually the list of options includes two to five probable, yet incorrect, options termed distractors. In medical education, many times the stem is situated within a clinical scenario or vignette. Guidelines for preparation of multiple choice questions are as follows (Case & Swanson, 1998):

Characteristics of stem

- Prepare a short problem, followed by a clear lead-in.
- Use simple language.
- Avoid strange and complex terms.
- It is more appropriate to use direct questions rather than incomplete statements.
- Use concise words and avoid unnecessary or irrelevant information.
- Ensure that the stem poses a clear question, with the possibility of arriving at an answer without looking at the options.
- Ensure that the number of words per item (WPI) in an item vignette or scenario does not exceed 100 WPI.
- It is more appropriate for questions about definitions to include the term in the stem, not the options.
- Hints that point out the correct option should be avoided.
- Usage of abbreviations is discouraged, but if needed should be followed by the full term.

Characteristics of the lead-in

- It is more appropriate to be the last sentence in the stem.

Characteristics of options (possible answers)

- Ensure that all options are plausible to the stem.
- Prepare the options in a similar format (e.g., all are sentences, all are phrases, etc.).
- Use generic names of drugs.
- Ensure that all options are homogeneous (i.e., all are drugs, all are adverse effects, all are dose regimens, etc.)
- Enumerate the options using capital letters (A, B, C, D, E) instead of lower-case letters (a, b, c, d, e).
- Do not exceed 35–40 words per item in the question line and options together.
- Avoid too long, tricky, or complicated options that need time for reading and understanding.
- Make sure that all choices are logically compatible and grammatically consistent with the stem.
- Try to make the length of all options approximately the same.
- Avoid options that include "none of the above" or "all of the above."
- List the options in logical (arrange numbers in ascending or descending form) or alphabetical order.

- Avoid presenting a key word or phrase only in the stem and the correct option, or giving more information and more details in the correct option.
- Avoid using absolute terms such as "always," "never," and "all," or vague terms such as "seldom," "frequently," etc.

Characteristics of distractors

- Prepare distractors that are homogeneous with each other and with the correct answer.
- The distractor should be grammatically comparable, logically compatible, and should have relatively the same length as the correct answer.
- Use plausible distractors with none standing out as being obviously incorrect.

Extended matching items

Extended matching items (EMIs) are one of the approaches to context-rich questions (EMQs or EMIs) (Case & Swanson, 1993). They are characterized by having a set of short clinical vignettes or scenarios and a list of options that cover specific aspects (e.g., treatments, adverse drug reactions, etc.). The number of options used can range from 5 to 26, although Swanson, Holtzman, and Allbee (2008) mentioned 8 options as a suitable number that makes more efficient use of testing time. Out of the options given, some may match more than one vignette, while others may not be appropriate to all.

Construction guidelines

Construction of EMIs includes four components: theme, options list, lead-in statement, and at least two item stems. Case and Swanson (1998) proposed the following characteristics for the components of EMIs:

Characteristics of the theme

- The question set should have a homogeneous, coherent theme (e.g., treatment therapies, adverse drug reactions, dose regimens, etc.)

Characteristics of the options

Options are a list of about eight possible answers. Students should select one of these options as the answer for the question and write it on the answer sheet.

- There should be grammatical comparability and logical compatibility with the stem/lead-in.
- Language should be homogeneous through all options.
- No use of trade names of drugs.
- Length of all options should be approximately the same.
- Options should not be too long or complicated.
- Options should be listed in logical or alphabetical order.
- All options should be mutually exclusive.
- All options should be plausible.
- There should be only one best answer for each item to be matched.
- Each set should consist of six or more options.

Characteristics of the lead-in

Lead-ins outline the scenario and ask the question to be matched with the options. There should be clear instructions specifying whether an option can be used more than once.

- Lead-in should clearly state the basis for matching the stems with the options.

Characteristics of the stems

Stems are clinical problems, or vignettes. There may be more than one clinical problem or vignette for each theme.

- Stems should match with a single theme.
- Stems should focus on important concepts and assess knowledge.
- Unnecessary information should not be included.
- Unnecessary complication and misleading stems are discouraged.
- There should be more options than stems.
- Stems included within one set should be of similar construction.
- Should be answerable without a need for the options.

True-false

In this type of question, a statement is made and students are asked to determine if it is true or false. This chapter does not elaborate on this type of question, as it is recommended to be avoided because the probability of guessing the correct answer in true or false questions is high.

Short answer questions

Short answer questions (SAQs) are open-ended questions that require students to create short answers to short questions sampled from a large part of the curriculum (Wakeford & Roberts, 1984). They carry greater objectivity and reliability and a more extended range of subject areas tested (Sabherwal, 1995). SAQs are commonly used in examinations to assess the basic knowledge and understanding of a topic before more in-depth assessment questions are asked on the topic. Unlike MCQs, SAQs require more time to answer, and consequently fewer questions can be asked in an hour of testing. This will limit the sampling and negatively affect the reliability of the test. In addition, marking of SAQs needs experts in the content of the question. Therefore, questions need to be written in clear, unambiguous language accompanied by a well-defined answer key to facilitate accurate marking (Schuwirth & van der Vleuten, 2005).

SAQs are commonly used to assess the basic knowledge and understanding of a topic before more in-depth assessment questions are asked.

Unlike MCQs, SAQs require more time to answer, consequently limited sampling and lower reliability.

Marking of SAQ needs experts in the content of the question.

SAQs should be accompanied by a well-defined answer key to facilitate accurate marking.

Double marking is encouraged in SAQs. However, for higher reliability of scoring, each marker correcting the same question for all candidates is preferred over having all questions for one group of candidates corrected by one marker and all questions for another group corrected by another marker (Schuwirth & Van Der Vleuten, 2004).

Construction guidelines

Construction of good SAQs requires forming a brief, highly directed question intended to obtain a reliable, constructed response from the student. Usually answers consist of a few words or short phrases. The model answer key is designed in a way presenting all possible correct answers.

Characteristics of the stem

- Test basic knowledge by designing the question for recalling specific names or facts.
- Insure that the question is focused enough to limit the number of possible correct answers to the least number of words, one if possible.
- Ensure that you are specific on how many constitute a correct answer (i.e., list three, or name any two, etc.).
- Formulate the question in a way that the intended answer becomes the only possible answer.
- Formulate the question in a way that requires one single word, number, or brief phrase answer.
- Ensure that the required answer is limited to a few words.
- If the question starts with a list, then the number to be listed should be limited to about six.
- Write the stem in your own words.
- Make sure that the stem is complete enough to ensure the clarity of the meaning.

Essay questions

Essay questions are defined by Stalnaker (1951, p. 495) as "A test item which requires a response composed by the examinee, usually in the form of one or more sentences, of a nature that no single response or pattern of responses can be listed as correct, and the accuracy and quality of which can be judged subjectively only by one skilled or informed in the subject."

Based on this definition, an essay question should meet the following criteria:

1. Students should compose rather than select their answer.
2. Answers allow different patterns, but must consist of more than one sentence.
3. Marking requires subjective judgment and therefore needs experts in the content of the question to judge the accuracy and quality of the answers.

Essays pose questions that require the synthesis and communication of content and often require critical thinking skills such as comparison, analysis, and judgment. Essay questions are the most appropriate method when students are required to organize, integrate, and express ideas. Unlike MCQs and SAQs, essay questions require more time to answer, and consequently fewer questions can be asked in an hour of testing. This will limit the sampling and negatively affect the reliability of the test. The only possible way to enhance the process of marking, and consequently improve reliability, is structuring, that is, to put the question in a specific format (but not overstructuring). However, the limited sampling and time-consuming scoring of the essay question is counterbalanced by the profound information obtained about student understanding.

Construction guidelines

- The question should make clear what is being measured and how the answer will be evaluated.
- The terminology used in the question should clarify and limit the task (e.g., "describe," rather than "discuss," and "in one sentence").
- Each question should be allowed sufficient time.
- The question should have clear criteria for marking (e.g., scoring key, model answers).

Modified essay questions

Modified essay questions (MEQs) were developed by Hodgkin and Knox (1975) for the examination of the Royal College of General Practitioners. These questions consist of a short clinical scenario followed by a series of questions with a structured format for scoring. Modified essay questions primarily assess the student's factual recall, but a well-written MEQ can go further in assessing, in addition to factual recall, the student's approach to solving a problem, reasoning skills, and understanding of concepts. MEQs have been adopted successfully to evaluate the five levels of cognitive processing (knowledge, comprehension, analysis, synthesis, and evaluation) (Bloom et al., 1956; Feletti, 1980; Feletti & Gillies, 1982; Feletti & Smith, 1986; Newble, Hoare, & Elmslie, 1981; Weinman, 1984).

Construction guidelines

Although MEQs are flexible, still they need careful construction and preparation of model answers, in addition to trained examiners to avoid interrater variability (Feletti & Smith, 1986; Feletti, 1980). Below are guidelines for construction:

- Base the MEQ on a factual case history presented in stages.
- Consult the course objectives to decide on the level and nature of the competencies to be assessed.
- The number of questions that require only factual information should be minimized.
- Cumulative error should be avoided.
- It is not required for the questions or cases to be of the same length.

OBJECTIVE STRUCTURED CLINICAL EXAMINATION

Objective structured clinical examinations (OSCEs) were developed by Harden, Stevenson, Downie, and Wilson (1975) as a tool to assess the clinical competence of medical students. This type of examination is based on several stations designed to assess a particular competency using predetermined guidelines. The OSCE is primarily used to assess basic clinical skills. Students are assessed as they rotate through the different "stations" on distinct focused activities that represent different aspects of clinical competence. At each station demonstration of specific skills can be observed and measured. OSCE stations can incorporate the assessment of interpretation, patient and nonpatient related skills, and technical skills like management problems and administrative skills. All students are exposed to the same stations, where they may encounter structured oral examination, a standardized patient, a high- or low-fidelity simulation, visual information, or a written task. Students are asked to respond through presenting a specific skill, simulating part of a patient encounter, or answering questions based on the presented material. Usefulness of OSCEs depends on many factors including the number of stations, the design or construction of stations, the allocation of time for the completion of each station, the time allocated for training the standardized patients, and the total cost (Gupta, Dewan, & Singh, 2010). Reliability of OSCEs is a function of sampling and therefore of the number of stations and competences tested (Tofade, Elsner, & Haines, 2013). A checklist or a combination of a checklist and a rating scale is used for scoring. However, results equivalent to those generated through checklists can be obtained using global ratings (Abate, Stamatakis, & Haggett, 2003; Kirkpatrick, 2009; Noble, O'Brien, Coombes, Shaw, & Nissen, 2011). Observers are used to score students. However, despite all this, till now no standards have been set as minimally accepted for passing OSCEs, and this was identified as a major problem in the assessment of OSCEs (Sturpe, 2010).

Construction guidelines

It is reported in the literature that when written examinations are complemented with OSCEs, this resulted in a more comprehensive assessment of problem-based learning (Salinitri, O'Connell, Garwood, Lehr, & Abdallah, 2012). In addition, incorporation and assessment of areas unique to the program's mission such as emergency preparedness and health policy can be done more effectively and efficiently through a well-designed OSCE, as compared to other testing methods. However, despite all these benefits of OSCEs, still only a few schools of pharmacy conduct OSCEs in an optimal manner, and most do not follow the best practices in OSCE construction and administration (Sturpe, 2010). Following are some guidelines for OSCE construction:

- The OSCE circuit is generally constructed of a number of stations clustered into a series of rooms and may include one or two rest stations.
- Depending on the situation, the number of stations may be as few as 8, to as many as more than 20.
- The number recommended for optimum reliability of measure of the performance is 14–18.
- Time allocated for completion of the OSCE station may range from 5 to 30 min depending on the complexity of the task.
- Time allowed between stations is about 2–5 min, which may be used to give further information explaining the next station.
- Students should be assessed using a standardized checklist or global rating scales, and in some cases through evaluation of their narrative responses.

PORTFOLIOS

Portfolios are a tremendously flexible, comprehensive educational means of collecting and accumulating evidence of achievement of competence over time; they can be tailored to suit multiple purposes, settings, and kinds of learners. Portfolios were defined in 1990 by the Northwest Evaluation Association as follows: "A portfolio is a purposeful collection of student work that exhibits the student's effort, progress, and achievement in one or more areas. The collection must include student participation in selecting contents, the criteria for selection, the criteria for judging merit, and evidence of student self-reflection" (Barrett, 2000). It is especially helpful when used as a longitudinal tool for the assessment of competence. Popularity of this assessment tool has increased with the increased interest in competency-based education.

Portfolios may consist of continuous quality-improvement projects, logbooks, rating scales, encounter cards, learning diaries, essays, multisource feedback instruments, etc. This makes the portfolio a real collection of assessment tools. It is mentioned in the literature that portfolios, besides offering evidence of learning, encourage students to integrate and assess evidence of their own learning (Epstein & Hundert, 2002). However, several points need to be cautiously considered when using portfolios, including the training of students and assessors, and the quality and quantity of evidence (i.e., what constitutes sufficient evidence). It may be these variabilities in how portfolios are structured and assessed that have led some researchers to judge their reliability as low (Al-Wardy, 2010), and others to go further and judge their educational effect in the undergraduate settings as limited (Buckley et al., 2009). In addition, some students are not accustomed to the use of portfolios and do not have enough time to become familiar with them and use them efficiently. Uses of portfolios are further weakened by the absence of both formal requirements of external assessment of the quality of the evidence and of the portfolios themselves (Wright, Loftus, Christou, Eggleton, & Norris, 2006). In spite of all this, student portfolios remain a useful qualitative method for assessing foundational knowledge, given they are conducted in a proper way.

When designing a portfolio for assessment, it is important to be clear not only on its purpose, but also on the role of the learner in collecting the material, the degree of reflection desired, the medium (e.g., paper or online), and on how expectations and standards will be set (Bryant & Timmins, 2002).

Implementation guidelines

Although most colleges and schools of pharmacy in advanced countries have a portfolio system in place, the proper way of conducting portfolios remains a problem in most of them, and consequently few are using portfolio assessment to fulfill accreditation requirements (Sundberg, 2002). Following are some general guidelines for effective implementation of portfolios (Bryant & Timmins, 2002):

- There should be effective training of teachers, administrators, and students on the portfolio approach to assessment.
- Students should have to learn to collect, select, and reflect on work that is central to the portfolio process (i.e., work that best shows what they have learned throughout the module or class).
- Sufficient time and effort should be allocated to deliver a meaningful portfolio assessment.
- Teachers must work as a team to plan for the implementation of portfolio assessment.
- Understanding and approval of the parents and the educational community is necessary for effective implementation of portfolio assessment.
- Teachers should play an active role as facilitators of the portfolio process.
- Teachers should facilitate the documentation of the learning process and achievements of the student, in addition to the analyses of the teaching and learning experiences to help students plan how to learn.
- There should be self-evaluation of learning as an essential part of the portfolio assessment.

ORAL TESTS

Oral tests can be described as a conversation between students and examiners, which can cover several general topics or can be a case or paper presentation. It is a setting in which examiners assess in one-on-one conversation whether students have acquired the learning outcomes of the course. It has the advantage of providing an examiner or panel of examiners an opportunity to ask a student a series of questions, with the ability to react to his responses while assessing him. Many faculties use oral tests in exceptional individual situations, not as a standard method of assessment. As oral examination is an unstructured approach to testing, it has low reliability in the sense that reproducibility of assessment is difficult, and also it is case or topic specific, which means it is difficult to generalize the result beyond the specific case applied (Finberg & Lloyd, 1983).

Construction guidelines

Challenges in constructing oral tests stem from the need to standardize the test so that students can be compared fairly, while at the same time allowing enough flexibility so that examiners can tailor the test to each student. However, in general, four things need to be considered while constructing oral tests, in order to achieve acceptable consistency in rating differences among tested students and attain the highest possible interjudge reliability coefficients, which indicates good reliability of oral tests (Le Mahieu, Gitomer, & Eresh, 1995):

- Examiners: examiners must be trained to keep differences in administration and scoring of oral tests to a minimum. However, as a human being each examiner will have unique perceptions and expectations as to what is satisfactory and what is unsatisfactory performance. Therefore, it is recommended to have several examiners providing independent assessment and thereafter make statistical corrections, which may help in eliminating the severity and bias variations between examiners. Also, it is necessary that all examiners use the same rating scale.
- Content: This can be a case, clinical scenario, problem, project, guided question, or any other stimuli in which the content is presented to students to demonstrate their knowledge and skills. It is recommended to prepare the content according to standard guidelines, in addition to using the same standardized content to test all students.
- Tasks or skills: There are a number of skills that can be tested using oral testing: e.g., technical skills, management, interpretation, or problem solving. Setting guidelines for task distribution among tested students is a necessary consideration.
- Administrative differences: These are times (day or night), locations at which students are tested, days of the week, or any other administrative factor. It is recommended that these factors should be controlled for better consistency.

SELECTING THE APPROPRIATE ASSESSMENT TOOL

DIRECT ASSESSMENT TOOLS

When selecting an assessment tool, the first thing needed to be considered is the curricular outcomes of the program, since usage of that assessment tool is intended to determine the progress of students towards those outcomes (Harden, Crosby, Davis, & Friedman, 1999). In fact, in addition to curricular outcomes, many other factors are important to consider, but the foremost is that the assessment tool should be valid and reliable. Validity means that tools should actually measure what is intended to be measured, while reliability means that scores are reproducible either across different populations of students, across repeated measurements of the same student, or across scorers (Schuwirth & van der Vleuten, 2011). However, it is not necessary for every assessment tool that can generate a valid and reliable measure to be appropriate for every situation. That means an assessment tool may be, for example, suitable for knowledge assessment, but not for skills, and consequently, as noted by some researchers, different assessment tools need to be chosen within a particular assessment plan (Epstein, 2007; Schuwirth & Van Der Vleuten, 2004) (Table 1).

INDIRECT ASSESSMENT TOOLS

Various factors need to be considered before selecting either a direct assessment tool (such as written exams, oral exams, OSCEs) or an indirect assessment tool (such as students' reflections on learning, surveys among stakeholder, or focus groups) to measure learning in a pharmacy program. One of the

Table 1 Guiding Criteria for Assessment Tool Selection

Assessment Tool	Assessment Ability	
	Good	**Limited**
1. Knowledge-Based Competencies		
MCQs	Knowledge and application of knowledge	Communication skills
	Diagnostic reasoning	Collaboration
		Ethical behavior
		Leadership
		Organizational skills
SAQs	Breadth and depth of factual knowledge	Behavior in clinical settings
	Clinical application of knowledge and diagnostic reasoning	Written and oral communication skills
	Problem-solving skills	Collaborative abilities
		Professionalism
Essay	Medical expertise	Performance in actual practice
	Organizational and writing skills	Practice behaviors
	Ability to synthesize information	Clinical skills and procedures
	Written communication	Collaborative skills
	Managerial knowledge base	
	Approaches to health advocacy	
	Scholarly knowledge base	
	Professional knowledge base	
Oral tests	Integration of facts	Breadth of knowledge
	Formation and prioritization of differential diagnoses	Procedural skills
	Development of management plans	Collaboration, teamwork and leadership
	Difficult decision-making	Actual performance in real situations
2. Procedural Skills Competencies		
OSCEs	History-taking skills	Complex ethical and professional behaviors
	Physical examination skills	Collaborative interactions
	Physician-patient communication skills	Teaching and research skills
	Diagnostic reasoning	A large spectrum of knowledge in different areas
	Patient management and treatment planning	
	Knowledge base within a specific context	

Continued

Table 1 Guiding Criteria for Assessment Tool Selection—cont'd

Assessment Tool	Assessment Ability	
	Good	Limited
Portfolio	Complex performance and integrative competencies Documentation of procedural activities Scholar competencies of lifelong learning Research and teaching Demonstrates evidence of collaboration and teamwork Performance in authentic situations Providing ongoing formative assessment	Situations in which all learners must demonstrate the same competency in a standardized way Situations where summative decisions are being taken and high reliability is required

important factors to consider is the view of accreditors, as they value direct assessment tools more than indirect because the first is a direct observation while the latter is just a reflection on learning (Schuwirth, Vleuten, & Donkers, 1996). However, although assessment tools that offer indirect measures alone may not be able to cover the whole measured trait, that does not mean they should not be used at all, as they can play a beneficial complementary role that may enhance the validity of additional data through providing additional support to the direct assessment tool (Schuwirth et al., 1996; Schuwirth & Van Der Vleuten, 2004). Therefore it can be concluded that for achieving the greatest benefit, an appropriate mix of both direct and indirect measurement tools can be used to assess a pharmacy program.

FACTORS GUIDING SELECTION FEASIBILITY

When considering the feasibility of using single or a blend of direct and indirect measurement tools, selection of the appropriate methods may depend on various factors, discussed in the following text.

Cost considerations

Regardless of the assessment tool validity or reliability, cost may become in many cases the deciding factor on whether or not to adopt a specific assessment tool by a college of pharmacy. Even if the assessment tool is financially affordable, cost concerns will exist in terms of whether the information provided by the assessment tool is worth the money it costs, and in the end a cost-benefit analysis may become necessary to decide whether or not to adopt a specific assessment tool.

Institutional culture

The ranking of assessment in the priority list of an institution is another important factor to consider before deciding on adoption of a specific assessment tool. Whether assessment has a top or bottom ranking in the institution culture can provide a good indication of the level of support you may expect from the dean of the college and other upper-level administration, and this consequently can determine the financial feasibility of an assessment plan. In addition, the willingness of the faculty member to become engaged in a specific assessment plan is an important factor, and of similar importance is the willingness of students. In other words, how receptive will students be to the assessment activity? It is reported by Sundre and Kitsantas (2004) that student motivation, or lack of motivation, is one of the biggest threats to assessment validity. Therefore, regardless of the assessment tool chosen, it is important to care about creating an environment that motivates students as well as staff to value and consequently actively participate in the assessment activities.

Curriculum considerations

The last but not least important factor in the selection of assessment tools is the curriculum itself: that is, whether the structure of the curriculum lends itself better to embedded assessment in the instructive or teaching classroom, in experimental or practical settings, or in an integrated block system not tied to courses. This structural consideration has an important role in selecting a specific assessment tool.

SELECTION OUTLINES

Appropriate selection of assessment tools to evaluate student learning is not an easy task and many points need to be considered. In addition, it is important to make sure while thinking about assessment tool selection that the learning outcomes to be measured form the principle that rules or drives assessment tool selection, and not the opposite. In other words, the assessment tool should not affect the design of the learning outcomes, but instead remain as a simple reflection of what is achieved from those outcomes. Unfortunately, although available assessment tool options are now far more numerous than in the past, this may have complicated tool selection even more, with a higher need for being critical while considering the previously discussed factors that affect appropriate assessment tool selection. That is to say, the cost, the available human resources, the culture of the institution, and the design of the curriculum all need to be considered and critically balanced before simply picking one or another assessment tool.

GENERAL CRITERIA OF ASSESSMENT TOOLS

During development and scoring of assessment tools some criteria need to be considered. Among these are educational impact (what are the effects of the assessment tool on teaching and learning?); validity (does it measure what it is supposed to be measuring?); reliability (does it consistently measure what it is supposed to be measuring?); acceptability (is it acceptable to learners, teachers, and other stakeholders?); and cost. However, the weight of these criteria is not always the same for a specific assessment tool, but rather is dependent on the purpose for which the tool was used. For example, if the purposes of assessment are certification or selection (summative purposes) of students, then more weight should be given to reliability; while if the purposes are diagnosis and improvement (formative purposes), more weight should be given to educational impact (Table 2).

Table 2 General Criteria of Assessment Tools

Tool	Development	Scoring	Administration	Face Validity	Standardization
MCQs	Time-consuming Difficult	Objective Simple Quick	Simple	Low	Most standardized
SAQs	Time-consuming Easier than MCQs	Time-consuming Creation of comprehensive answer key is difficult Well-designed questions can be scored objectively	Simple	Lower than performance-based assessment	Unstandardized
Essay Questions	Simple	Time-consuming Reliability is difficult	Simple	Low	Unstandardized
OSCE	Time-consuming		Complex	High	Standardizable
Portfolios	Time-consuming	Time-consuming		Validity and reliability depend on the instruments used to gather data	Difficult to standardize

ASSESSMENT AUTOMATION

Over the last decades the number of students has continued to increase, and consequently so have the workload and amount of time academic staff spend in assessing their students. Hence, movement towards automated assessment has increased as an approach to decrease time spent on students' assessment. Another reason for getting automated assessment more and more involved in student assessment is the increased induction of formative assessment in many academic institutions, as a beneficial assessment method for supporting students in their learning through quick feedback that helps continuous review and improvement of the learning procedure (Al-Smadi, Guetl, & Kappe, 2010; Gutl, 2008). For these reasons and others, usage of technology in student assessment has started to rise to the extent that some researchers have suggested automatic or semiautomatic assessment to be an integral part of educational institutions. However, since it is not feasible or practical for all types of curricula or courses to be assessed using technological tools (Harvey & Mogey, 1999), many things need to be considered before making a decision on the best ways to assess a particular outcome and deciding whether going for technology is the best way to do the assessment.

In spite of the rise in the usage of automated assessment, still it is confused with computer-assisted assessment. However, the distinct difference between the two is that while computer-assisted assessment is conducted using computers but not necessarily automatically, in the case of automated assessment it must be conducted electronically and automatically using a computer program or software system (Symeonidis, 2006). Due to this confusion, some researchers have tried to define automated assessment, describing it as "The identification, evaluation, assessment, documentation and feedback based on the new electronic information and communication technologies." Another definition was given by the Joint Information Systems Committee (2006), which described automated assessment as "The end-to-end electronic assessment processes where ICT (information and communication technology) is used for the presentation of assessment activity and the recording of responses. This includes the end-to-end assessment process from the perspective of learners, tutors, learning establishments, awarding bodies and regulators, and the general public."

RATIONALE OF ASSESSMENT AUTOMATION

Automization of assessment will neither automatically solve assessment challenges nor guarantee sound assessment practices. This is because the technology used in automated assessment will not serve as more than a tool that needs proper evaluation and selection, in addition to wise implementation, to result in a meaningful savings in both time and resources. Therefore there is heavy debate on the rationality of purchasing such expensive technology. AL-Smadi and Gutl (2008) presented a practical and educational rationale behind using this technology. From a practical point of view, with the increasing numbers of students joining higher education institutions each year and the approximately constant number of academic staff in those institutions, keeping the practice of paper-based assessment will mean teachers must spend most of their time busy with assessing their students instead of focusing on educational development and active support of student learning. Therefore the use of technology in assessment will help in enrolling greater numbers of students, using the same number of teaching staff without compormising the quality of academic support given to the students (AL-Smadi & Gutl, 2008).

The educational rationale of automated assessment has become more and more evident with the increased adoption of formative assessment in higher education to enhance continuous improvement of the learning process. Formative assessment warrants the need for quick feedback, to improve both teaching and learning, and consequently the need for automization and technology involvement. AL-Smadi and Gutl (2008) claimed that it is essential for good support of formative assessment to use automated assessment.

Other rationales mentioned by AL-Smadi and Gutl (2008) for using technology in assessment was the accreditation purpose. Automated assessment, if well integrated in the curriculum, provides fair, reliable, efficient, and effective assessment (AL-Smadi & Gutl, 2008).

AUTOMATION TOOLS

Tools used in student assessment vary from simple tools such as spreadsheets (e.g., Excel), which have the ability to perform simple tasks like curricular mapping or web-based data collection, to advanced comprehensive assessment tools which, in addition to curricular mapping, can assist in competency documentation, strategic planning, and productivity. The advanced comprehensive systems have the advantages of being designed specifically to meet accreditation needs. An example of these systems in pharmacy education is the Assessment and Accreditation Management System (AAMS), which was developed jointly between the American Association of Colleges of Pharmacy (AACP) and the Accreditation Council for Pharmacy Education (ACPE).

CHALLENGES TO TECHNOLOGY IMPLEMENTATION

Although assessment automation can help in many aspects such as accreditation purposes, if not well integrated into the college program, it can also be a burden to the faculty, students, and other stakeholders. Therefore, several challenges need to be considered before deciding to implement such technology. Some of these challenges are:

- Resistance to the use of technology, which may be due to lack of technology skills or simply because technology is not a preference.
- Negative experience with technology.
- Some types of assignments may be difficult to be graded using technology.
- Choosing of a suitable time for data collection or survey dissemination may be challenging (e.g., exam weeks for students and vacation time for preceptors).
- Overburden of students, academic staff, or other stakeholders, with too many requests for survey filling, or other type of data collection requests, may negatively impact response rate and data reliability.
- Risk of technical failure, which accompanies all technology and may be disruptive, particularly during presentations, exams, or performance-based assessments. This may necessitate presence of a ready back-up plan.

TECHNOLOGY SELECTION

Selection of the right technology is a critical step for the success of assessment automation. Wrong selection and implementation of technology can result in overwhelming the faculty program with unnecessary data that is disconnected from the outcomes. Therefore for the appropriate selection and implementation of automation technology, the following considerations need to be satisfied:

- Easy access of the technology.
- Chosen software should include all various necessary tools.
- The software should be easily integrated with the existing technologies.
- The software should include many reporting options.
- Technology support should be available at both vender and faculty level.
- Cost of the technology should be reasonable and within the faculty budget.

ADVANTAGES OF ASSESSMENT AUTOMATION

- It is necessary before listing the advantages of assessment automation to remind the reader that not all these advantages can be achieved with all types of technology, and more importantly inappropriate selection and implementation of technology may lead to the loss of these advantages altogether (Bournemouth, 2010; Winkley, 2010).
- Software tools, unlike nonautomated tools, have the advantage of being used several times as needed. This can save time wasted in preparing assessments every time they are needed.
- Software can provide immediate feedback, so the students can use the time to prepare themselves for the next assessments and hence improve their learning process.
- Flexibility of software makes it easy to provide several assessments at different places.

- Statistical analysis becomes easier with automated assessments and this can enhance evaluation and improvement based on statistical information.
- Automation can increase assessment validity through rich information as well as interaction with this information.
- Assessment automation when appropriately implemented can reduce workload on the academic staff as well as the administration effort on the administrative personnel.
- Automation can reduce printing and storage of documents (e.g., exams and rubric) to a minimum, and hence it is more eco- and space-friendly.

DISADVANTAGES OF ASSESSMENT AUTOMATION

According to Bournemouth (2010) the main disadvantages and limitations of assessment automation are:

- It is very expensive to acquire and implement the technology for assessment automation, and it also is time consuming as it needs practice and special skills.
- Risk of failure of the hardware and software of the system is always there, so there is a need for continuous monitoring, especially during examinations.

CONCLUSION

Conduction of student assessment in pharmacy education is no longer a haphazard process, but rather a well-defined process with systematic approaches paying great attention to learning through assessment. This is achieved through development and implementation of appropriate assessment tools. Therefore, this chapter tried to help the reader understand the benefits and drawbacks of selecting one or another assessment tool, while at the same time evaluating the feasibility of implementing that specific tool. Also, it tried to present simple guidelines for developing different assessment tools. The assessment tools covered vary greatly in purpose, scope, function, and criteria because there is no valid assessment tool or method that can measure all aspects of pharmacy education. At the same time, all assessment tools have their deficiencies and limitations which, unfortunately, may only be possible to identify after their actual implementation. The assessment tool should provide sufficient evidence to enable evaluators to judge "beyond reasonable doubt" that a student is competent. The assessment tool used should be applicable within a specific college setting (i.e., workplace and working practice). It is acceptable practice to use more than one assessment tool to assess a single component in a program, as long as the assessment tools used complement each other. This practice improves assessment reliability.

REFERENCES

Abate, M. A., Stamatakis, M. K., & Haggett, R. R. (2003). Excellence in curriculum development and assessment. *American Journal of Pharmaceutical Education*, *67*(3), 89.

Al-Smadi, M., Guetl, C., & Kappe, F. (2010). Peer assessment system for modern learning settings: towards a flexible e-assessment system. *International Journal of Emerging Technologies in Learning*, *5*(SI2).

AL-Smadi, M., & Gutl, C. (2008). In *Past, present and future of e-assessment: towards a flexible e-assessment system. Special track on computer-based knowledge & skill assessment and feedback in learning settings (CAF 2008), ICL 2008, Villach, Austria, September.*

Al-Wardy, N. M. (2010). Assessment methods in undergraduate medical education. *Sultan Qaboos University Medical Journal*, *10*(2), 203.

Barrett, H. C. (2000). Create your own electronic portfolio. *Learning and Leading with Technology*, *27*(7), 14–21.

Bloom, B. S., et al. (1956). Taxonomy of educational objectives: the classification of educational goals. In *Handbook I: Cognitive domain*. New York, NY: David McKay.

Boston, C. (2002). *The concept of formative assessment*. ERIC: Digest.

Bournemouth. (2010). *E-assessment (Bournemouth University)*. [cited 21 August 2017]. Available from: http://www.bournemouth.ac.uk/eds/e-assessment/index.html.

Bryant, S. L., & Timmins, A. A. (2002). *Using portfolio assessment to enhance student learning*. Hong Kong, China: The Hong Kong Institute of Education.

Buckley, S., Coleman, J., Davison, I., Khan, K. S., Zamora, J., Malick, S., et al. (2009). The educational effects of portfolios on undergraduate student learning: A best evidence medical education (BEME) systematic review. BEME guide no. 11. *Medical Teacher*, *31*(4), 282–298.

Buzzetto-More, N. A., & Alade, A. J. (2006). Best practices in e-assessment. *Journal of Information Technology Education*, *5*(1), 251–269.

Case, S. M., & Swanson, D. B. (1993). Extended-matching items: A practical alternative to free-response questions. *Teaching and Learning in Medicine: An International Journal*, *5*(2), 107–115.

Case, S. M., & Swanson, D. B. (1998). *Constructing written test questions for the basic and clinical sciences*. Philadelphia: National Board of Medical Examiners.

Centre for the Study of Higher Education (CSHE) [Internet]. (2002). In *Core principles of effective assessment Centre for the Study of Higher Education*. [cited 23 November 2016]. Available from: http://melbourne-cshe.unimelb.edu.au/__data/assets/pdf_file/0010/1770697/CorePrinciples.pdf.

Crisp, G. (2009). In *Towards authentic e-assessment tasks Ed Media: World Conference on Educational Media and Technology June 22* (pp. 1585–1590): Association for the Advancement of Computing in Education (AACE).

Editorial. (1976). Assessments in medical school. *Medical Education*, *10*(2), 79–80.

Epstein, R. M. (2007). Assessment in medical education. *The New England Journal of Medicine*, *2007*(356), 387–396.

Epstein, R. M., & Hundert, E. M. (2002). Defining and assessing professional competence. *Journal of the American Medical Association*, *287*(2), 226–235.

Feletti, G. I. (1980). Reliability and validity studies on modified essay questions. *Academic Medicine*, *55*(11), 933–941.

Feletti, G. I., & Gillies, A. H. (1982). Developing oral and written formats for evaluating clinical problems-solving by medical undergraduates. *Academic Medicine*, *57*(11), 874–876.

Feletti, G. I., & Smith, E. K. (1986). Modified essay questions: are they worth the effort? *Medical Education*, *20*(2), 126–132.

Finberg, L., & Lloyd, J. S. (1983). Suggested guidelines for ideal oral examinations. In J. S. Lloyd (Ed.), *Oral examinations in medical specialty board certification*. Chicago, IL: American Board of Medical Specialties.

Garrison, C., & Ehringhaus, M. (2007). *Formative and summative assessments in the classroom*. [cited 23 November 2016] Available from: http://www.amle.org/publications/webexclusive/assessment/tabid/1120/Default.aspx.

Gupta, P., Dewan, P., & Singh, T. (2010). Objective structured clinical examination (OSCE) revisited. *Indian Pediatrics*, *47*(11), 911–920.

Gutl, C. (2008). Moving towards a fully-automatic knowledge assessment tool. *International Journal of Emerging Technologies in Learning*, *3*(1).

Hamdorf, J. M., & Hall, J. C. (2001). The development of undergraduate curricula in surgery: III. Assessment. *ANZ Journal of Surgery*, *71*(3), 178–183.

Harden, J. R., Crosby, M. H., Davis, M., & Friedman, R. M. (1999). AMEE Guide no. 14: Outcome-based education: Part 5—from competency to meta-competency: a model for the specification of learning outcomes. *Medical Teacher*, *21*(6), 546–552.

Harden, R. T., Stevenson, M., Downie, W. W., & Wilson, G. M. (1975). Assessment of clinical competence using objective structured examination. *British Medical Journal*, *1*(5955), 447–451.

Harlen, W. (2007). *Assessment of learning*. London: Sage.

Harvey, J., & Mogey, N. (1999). Pragmatic issues when integrating technology into the assessment of students. In S. Brown, P. Race, & J. Bull (Eds.), *Computer-assisted assessment in higher education* (pp. 7–20). London: Kogan Page Ltd.

Hodgkin, K., & Knox, J. D. E. (1975). *Problem centered learning*. London: Churchill Livingstone.

Kirkpatrick, J. (2009). The Kirkpatrick four levels: A fresh look after 50 years 1959-2009. *Training Magazine*.

Le Mahieu, P., Gitomer, D., & Eresh, J. (1995). Portfolios in large-scale assessments: Difficult but not impossible. *Educational Measurement: Issues and Practice*, *14*(3), 11–28.

Liyanage, C. A., Ariyaratne, M. H., Dankanda, D. H., & Deen, K. I. (2009). Multiple choice questions as a ranking tool: a Friend or foe? *South East Asian Journal of Medical Education*, *3*(1), 62.

Lorin, W., & David, R. A. (2001). *Taxonomy for learning, teaching, and assessing*. New York: Longman.

Miller, G. E. (1973). Educational strategies for the health professions. In *Developments of educational programmes for the health professionals. WHO Public Health Papers No. 52*.

Miller, G. E. (1990). The assessment of clinical skills/competence/performance. *Academic Medicine*, *65*(9), S63–7.

Miller, A. H., Imrie, B. W., & Cox, K. (1998). *Student assessment in higher education: A handbook for assessing performance*. London: Kogan Page Ltd.

Newble, D. I., Hoare, J., & Elmslie, R. G. (1981). The validity and reliability of a new examination of the clinical competence of medical students. *Medical Education*, *15*(1), 46–52.

Noble, C., O'Brien, M., Coombes, I., Shaw, P. N., & Nissen, L. (2011). Concept mapping to evaluate an undergraduate pharmacy curriculum. *American Journal of Pharmaceutical Education*, *75*(3), 55.

Sabherwal, U. (1995). Short Answered Questions. In R. Sood, V. K. Paul, P. Sahni, S. Mittal, O. P. Kharbandra, & B. V. Adkoli (Eds.), *Assessments in Medical Education: Trend and Tools* (pp. 27–31). New Delhi: KL Wig Centre for Medical Education and Technology.

Salinitri, F. D., O'Connell, M. B., Garwood, C. L., Lehr, V. T., & Abdallah, K. (2012). An objective structured clinical examination to assess problem-based learning. *American Journal of Pharmaceutical Education*, *76*(3), 44.

Schuwirth, L. W., & Van Der Vleuten, C. P. (2004). Different written assessment methods: What can be said about their strengths and weaknesses? *Medical Education*, *38*(9), 974–979.

Schuwirth, L. W. T., & van der Vleuten, C. P. (2005). In J. Dent & R. Harden (Eds.), *Written assessments* (pp. 311–322). New York: Elsevier Churchill Livingstone.

Schuwirth, L. W., & van der Vleuten, C. P. (2011). General overview of the theories used in assessment: AMEE guide no. 57. *Medical Teacher*, *33*(10), 783–797.

Schuwirth, L. W., Verheggen, M. M., Van der Vleuten, C. P., Boshuizen, H. P., & Dinant, G. J. (2001). Do short cases elicit different thinking processes than factual knowledge questions do? *Medical Education*, *35*(4), 348–356.

Schuwirth, L. W., Vleuten, C. V., & Donkers, H. H. (1996). A closer look at cueing effects in multiple-choice questions. *Medical Education*, *30*(1), 44–49.

Stalnaker, J. M. (1951). The essay type of examination. In E. F. Lindquist (Ed.), *Educational measurement* (pp. 495–530). Menasha, WI: George Banta.

Sturpe, D. A. (2010). Objective structured clinical examinations in doctor of pharmacy programs in the United States. *American Journal of Pharmaceutical Education*, *74*(8), 148.

Sundberg, M. D. (2002). Assessing student learning. *Cell Biology Education*, *1*(1), 11–15.

Sundre, D. L., & Kitsantas, A. (2004). An exploration of the psychology of the examinee: Can examinee self-regulation and test-taking motivation predict consequential and non-consequential test performance? *Contemporary Educational Psychology*, *29*(1), 6–26.

Swanson, D. B., Holtzman, K. Z., & Allbee, K. (2008). Measurement characteristics of content-parallel single-best-answer and extended-matching questions in relation to number and source of options. *Academic Medicine*, *83*(10), S21–4.

Symeonidis, P. (2006). *Automated assessment of Java programming coursework for computer science education*. Unpublished doctoral dissertationThe University of Nottingham, School of Computer Science and Information Technology.

Tofade, T., Elsner, J., & Haines, S. T. (2013). Best practice strategies for effective use of questions as a teaching tool. *American Journal of Pharmaceutical Education*, *77*(7), 155.

University of Northern Iowa. (2006). *A Definition of Assessment from the Higher Learning Commission*. [cited 23 November 2016]. Available from: http://www.uni.edu/assessment/definitionofassessment.shtml.

Vinu, E. V., & Kumar, S. (2015). A novel approach to generate MCQs from domain ontology: Considering DL semantics and open-world assumption. *Web Semantics: Science, Services and Agents on the World Wide Web*, *34*, 40–54.

Wakeford, R. E., & Roberts, S. (1984). Short answer questions in an undergraduate qualifying examination: a study of examiner variability. *Medical Education*, *18*(3), 168–173.

Walvoord, B. E. (2010). *Assessment clear and simple: A practical guide for institutions, departments, and general education*. San Francisco: John Wiley & Sons.

Weinman, J. (1984). A modified essay question evaluation of pre-clinical teaching of communication skills. *Medical Education*, *18*(3), 164–167.

Winkley, J. (2010). *E-assessment and innovation. Becta—leading next generation learning*. [cited 21 August 2017]. Available from http://emergingtechnologies.becta.org.uk/index.Bibliographyphp?section=etr&rid=15233.

Wright, D., Loftus, M., Christou, M., Eggleton, A., & Norris, N. (2006). *Healthcare professionals education & training: How does pharmacy in great Britain compare?* London: Royal Pharmaceutical Society.

FURTHER READING

Imrie, B. W., Cox, K., & Miller, A. (2014). *Student assessment in higher education: A handbook for assessing performance*. London: Routledge.

CHAPTER

12 COMPETENCY-BASED PHARMACY EDUCATION: AN EDUCATIONAL PARADIGM FOR THE PHARMACY PROFESSION TO MEET SOCIETY'S HEALTHCARE NEEDS

Maram G. Katoue*, Terry L. Schwinghammer†

**Kuwait University Faculty of Pharmacy, Kuwait City, Kuwait, †West Virginia University School of Pharmacy, Morgantown, WV, United States*

INTRODUCTION

The healthcare needs of countries across the globe vary widely, as do the manner and quality of health professions education. Competency-based education (CBE) was developed to instill in graduates the competencies required to provide patient care services that meet societal needs, regardless of country or region. This model represents a shift from traditional educational programs that have been rigid, static, and unresponsive to advances in healthcare and changing societal and patient needs.

COMPETENCY-BASED EDUCATION: DEFINING KEY CONCEPTS

The core concept of CBE is development of health workforce competencies that enable practitioners to care for patients effectively. Competencies encompass the knowledge, skills, attitudes, and behaviors that individuals acquire and develop through education, training, and work experience (Brown, Gilbert, Bruno, & Cooper, 2012). Practice competence represents the full repertoire of competencies and reflects the ability to perform duties accurately, make correct decisions, and interact properly with patients and colleagues (Brown et al., 2012; The Council on Credentialing in Pharmacy (CCP), 2010). Practitioner competence needs to be understood as being *multidimensional*, *dynamic*, *contextual*, and *developmental* (Frank et al., 2010; Koster, Schalekamp, & Meijerman, 2017). It involves multiple components that must be integrated; it is affected by the practice setting and specific circumstances and can either further develop or diminish over time.

Pharmacy Education in the Twenty First Century and Beyond. https://doi.org/10.1016/B978-0-12-811909-9.00012-5

"Competency frameworks" represent the complete set of competencies considered essential for practice performance (Brown et al., 2012). A "competency cluster" is a group of closely related competencies within the overall framework (Whiddett & Hollyforde, 2003). "Competency standards" describe the skills, attitudes, values, beliefs, and other attributes attained by an individual from education, training, and clinical experience, which collectively enable the individual to practice effectively in the pharmacy profession (Pharmaceutical Society of Australia, 2010).

CBE is closely related to outcome-based education (OBE), which is an educational philosophy advanced in the 1980s emphasizing learner outcomes rather than the pathways or processes used to attain them (Frank et al., 2010). In OBE, educational content is targeted toward what all students should be able to do upon completion of their learning experiences (Harden, 1999). The construction of an OBE curriculum begins by defining the learning outcomes; the curricular content and instructional and assessment methods are all determined based on these outcomes (Harden, 1999). CBE also begins by defining the expected outcomes; these are the abilities graduates need for practice (Frank et al., 2010). However, CBE goes beyond learning outcomes and enhances the ability of students and practitioners to integrate their knowledge, skills, attitudes, and values to achieve an expected level of professional performance (Ten Cate, Snell, & Carraccio, 2010).

FEATURES OF COMPETENCY-BASED EDUCATION

Competency-based approaches have four main characteristics: (1) a focus on curricular outcomes, (2) an emphasis on abilities, (3) a de-emphasis of time-based training, and (4) promotion of learner-centeredness (Frank et al., 2010; Gruppen et al., 2016). In CBE, the curriculum focuses on outcomes while inculcating the essential practice competencies in learners to fulfill the needs of those served by graduates (Frank et al., 2010). It may offer a more flexible completion timeframe than traditional semester- and year-based programs (Frank et al., 2010). This can be more efficient and engaging to learners because they can progress at their own pace while building upon prior competencies (Chuenjitwongsa, Oliver, & Bullock, 2016; Iobst et al., 2010). Lastly, CBE is learner-centered because it fosters learner responsibility for personal development by mapping a pathway from one milestone to another on the way to achieving competence (Frank et al., 2010).

THE NOVICE-EXPERT CONTINUUM

Becoming a competent practitioner is an ongoing process. Competence is a developmental stage in the continuum of improving performance (Dreyfus & Dreyfus, 1980). In the Dreyfus model for skills acquisition that was originally developed for airline pilot training, a learner starts acquiring skills as a novice and progresses to ultimately achieve expertise (Dreyfus & Dreyfus, 1980). The five stages of adult skills acquisition are: (1) novice, (2) advanced beginner, (3) competent, (4) proficient, and (5) expert. A mastery level beyond expertise on this spectrum has also been proposed (Carraccio, Benson, Nixon, & Derstine, 2008). This model has been modified and adapted to describe skills acquisition in medical (Carraccio et al., 2008; Ten Cate et al., 2010) and dental (Chuenjitwongsa et al., 2016) education. According to Chuenjitwongsa et al. (2016), at the start of a professional curriculum students are in the *novice* stage. Their learning and training depend on well-structured strategies and direct support from educators. At this stage, students develop basic knowledge, skills, and values essential for practice. They then progress to the *beginner* stage in which they start to apply their

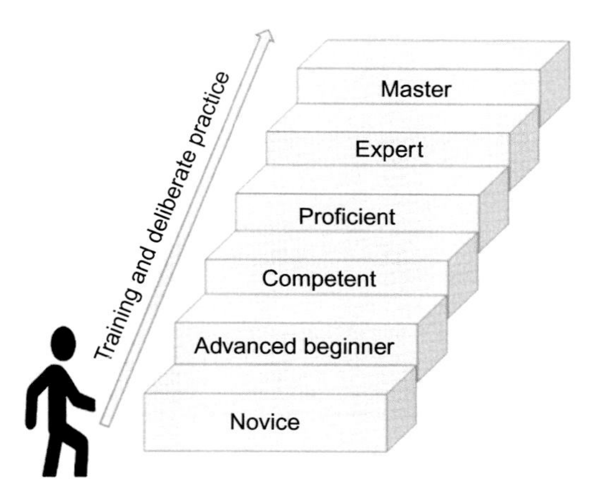

FIG. 1

Spectrum of skills acquisition.

Based on Dreyfus, S. E., & Dreyfus, H. L. (1980). A five stage model of the mental activities involved in directed skill acquisition, research paper. *Berkeley, CA: California University Berkeley Operations Research Center.*

knowledge and skills to different contexts. By the time of graduation, students are expected to be in the *competent* stage, where they can practice independently and assume responsibility for their continued professional growth. After a few years of practice following attaining a practice licensure or specialist training, they reach the *proficient* stage, with more in-depth understanding and skills to deal with a broader range of professional problems. It may take a decade or longer after starting the professional program to reach the *expert* stage, at which point practitioners have the capacity of integration and internalization of professional practice. Throughout this continuum, individuals use appropriate training and deliberate practice to gradually enhance their performance. Deliberate practice aims to improve a specific aspect of performance through intense repetitive performance of a cognitive or psychomotor skill, combined with rigorous skills assessment and informative feedback (Ericsson, 2008). Thus, competence is a transitional state toward expertise, and individuals advance along this continuum by focused training and deliberate practice (Fig. 1).

ASSESSING THE LEARNER'S PERFORMANCE

An assessment is the formal process of evaluating a learner's performance on an individual outcome (Jungnickel, Kelley, Hammer, Haines, & Marlowe, 2009). Implementation of CBE requires valid assessment tools to evaluate students progress based on their demonstrated performance of these competencies and to ensure a standard minimum acceptable level of outcomes for all graduates (Frank et al., 2010). Competence is evident by the eventual entrustment of learners/trainees to perform their expected professional activities (Ten Cate et al., 2010). Entrustable Professional Activities (EPAs) are units of professional practice (defined as specific tasks or responsibilities) that trainees are entrusted to perform without direct supervision once they have acquired sufficient competence (Ten Cate, 2013; Ten Cate et al., 2015). While competencies are descriptors of practitioners, EPAs are descriptors of

BOX 1

Key messages

1. Competency-based education (CBE) was developed to instill in graduates the competencies required to provide patient care services that meet societal needs.
2. Competencies encompass the knowledge, skills, attitudes, and behaviors that individuals acquire and develop through education, training, and work experience.
3. The main features of CBE include: a focus on curricular outcomes, an emphasis on abilities, a de-emphasis of time-based training, and promotion of learner-centeredness.
4. Deliberate practice aims to improve a specific aspect of performance through intense repetitive performance of a cognitive or psychomotor skill, combined with rigorous skills assessment and informative feedback.
5. Entrustable Professional Activities (EPAs) are units of professional practice (defined as specific tasks or responsibilities) that trainees are entrusted to perform without direct supervision once they have acquired sufficient competence.

work and usually require the integration of multiple competencies in an integrated, holistic manner (Ten Cate, 2013). Competencies and EPAs relate to each other as two dimensions of a grid in which each EPA can be linked back to a number of competencies (Ten Cate et al., 2010) (Box 1).

EVOLUTION OF COMPETENCY-BASED EDUCATION

COMPETENCY-BASED EDUCATION IN HEALTH PROFESSIONS EDUCATION

The growing interest in CBE in health professions education has resulted from a perceived need to prepare practitioners capable of meeting the demands of a changing healthcare landscape (Gruppen et al., 2016). CBE is used in many countries in medical training, including physician residency training and board certification (Albanese, Mejicano, Anderson, & Gruppen, 2010; Iobst et al., 2010; Ten Cate, 2013). It is a requirement for graduate medical education accreditation in North America and Europe (Gruppen, 2015; Iobst et al., 2010). A number of key medical organizations have developed competency frameworks. The best known are the United States Accreditation Council for Graduate Medical Education (ACGME) Outcome Project, the Canadian Medical Education Directives for Specialists (CanMEDs) framework of the Royal College of Physicians and Surgeons of Canada, the Good Medical Practice framework from the United Kingdom, and the Australian Curriculum Framework for Junior Doctors from Australia (Frank & Danoff, 2007; General Medical Council, 2013; Graham et al., 2007; Swing, 2007). These frameworks form the foundation of training for the majority of medical learners in the Western world.

The CanMEDs competency framework, which has been adopted in many countries, defines seven physician roles (medical expert, communicator, collaborator, health advocate, manager, scholar, and professional) (Frank & Danoff, 2007). The ACGME and the American Board of Medical Specialties jointly agreed on six core competencies for board certification and maintenance of certification of physicians (Albanese et al., 2010). These competencies were established in six domains: (1) patient care, (2) medical knowledge, (3) practice-based learning and improvement, (4) interpersonal and communication skills, (5) professionalism, and (6) systems-based practice (Albanese et al., 2010). The EPAs that frame competencies in the context of clinical workplace activities have been used widely to structure learning, training, and assessment in postgraduate medical education (Ten Cate & Scheele, 2007).

CBE has also been adopted by other healthcare professionals. In dentistry, undergraduate dental education has been shifting from a discipline-based, teacher-centered curriculum to CBE to provide competent dentists capable of serving societal needs (Chuenjitwongsa et al., 2016). Several key organizations developed competency frameworks and standards of practice for dentists in the United States, Australia, and Europe (American Dental Education Association, 2008; Australian Dental Council, 2016; Cowpe, Plasschaert, Harzer, Vinkka-Puhakka, & Walmsley, 2010). Published literature describes the implementation of CBE in specific areas such as conservative dentistry (Yip, Smales, Newsome, Chu, & Chow, 2001).

CBE has also been integrated into nursing education to improve the quality of care provided by graduating nurses (Fan, Wang, Chao, Jane, & Hsu, 2015). Leading nursing organizations in the United Kingdom and United States have developed performance competencies for registered nurses (The American Nurses Association, 2013; The Nursing and Midwifery Council, 2010). The competency-based approach has been found effective in enhancing student learning and attainment of core nursing competencies (Fan et al., 2015). CBE has been incorporated into the education and training of other health workers such as midwives and physician assistants (Fullerton, Thompson, & Johnson, 2013; Mulder, Ten Cate, Daalder, & Berkvens, 2010).

COMPETENCY-BASED EDUCATION IN PHARMACY

As key healthcare professionals, pharmacists must master a set of professional competencies to meet patients' health needs effectively. CBE has been described in the pharmacy literature since the 1970s (Knapp & Supernaw, 1977; Krautheim, 1975) but renewed interest in pharmacy education was stimulated only recently by widespread acceptance in medical education (Medina, 2017). The educational outcomes in the United States Accreditation Council for Pharmacy Education (ACPE) Standards 2016 emphasize development of students' professional knowledge, skills, abilities, behaviors, and attitudes, including practice competencies (ACPE, 2015). The American Association of Colleges of Pharmacy (AACP) is also focusing attention on core EPAs for new pharmacy graduates (Haines et al., 2016, 2017).

INTERNATIONAL PHARMACY COMPETENCY FRAMEWORKS

A number of professional organizations have developed competency-based frameworks for pharmacists. These frameworks have been used for development of CBE curricula, accreditation criteria, and professional registration/licensure to practice pharmacy (CCP, 2009; Nash, Chalmers, Brown, Jackson, & Peterson, 2015).

In the United States, the AACP Center for the Advancement of Pharmacy Education (CAPE) educational outcomes were developed in the early 1990s and periodically revised to guide curriculum planning, delivery, and assessment. The CAPE outcomes are constructed around four domains: (1) foundational knowledge, (2) essentials for practice and care, (3) approaches to practice and care, and (4) personal and professional development (CAPE, 2013). These 4 domains are divided into 15 subdomains to detail the competencies that a graduate of a professional degree program in pharmacy must achieve prior to entering practice. The CAPE educational outcomes are included as Standards 1 through 4 in the ACPE 2016 accreditation standards for Doctor of Pharmacy (PharmD) programs

(ACPE, 2015). The National Association of Boards of Pharmacy (NABP) is an independent organization that administers the North American Pharmacist Licensure Examination (NAPLEX®), which all students graduating from accredited professional degree programs in pharmacy must pass to obtain licensure to practice as a pharmacist (NABP, 2017a). The NAPLEX Blueprint includes detailed competency statements that reflect the knowledge, judgment, and skills expected to be demonstrated by entry-level pharmacists. The CAPE Educational Outcomes, ACPE Standards, and the NAPLEX Blueprint correlate with each other (CCP, 2009).

The Pharmacy Education Taskforce (PET) is a collaboration of the International Pharmaceutical Federation (FIP), the World Health Organization (WHO), and the United Nations Educational, Scientific and Cultural Organization (UNESCO) (Anderson et al., 2009; FIP, 2012). The coalition published a global competency framework to achieve worldwide harmonization of competencies for the pharmacy profession (Anderson et al., 2009). The scope of this framework covers foundation level (or early years) practice and the competencies of the outcomes of registration (licensing) levels of initial career education and training. In this framework, the competencies are organized into four clusters: (1) pharmaceutical public health, (2) pharmaceutical care, (3) organization and management, and (4) professional/personal competencies, with a set of corresponding behaviors illustrated under each competency cluster (FIP, 2012).

In Canada, the Association of Faculties of Pharmacy of Canada (AFPC) developed educational outcomes for first professional degree (entry-to-practice) pharmacy programs (AFPC, 2010). These were constructed to graduate medication therapy experts capable of integrating knowledge, skills, and attitudes from seven educational outcomes defined under the roles of: care provider, communicator, collaborator, manager, advocate, scholar, and professional. The National Association of Pharmacy Regulatory Authorities (NAPRA), which represents all pharmacy licensing authorities in Canada, developed professional competencies for Canadian pharmacists at entry to practice (NAPRA, 2014). The competencies within this framework are distributed into nine categories: (1) ethical, legal, and professional responsibilities, (2) patient care, (3) product distribution, (4) practice setting, (5) health promotion, (6) knowledge and research application, (7) communication and education, (8) intra- and interprofessional collaboration, and (9) quality and safety, along with detailed key competencies (outcome objectives) and enabling competencies (subelements) outlined under each category.

In the United Kingdom, the General Pharmaceutical Council (GPhC) issued standards for the initial education and training of pharmacists (GPhC, 2011). Standard 10 outlines the outcomes for the initial education and training of pharmacists, including the expectations of a pharmacy professional, skills required in practice, educational context, and assessment methods. The Competency Development and Evaluation Group (CoDEG) is a collaborative network of pharmacists, including academics and practitioners, who develop frameworks to support pharmacy practitioners and ensure their suitability to practice at all levels in the United Kingdom. The CoDEG issued a general level competency framework for pharmacy practitioners that supports the development of an individual practitioner from registration to a general practice level (CoDEG, 2007). The competencies within this framework are organized in four clusters: (1) delivery of patient care, (2) personal attributes, (3) problem solving, and (4) management and organization. The CoDEG also issued an advanced and consultant level framework for pharmacists that involves six clusters: (1) expert professional practice, (2) building working relationships, (3) leadership, (4) management, (5) education, training, and development, and (6) research and evaluation, with each cluster being divided into individual competencies (CoDEG, 2009).

The Pharmaceutical Society of Ireland (PSI) developed a core competency framework for pharmacists based on the PET global competency framework tailored to the Irish context after consultation with pharmacists and other stakeholders (PSI, 2013). The framework covers six domains and was intended to reform the education and training of pharmacists, both in terms of the qualifications for practice and also for continuing professional development of registered pharmacists.

Attempts have also been made to harmonize pharmacy competencies across the European Union (EU) countries. A European pharmacy competency framework was developed based on Delphi-consultations with pharmacists, students, and pharmacy faculty. The framework consists of 50 competencies organized in 11 domains (European Expertise Centre for Pharmacy Education and Training, 2016).

In Australia, a national competency standards framework for pharmacists was developed through a profession-wide consultative forum involving several organizations. The competency standards were organized into eight domains covering various aspects of professional practice (Pharmaceutical Society of Australia, 2010). An advanced pharmacy practice framework for Australia was subsequently developed based on the CoDEG advanced and consultant level framework to complement the national competency standards framework (Jackson et al., 2015).

In summary, the development of foundation and advanced level competency frameworks has been increasing worldwide. In some countries, frameworks were created after wide consultation with pharmacists and other stakeholders. In others, frameworks were adapted from established frameworks after modifications to meet local needs. The diversity of the pharmacy frameworks developed in different countries illustrates that no "gold standard" exists for a competency framework (Koster et al., 2017). As long as the framework covers all aspects essential for professional competence and is internally consistent, it can be used as a guide for the analysis, development, and structuring of a curriculum (Koster et al., 2017). As new pharmacy practice roles and models emerge, the accreditation organizations will require ongoing attention to the new practice competencies that will be required (CCP, 2009). Accordingly, these competency frameworks should be reviewed and updated periodically by the issuing organizations to keep pace with the evolving role of pharmacists within healthcare.

DESIGN AND IMPLEMENTATION OF A COMPETENCY-BASED PHARMACY CURRICULUM

In CBE, the health needs of society determine the competencies required of graduating practitioners in a profession (Chuenjitwongsa et al., 2016; Frank et al., 2010). These competencies in turn inform the choice of curricular content, teaching and learning methods, assessment strategies, and educational environment (Gruppen et al., 2016). In medical education, Frank et al. (2010) report that planning CBE curricula starts by identifying the abilities the graduates need to obtain, which can then be defined as required competencies and their components. This is followed by determining milestones that learners must reach as they attain the competencies. Educational activities and instructional methods are then selected to facilitate acquisition of the abilities by learners, and appropriate assessment methods are devised to measure learners progress along the milestones. Programmatic assessment must be conducted to continually refine the curriculum.

Koster et al. (2017) delineated a similar stepwise approach to the implementation of a competency-based pharmacy curriculum. Their approach includes: identifying the required competencies and constructing the curriculum accordingly; selecting the assessment methods; establishing a teaching-learning environment that is congruent with both the outcomes and assessment methods; and evaluating the curriculum.

IDENTIFYING THE REQUIRED COMPETENCIES AND CONSTRUCTING THE CURRICULUM

An existing competency framework can be used as a starting point to identify the required competencies (Koster et al., 2017). However, the framework must be adapted to local needs based on an educational needs assessment by consulting stakeholders to align the competencies to local healthcare needs. Stakeholders may include faculty members, current students, pharmacy graduates, practicing pharmacists, professional and regulatory bodies, and patients. This step involves applying the principles of the needs-based professional educational model (Anderson et al., 2009, 2014). In this model, the development of an optimal educational system progresses through a cycle that involves determining local needs, defining the services required to meet those needs, identifying the competencies to be acquired by all practitioners, and then using these criteria to develop a comprehensive educational system that ensures that local and national needs are met (Fig. 2) (Anderson et al., 2009, 2014).

As the pharmacy profession evolves from providing product-oriented to patient-oriented services, pharmacy schools must alter their curricular emphases to develop competencies that prepare students to provide direct patient care services (Hill, Delafuente, Sicat, & Kirkwood, 2006). Therefore, areas such as pharmacotherapeutics, patient counseling, and communication skills must be emphasized in the curriculum (Koster et al., 2017). The curriculum must also be designed to prepare students to become competent pharmacists who can practice effectively within the local healthcare system.

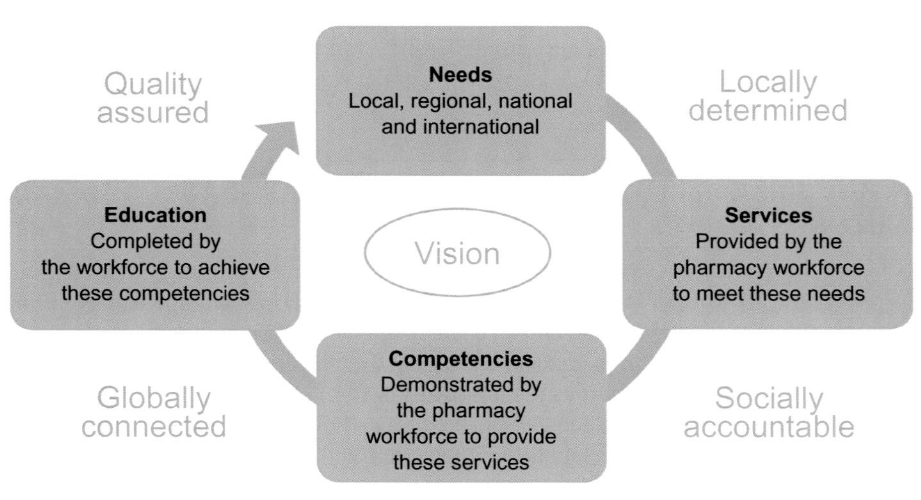

FIG. 2

The FIP needs-based educational model.

Reproduced with permission from Anderson, C., Bates, I., Brock, T., Brown, A., Bruno, A., Gal, D., et al. (2014). Highlights from the FIPEd global education report. American Journal of Pharmaceutical Education, *78(1), 4.*

BOX 2

Key messages

1. Several pharmacy competency frameworks have been developed and used in developed countries to support construction of CBE curricula, accreditation criteria of pharmacy programs, and professional pharmacy registration/licensure.
2. The approach to the design and implementation of a competency-based pharmacy curriculum involves: identifying the required competencies and constructing the curriculum accordingly; selecting the assessment methods; establishing a teaching-learning environment; and evaluating the curriculum.
3. As the pharmacy profession evolves from providing product-oriented to patient-oriented services, pharmacy schools must alter their curricular emphases to develop competencies that prepare students to provide direct patient care services. Therefore, areas such as pharmacotherapeutics, patient counseling, and communication skills must be emphasized in the curriculum.
4. Student progression through the curriculum can be assessed by defining intermediate stages or "milestone" in their development path toward attainment of the competencies.

In constructing the curriculum, the required competencies and learning outcomes must be considered while allowing for some specialization (Koster et al., 2017). The competencies are mapped against the curriculum elements (i.e., modules, courses) that are divided into discrete lessons. Students progression through the curriculum can be assessed by defining intermediate stages or "milestone" in their development path toward attainment of the competencies (Koster et al., 2017). Careful attention must be given to the horizontal and vertical integration of content knowledge and skills as the curriculum advances (Koster et al., 2017; Pearson & Hubball, 2012). Students must progress from learning content knowledge and skills in isolation to integration of skills with course content in clinically relevant tasks that gradually increase in complexity as they advance through the curriculum (Pearson & Hubball, 2012) (Box 2).

SELECTING THE ASSESSMENT METHODS

Appropriate assessment methods must be selected to evaluate student progress toward achieving the competencies (Koster et al., 2017). Clinical competency must be assessed at relevant stages to determine the extent to which students can apply knowledge in practice situations. Both summative and formative assessments are required; in summative assessment (or assessment *of* learning), each student is evaluated against a standard at the end of each curricular element to ensure that he or she has fulfilled the curricular requirements (Koster et al., 2017). A competency-based assessment process measures student performance against previously defined standards of competence rather than on comparisons with other learners (Gruppen, 2015; Hill et al., 2006). Formative assessment (or assessment *for* learning) is intended to evaluate student progress and provide feedback to support and enhance learning (Koster et al., 2017; Norcini & Burch, 2007). Results of formative assessment can help students recognize their strengths and weaknesses and also help teachers identify problematic areas for students and areas for improvement in their teaching (Koster et al., 2017). A limited number of well-chosen summative assessments should be used to prevent burnout of students and teachers and should be balanced with frequent formative assessments (Koster et al., 2017).

In addition to course-specific assessments, "milestone" or "longitudinal" assessments can be administered at critical points in the curriculum, such as at the end of each academic year, just before

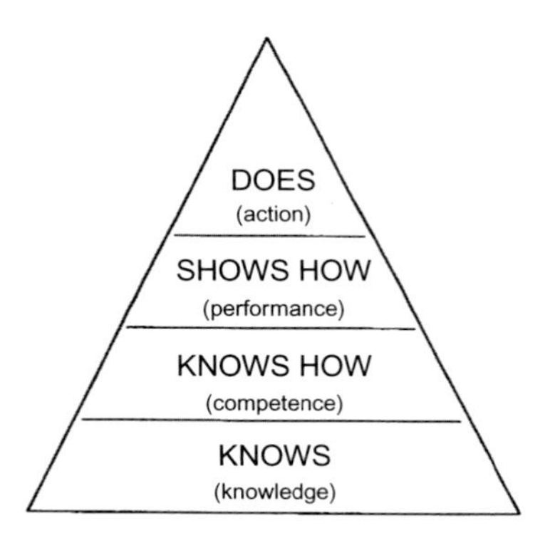

FIG. 3

Miller's framework for clinical assessment.

Reproduced with permission from Miller, G. E. (1990). The assessment of clinical skills/competence/performance. Academic Medicine, *65(Suppl. 9), S63–67.*

starting experiential training, or at the end of the curriculum (Beck, 2000). These assessments are used to assure that students are integrating learning over time and across multiple courses (Beck, 2000). In the United States, the Pharmacy Curriculum Outcomes Assessment (PCOA) examination is a comprehensive test administered by NABP that is required for all pharmacy students approaching completion of their didactic curriculum to assess their readiness to start the advanced pharmacy practice experiences (APPEs) (NABP, 2017b).

Assessment of competency is a complex task, and multiple approaches should be used that employ both self- and performance-based assessments (Nash et al., 2015). According to Miller's pyramid of assessment, each method must be carefully chosen to assess the desired outcome/competency (Fig. 3) (Miller, 1990). For example, multiple choice questions, essays, and oral examinations can test factual recall and applied knowledge, reflecting the "knows" and "knows how" levels of Miller's pyramid (Miller, 1990; Wass, Van der Vleuten, Shatzer, & Jones, 2001). Students being asked to perform a skill in an objective structured clinical examination (OSCE) are being assessed at the "shows how" level. Workplace or in-training assessments that measure individuals' actual performance mirror the "does" level. Assessment formats must increase in complexity from simple, isolated assessments to more integrated, complex assessment formats as the curriculum progresses (Koster et al., 2017).

Because the purpose of competency-based pharmacy education (CBPE) is to develop students' abilities (Frank et al., 2010), authentic assessment methods that mimic aspects of their future professional practice are recommended to ensure that students achieve the required competencies (Chuenjitwongsa et al., 2016; Koster et al., 2017). Assessments should evaluate students' abilities to deal with problems from the real-world setting. They can include patient cases, OSCEs, patient/computer simulations, EPAs, and other methods that enhance student learning, motivation, and preparation for future practice (Beck, 2000).

Ideally, the acquisition of competencies that integrate knowledge, skills, and attitudes required for professional practice should be assessed in actual workplace environments (Ten Cate et al., 2015). Direct observation of learners providing patient care remains a cornerstone of the CBE assessment process (Iobst et al., 2010). In the United States, mapping the performance of students in experiential courses to the competencies required to practice pharmacy is a requirement of accreditation standards of schools of pharmacy (ACPE, 2015). Accordingly, competency-based assessment tools based on CAPE educational outcomes have been developed to assess student clinical performance during APPEs (Hill et al., 2006; Ried, Doty, & Nemire, 2015).

Because competencies may be too theoretical to validly assess, EPAs have been used because they are executable within a given time, observable, measurable, limited to qualified personnel, and suitable for focused entrustment decisions (Ten Cate et al., 2015). In the medical education literature, five levels of entrustment for EPAs have been described for trainees, ranging from acting under full supervision to providing supervision to a junior learner (Ten Cate, 2013; Ten Cate & Scheele, 2007; Ten Cate et al., 2010). Numerous workplace assessment instruments have been used to evaluate medical trainees and arrive at entrustment decisions, including written and oral examinations, skills testing via OSCEs, case-based discussions, practice observations, presentations, case reports, and product evaluations (e.g., discharge summaries, letters, and prescriptions) (Ten Cate et al., 2015; Wass et al., 2001). Some of these methods could be extrapolated to workplace assessment in clinical pharmacy settings.

Influenced by their use in medical education for assessing trainees' preparation for practice, EPAs have gained recent attention in pharmacy education in the United States. A 2016 report by the AACP Academic Affairs Committee defined a set of "Core Entrustable Practice Activities for New Pharmacy Graduates" that all graduates should be entrusted to perform without direct supervision after graduation (Haines et al., 2016). These essential activities and tasks include six core domains, each with a number of supporting tasks: (1) patient care provider, (2) interprofessional team member, (3) population health promoter, (4) information master, (5) practice manager, and (6) self-developer (Haines et al., 2017). These core EPAs are observable tasks that translate multiple competencies into meaningful activities to facilitate their assessment (Haines et al., 2016). They were developed to define pharmacy practice and interpret the CAPE 2013 Educational Outcomes and ACPE 2016 Standards to ensure that graduates are practice- and team-ready upon graduation (Haines et al., 2016, 2017).

Finally, student portfolios have been used to document, organize, and support competency-based development and assessment (Skrabal, Turner, Jones, Tilleman, & Coover, 2012; Ten Cate et al., 2015). However, because portfolios may only assess "performance" (actual acts) rather than "competence" (capability to perform) (Chuenjitwongsa et al., 2016), they should preferably be used along with other assessment strategies to assess the "does" level of Miller's pyramid (Fig. 3) (Wass et al., 2001). Further work is needed to develop and validate competency-based assessment methods (Hill et al., 2006) (Box 3).

BOX 3

Key messages

1. A limited number of well-chosen summative assessments should be used to prevent burnout of students and teachers and should be balanced with frequent formative assessments.
2. "Milestone" or "longitudinal" assessments can be administered at critical points in the curriculum, such as at the end of each academic year, just before starting experiential training, or at the end of the curriculum.
3. Assessment of competency is a complex task, and multiple approaches should be used that employ both self- and performance-based assessments.
4. Direct observation of learners providing patient care remains a cornerstone of the CBE assessment process.

ESTABLISHING A TEACHING-LEARNING ENVIRONMENT

An effective teaching-learning environment promotes deep, self-regulated learning and should be constructively aligned with the assessment methods (Koster et al., 2017). Constructive alignment means that the learning outcomes are first defined and then used to align the teaching methods with assessments to best attain those outcomes (Biggs, 1996).

In CBE, student-centered learning is emphasized (Chuenjitwongsa et al., 2016). Students must take responsibility for their own learning and performance improvement to achieve competence, utilizing all learning opportunities and resources available to them (Gruppen, 2015). Learner-centeredness shifts the focus from teaching to learning (Gruppen et al., 2016). This redefines the roles of teachers and students and the design of the educational activities and assessment tasks (Koster et al., 2017). The job of the teacher changes from being a source of expert knowledge to a facilitator and learning coach (Gruppen et al., 2016). There is a transition from full reliance on external guidance (from the teacher), through shared guidance (by the student together with the teacher), to internal guidance (by the student alone) (Iobst et al., 2010; Ten Cate, Snell, Mann, & Vermunt, 2004). This paradigm shift from teaching to learning also helps students to develop competencies in lifelong and self-directed learning, self-reflection, and self-assessment (Iobst et al., 2010; Jungnickel et al., 2009). Students who assume responsibility for their own learning and personal development are better prepared to pursue their professional lives independently (Ten Cate et al., 2004).

Students must receive ample feedback to identify their strengths and weaknesses and to tailor their learning accordingly (Gruppen, 2015; Gruppen et al., 2016; Iobst et al., 2010). Learners must seek out feedback and apply it to their learning to enhance performance, and teachers must offer it frequently. Feedback must be specific, timely, consistent with the learner's needs, and focused on important aspects of performance (Norcini & Burch, 2007). This requires creating safe learning environments with a "feedback culture" for learners, in which the roles and expectations are clearly defined for all participants (Gruppen, 2015; Iobst et al., 2010).

Learning strategies should actively involve students and allow them to apply knowledge and skills in clinically relevant activities (Koster et al., 2017). Traditional lectures can be used to impart foundational concepts and basic knowledge, but students need to be more than passive recipients of facts. Active learning strategies can improve knowledge retention; develop critical thinking, problem solving, and decision-making skills; and foster development of professionalism (Jungnickel et al., 2009). Some active learning methods include inquiry-based learning, case-based learning, problem-based learning, team-based learning, and role playing (Gleason et al., 2011; Jungnickel et al., 2009). These types of activities should be incorporated into classroom courses and practice experiences throughout the curriculum (Gleason et al., 2011; Jungnickel et al., 2009).

Students must also have opportunities to practice the integration of knowledge, skills, and attitudes in either simulated or actual practice settings with a gradual increase in the complexity of experiences as they advance through the curriculum (Beck, 2000; Koster et al., 2017). Simulation-based experiences involving interaction with actual or standardized patients can enhance skills such as patient assessment and patient- and physician-directed communication (Beck, 2000). Experiential training allows students to apply their skills in real clinical settings under preceptors' supervision. Experiential education promotes students to be active, motivated, and self-directed learners, which prepares them for future professional roles (Jungnickel et al., 2009).

CURRICULUM EVALUATION AND QUALITY IMPROVEMENT

A cycle of curriculum evaluation and refinement constitutes the last step of the curriculum design process (Koster et al., 2017). Quality improvement involves developing and conducting an action plan for improving the curriculum based on analysis of data collected after initial implementation (Beck, 2000). Curricular evaluation provides data on the success of students, instructors, courses, and the overall curriculum with regard to achievement of educational outcomes (Beck, 2000; Jungnickel et al., 2009). This should include both a short-term feedback loop, in which all curricular elements are evaluated on a regular (usually yearly) basis, and a long-term feedback loop, in which the curriculum is reviewed every 5 to 10 years (Koster et al., 2017). This internal review can be complemented by external evaluations or visitations.

Curriculum mapping involves mapping the different curricular elements (courses/modules) against existing frameworks for quality improvement (Koster et al., 2017). This process can be useful to evaluate the concordance between the intended/designed curriculum and the received curriculum (the curriculum as perceived by students) to help identify gaps, overlaps, and inconsistencies (Plaza, Draugalis, Slack, Skrepnek, & Sauer, 2007). It can also be valuable to compare student versus faculty perceptions of the delivery and achievement of professional competencies (Kelley & Demb, 2006).

The process of continuous refinement and optimization of the curriculum must be sanctioned by the institution's administration and requires frequent communication with all stakeholders (Koster et al., 2017). Continuity in curricular development and management can be maintained by appointing an education director (or vice dean or assistant/associate dean with a similar title) and establishing a curriculum committee that is authorized to implement change (Koster et al., 2017). Promoting faculty development regarding innovative educational approaches and encouraging a scholarly approach to teaching and assessment are also ways to sustain the school's focus on curricular improvement (Koster et al., 2017) (Box 4).

BOX 4

Key messages

1. Learner-centeredness shifts the focus from teaching to learning. This redefines the roles of teachers and students and the design of the educational activities and assessment tasks.
2. The job of the teacher changes from being a source of expert knowledge to a facilitator and learning coach. There is a transition from full reliance on external guidance (from the teacher), through shared guidance (by the student together with the teacher), to internal guidance (by the student alone).
3. Students must receive ample feedback to identify their strengths and weaknesses. Feedback must be specific, timely, consistent with the learner's needs, and focused on important aspects of performance.
4. Active learning strategies should be incorporated into classroom courses and practice experiences throughout the curriculum. Examples include inquiry-based learning, case-based learning, problem-based learning, team-based learning, and role playing.
5. Curriculum mapping involves mapping the different curricular elements (courses/modules) against existing frameworks for quality improvement. This process can be useful to evaluate the concordance between the intended/designed curriculum and the received curriculum (the curriculum as perceived by students) to help identify gaps, overlaps and inconsistencies.

COMPETENCY-BASED PHARMACY CURRICULA IN DIFFERENT COUNTRIES

Developed countries have been the leaders in CBPE because of increased attention to health system planning and investment in the development of pharmacy education and practice to provide patient-oriented pharmacy services (Anderson et al., 2012). This mirrors development of internationally recognized competency-based frameworks/standards in these countries. Nash et al. (2015) reviewed the literature on program-wide use of competency standards within undergraduate pharmacy education. Their review included 19 articles in which competency standards were used in curriculum design, mapping, and/or assessment. Thirteen papers were from the United States literature and the remainder were from the United Kingdom, Australia, and New Zealand. The use of competency frameworks in pharmacy education has also been reported in other countries such as Japan and Croatia (Kiuchi, Masuda, Kamei, Kogo, & Nakamura, 2013; Mestrovic et al., 2012).

Clinically oriented curricula in developed countries may not fit the needs in developing countries due to differences in pharmacy practice environment, job opportunities for graduates, and limited human and fiscal resources to support these curricula (Anderson et al., 2009). There have been attempts to develop pharmacy education to meet societal needs in some developing countries. In Zimbabwe, a workshop was held in 1999 for stakeholders in the pharmacy profession including academics, ministry of health officials, and representatives from professional and regulatory bodies to draft, review, and approve the undergraduate pharmacy curriculum at the University of Zimbabwe (Pharmacy Department, Faculty of Medicine, University of Zimbabwe, 1999). The goal of the curricular reform was to suit the training of pharmacists for serving local needs. In Thailand, the Thai Pharmacy Council established competency standards for pharmacy licensure examination in 2002 (Kapol, Maitreemit, Pongcharoensuk, & Armstrong, 2008). These standards have been the foundation for all pharmacy degree programs in the country. In Pacific-Island countries, a competency framework for the delivery of pharmacy services was developed by conducting consultations with academics, ministry of health officials, and health personnel (Brown et al., 2012). The framework was developed for training staff and monitoring their performance. To our knowledge, there is no published model for CBPE from developing countries. In the Eastern Mediterranean region, most of the literature related to CBPE describes the experiences of pharmacy students and practitioners regarding the education, training, or practice experiences relevant to specific competencies, rather than the implementation of competency frameworks as a basis for designing the pharmacy curriculum (Bajis, Chaar, Penm, & Moles, 2016). However, this model is currently under development in the design of pharmacy curricula in some countries in the region, such as Kuwait.

IMPLICATIONS OF COMPETENCY-BASED PHARMACY EDUCATION FOR THE PHARMACY PROFESSION

POTENTIAL BENEFITS OF CBPE

Successful implementation of CBPE may enhance the preparation of an appropriately trained and competent pharmacy workforce. Beneficial attributes reported in the medical education literature that can be extrapolated to pharmacy education include that CBE:

- Provides a clear definition of professional competence and the role of education in the acquisition, maintenance, and enhancement of competencies (Frank et al., 2010). This can provide confidence in graduates' capabilities and enhance public accountability because CBE provides objective evidence of learner/practitioner competence (Hawkins et al., 2015).

- Emphasizes development of abilities that prepare practitioners to serve their patients and communities, which should result in the delivery of better health care (Frank et al., 2010; Gruppen et al., 2016).
- Focuses on the role of assessment, including both formative and summative assessments in the learning process and in guiding professional development (Frank et al., 2010; Koster et al., 2017). Determining acceptable levels of performance for competencies can help unify society and faculty members expectations for acceptable levels of professional competence (Medina, 2017).
- Fosters the continuum of learning from undergraduate student to pharmacy resident to practitioner. Achieving and sustaining competence becomes the goal of education along the continuum of professional development from novice learner to expert professional (Chuenjitwongsa et al., 2016; GPhC, 2011).
- Promotes learner-centeredness to enhance learner engagement and development (Frank et al., 2010).
- De-emphasizes time-based credentialing in favor of flexibility for learners to progress toward competency acquisition at their own rates (Frank et al., 2010).

CHALLENGES ASSOCIATED WITH IMPLEMENTATION OF CBPE

Adopting CBE in pharmacy education poses several significant challenges, including:

- Difficulty in defining, developing, implementing, and assessing competencies (Frank et al., 2010; Hawkins et al., 2015). Competency definitions vary among countries, and dividing competencies further into small observable units of behavior (e.g., EPAs) can result in a large list of tasks/behaviors that is overwhelming to both learners and teachers (Frank et al., 2010).
- Endorsing the lowest common denominator or minimum acceptable standards; when learners focus on a range of competencies so comprehensively, they may only strive to reach the defined milestones or to pass the threshold performance assessment rather than pursue excellence (Chuenjitwongsa et al., 2016; Frank et al., 2010).
- Transforming the traditional time-based curriculum to one with a flexible timeframe (Frank et al., 2010). There are few models for CBE that accommodate individual, flexible student learning plans while respecting instructors' schedules and time allocation (Hawkins et al., 2015; Medina, 2017). Time flexibility may complicate management of poor student performance and academic progression (Medina, 2017). This could lead to more program dismissals because of poor time management by weak students (Medina, 2017). However, most medical programs that have adopted CBE maintain a time-based definition of the program length (Gruppen et al., 2016). This will likely also be the case for pharmacy programs intending to implement CBPE.
- Changing traditional curricula with longstanding histories to a new paradigm with a unique instructional design that focuses on outcomes (Frank et al., 2010).
- The need to employ new teaching techniques and assessment methods (Frank et al., 2010). CBE requires formative assessment and feedback (Gruppen, 2015; Gruppen et al., 2016; Iobst et al., 2010), but institutions may emphasize summative evaluation rather than formative assessments and feedback (Gruppen, 2015). Learners may not have adequate opportunities to be observed, to receive feedback, and to reflect on feedback received to translate it into improvements (Gruppen, 2015).

- Inadequate resources for implementation; CBE requires significant funding and other resources to meet the demands of teaching, assessment, and infrastructure, and perhaps an increased faculty workforce and faculty development requirements (Frank et al., 2010; Hawkins et al., 2015).

MEETING THE CHALLENGES OF CBPE IMPLEMENTATION

The decision to transform a traditional educational program into one using CBPE depends on the perceived need and urgency for change, institutional preparedness, and determination to support and facilitate the change process (Koster et al., 2017). Strong and supportive leadership is required to orchestrate the change process (Koster et al., 2017). The views of diverse stakeholders from within and outside academia must be considered when defining the required competencies and designing the curriculum (Frank et al., 2010; Koster et al., 2017). Careful planning and preparation of the curriculum and maintaining quality control are required to achieve success (Albanese et al., 2010). A competent and committed academic workforce is required to provide education and training at all levels (Anderson et al., 2009). Instructors themselves must have the appropriate training and clinical skills in order to produce competent graduates who can contribute effectively to patient care. Therefore, faculty development is critical to the effective implementation of a high-quality competency-based curriculum (Koster et al., 2017). Faculty members and adjunct faculty preceptors must understand and effectively use active learning strategies, formative assessment and feedback, and direct observation and assessment to deliver valid and reliable evaluations of learners (Iobst et al., 2010; Norcini & Burch, 2007).

CONCLUSIONS

Health professions are under pressure from various constituents to assure that their graduates are competent to enter practice. This has resulted in a growing interest in CBE in healthcare professions education, training, and professional development to gain public trust and demonstrate accountability for enhancing practice proficiency that meets societal health needs. The potential for implementing this model in pharmacy education is promising and has been the focus of recent attention. Various competency-based frameworks have been developed and used in different countries to support design of CBE curricula, accreditation criteria for pharmacy programs, and professional pharmacy registration/licensure. CBPE has been implemented primarily in developed countries but is also being investigated in some developing countries. Transformation of traditional pharmacy educational programs into CBPE offers several advantages but comes with substantial implementation challenges. Strong institutional leadership; appropriate design, implementation and management of the curriculum; efficient use of financial, physical, and human resources; and substantial investment in faculty development are necessary for these programs to be successful.

REFERENCES

Accreditation Council for Pharmacy Education. (2015). *Accreditation standards and key elements for the professional program in pharmacy leading to the Doctor of Pharmacy Degree (Standards 2016).* Retrieved from https://www.acpeaccredit.org/pdf/Standards2016FINAL.pdf.

Albanese, M. A., Mejicano, G., Anderson, W. M., & Gruppen, L. (2010). Building a competency-based curriculum: the agony and the ecstasy. *Advances in Health Sciences Education: Theory and Practice*, *15*(3), 439–454. https://doi.org/10.1007/s10459-008-9118-2.

American Association of Colleges of Pharmacy Center for the Advancement of Pharmacy Education. (2013). *CAPE 2013 educational outcomes.* Retrieved from http://www.aacp.org/resources/education/cape/Open%20Access%20Documents/CAPEoutcomes2013.pdf.

American Dental Education Association. (2008). *Competencies for the new general dentist.* Retrieved from http://www.adea.org/about_adea/governance/Pages/Competencies-for-the-New-General-Dentist.aspx.

Anderson, C., Bates, I., Beck, D., Brock, T. P., Futter, B., Mercer, H., et al. (2009). The WHO UNESCO FIP pharmacy education taskforce. *Human Resources for Health*, *7*, 45. https://doi.org/10.1186/1478-4491-7-45.

Anderson, C., Bates, I., Brock, T., Brown, A. N., Bruno, A., Futter, B., et al. (2012). Needs-based education in the context of globalization. *American Journal of Pharmaceutical Education*, *76*(4), 56. https://doi.org/10.5688/ajpe76456.

Anderson, C., Bates, I., Brock, T., Brown, A., Bruno, A., Gal, D., et al. (2014). Highlights from the FIPEd global education report. *American Journal of Pharmaceutical Education*, *78*(1), 4. https://doi.org/10.5688/ajpe7814.

Association of Faculties of Pharmacy of Canada. (2010). *Educational outcomes for first professional degree programs in pharmacy (entry-to-practice pharmacy programs) in Canada.* Retrieved from http://www.afpc.info/sites/default/files/AFPC%20Educational%20Outcomes.pdf.

Australian Dental Council. (2016). *Professional competencies of the newly qualified dentist.* Retrieved from http://www.adc.org.au/documents/Professional%20Competencies%20of%20the%20Newly%20Qualified%20Dentist%20-%20February%202016.pdf.

Bajis, D., Chaar, B., Penm, J., & Moles, R. (2016). Competency-based pharmacy education in the Eastern Mediterranean Region—a scoping review. *Currents in Pharmacy Teaching and Learning*, *8*(3), 401–428. https://doi.org/10.1016/j.cptl.2016.02.003.

Beck, D. E. (2000). Outcomes and experiential education. *Pharmacotherapy*, *20*(10 Pt 2), 297S–306S.

Biggs, J. (1996). Enhancing teaching through constructive alignment. *Higher Education*, *32*(3), 347–364. https://doi.org/10.1007/bf00138871.

Brown, A. N., Gilbert, B. J., Bruno, A. F., & Cooper, G. M. (2012). Validated competency framework for delivery of pharmacy services in Pacific-Island countries. *Journal of Pharmacy Practice and Research*, *42*(4), 268–272. https://doi.org/10.1002/j.2055-2335.2012.tb00186.x.

Carraccio, C. L., Benson, B. J., Nixon, L. J., & Derstine, P. L. (2008). From the educational bench to the clinical bedside: translating the Dreyfus developmental model to the learning of clinical skills. *Academic Medicine*, *83*(8), 761–767. https://doi.org/10.1097/ACM.0b013e31817eb632.

Chuenjitwongsa, S., Oliver, R. G., & Bullock, A. D. (2016). Competence, competency-based education, and undergraduate dental education: a discussion paper. *European Journal of Dental Education*. https://doi.org/10.1111/eje.12213.

Cowpe, J., Plasschaert, A., Harzer, W., Vinkka-Puhakka, H., & Walmsley, A. D. (2010). Profile and competences for the graduating European dentist —update 2009. *European Journal of Dental Education*, *14*(4), 193–202. https://doi.org/10.1111/j.1600-0579.2009.00609.x.

Dreyfus, S. E., & Dreyfus, H. L. (1980). *A five stage model of the mental activities involved in directed skill acquisition, research paper.* Berkeley, CA: California University Berkeley Operations Research Center.

Ericsson, K. A. (2008). Deliberate practice and acquisition of expert performance: a general overview. *Academic Emergency Medicine*, *15*(11), 988–994. https://doi.org/10.1111/j.1553-2712.2008.00227.x.

European Expertise Centre for Pharmacy Education and Training. (2016). *European pharmacy competency framework*. Retrieved from http://eec-pet.eu/pharmacy-education/competency-framework/.

Fan, J. Y., Wang, Y. H., Chao, L. F., Jane, S. W., & Hsu, L. L. (2015). Performance evaluation of nursing students following competency-based education. *Nurse Education Today*, *35*(1), 97–103. https://doi.org/10.1016/j.nedt.2014.07.002.

Frank, J. R., & Danoff, D. (2007). The CanMEDS initiative: implementing an outcomes-based framework of physician competencies. *Medical Teacher*, *29*(7), 642–647. https://doi.org/10.1080/01421590701746983.

Frank, J. R., Snell, L. S., Ten Cate, O., Holmboe, E. S., Carraccio, C., Swing, S. R., et al. (2010). Competency-based medical education: theory to practice. *Medical Teacher*, *32*(8), 638–645. https://doi.org/10.3109/0142159x.2010.501190.

Fullerton, J. T., Thompson, J. B., & Johnson, P. (2013). Competency-based education: the essential basis of pre-service education for the professional midwifery workforce. *Midwifery*, *29*(10), 1129–1136. https://doi.org/10.1016/j.midw.2013.07.006.

General Medical Council. (2013). *Good medical practice: working with doctors, working for patients*. Retrieved from http://www.gmcuk.org/Good_medical_practice___English_1215.pdf_51527435.pdf.

General Pharmaceutical Council. (2011). *Future pharmacists: standards for the initial education and training of pharmacists*. Retrieved from https://www.pharmacyregulation.org/sites/default/files/GPhC_Future_Pharmacists.pdf.

Gleason, B. L., Peeters, M. J., Resman-Targoff, B. H., Karr, S., Mcbane, S., Kelley, K., et al. (2011). An active-learning strategies primer for achieving ability-based educational outcomes. *American Journal of Pharmaceutical Education*, *75*(9), 186. https://doi.org/10.5688/ajpe759186.

Graham, I. S., Gleason, A. J., Keogh, G. W., Paltridge, D., Rogers, I. R., Walton, M., et al. (2007). Australian curriculum framework for junior doctors. *The Medical Journal of Australia*, *186*(Suppl. 7), S14–19.

Gruppen, L. D. (2015). Competency-based education, feedback, and humility. *Gastroenterology*, *148*(1), 4–7. https://doi.org/10.1053/j.gastro.2014.11.021.

Gruppen, L. D., Burkhardt, J. C., Fitzgerald, J. T., Funnell, M., Haftel, H. M., Lypson, M. L., et al. (2016). Competency-based education: programme design and challenges to implementation. *Medical Education*, *50*(5), 532–539. https://doi.org/10.1111/medu.12977.

Haines, S. T., Gleason, B. L., Kantorovich, A., Mccollum, M., Pittenger, A. L., Plaza, C. M., et al. (2016). Report of the 2015–2016 academic affairs standing committee. *American Journal of Pharmaceutical Education*, *80*(9), S20. https://doi.org/10.5688/ajpe809S20.

Haines, S. T., Pittenger, A. L., Stolte, S. K., Plaza, C. M., Gleason, B. L., Kantorovich, A., et al. (2017). Core entrustable professional activities for new pharmacy graduates. *American Journal of Pharmaceutical Education*, *81*(1), S2. https://doi.org/10.5688/ajpe811S2.

Harden, R. M. (1999). AMEE Guide No. 14: outcome-based education: part 1–an introduction to outcome-based education. *Medical Teacher*, *21*(1), 7–14. https://doi.org/10.1080/01421599979969.

Hawkins, R. E., Welcher, C. M., Holmboe, E. S., Kirk, L. M., Norcini, J. J., Simons, K. B., et al. (2015). Implementation of competency-based medical education: are we addressing the concerns and challenges? *Medical Education*, *49*(11), 1086–1102. https://doi.org/10.1111/medu.12831.

Hill, L. H., Delafuente, J. C., Sicat, B. L., & Kirkwood, C. K. (2006). Development of a competency-based assessment process for advanced pharmacy practice experiences. *American Journal of Pharmaceutical Education*, *70*(1), 1.

International Pharmaceutical Federation. (2012). *Pharmacy education taskforce: a global competency framework*. Retrieved from https://www.fip.org/files/fip/PharmacyEducation/GbCF_v1.pdf.

Iobst, W. F., Sherbino, J., Ten Cate, O., Richardson, D. L., Dath, D., Swing, S. R., et al. (2010). Competency-based medical education in postgraduate medical education. *Medical Teacher*, *32*(8), 651–656. https://doi.org/10.3109/0142159x.2010.500709.

Jackson, S., Martin, G., Bergin, J., Clark, B., Stupans, I., Yeates, G., et al. (2015). An advanced pharmacy practice framework for Australia. *Pharmacy*, *3*(2), 13. Retrieved from http://www.mdpi.com/2226-4787/3/2/13.

Jungnickel, P. W., Kelley, K. W., Hammer, D. P., Haines, S. T., & Marlowe, K. F. (2009). Addressing competencies for the future in the professional curriculum. *American Journal of Pharmaceutical Education*, *73*(8), 156.

Kapol, N., Maitreemit, P., Pongcharoensuk, P., & Armstrong, E. P. (2008). Evaluation of curricula content based on Thai pharmacy competency standards. *American Journal of Pharmaceutical Education*, *72*(1), 9.

Kelley, K. A., & Demb, A. (2006). Instrumentation for comparing student and faculty perceptions of competency-based assessment. *American Journal of Pharmaceutical Education*, *70*(6), 134.

Kiuchi, Y., Masuda, Y., Kamei, D., Kogo, M., & Nakamura, A. (2013). Advanced curriculum for clinical assessment and skill in new age pharmacist education. *Yakugaku Zasshi: Journal of the Pharmaceutical Society of Japan*, *133*(2), 231–241.

Knapp, K. K., & Supernaw, R. B. (1977). A systematic approach to the development of a competency-based Doctor of Pharmacy program. *American Journal of Pharmaceutical Education*, *41*(3), 290–295.

Koster, A., Schalekamp, T., & Meijerman, I. (2017). Implementation of competency-based pharmacy education (CBPE). *Pharmacy*, *5*(1), 10. Retrieved from http://www.mdpi.com/2226-4787/5/1/10.

Krautheim, D. (1975). Competency-based programs in pharmaceutical education: consideration of a model. *American Journal of Pharmaceutical Education*, *39*(5), 566–569.

Medina, M. (2017). Does competency-based education have a role in academic pharmacy in the United States? *Pharmacy*, *5*(1), 13. Retrieved from http://www.mdpi.com/2226-4787/5/1/13.

Mestrovic, A., Stanicic, Z., Hadziabdic, M. O., Mucalo, I., Bates, I., Duggan, C., et al. (2012). Individualized education and competency development of Croatian community pharmacists using the general level framework. *American Journal of Pharmaceutical Education*, *76*(2), 23. https://doi.org/10.5688/ajpe76223.

Miller, G. E. (1990). The assessment of clinical skills/competence/performance. *Academic Medicine*, *65*(Suppl. 9), S63–67.

Mulder, H., Ten Cate, O., Daalder, R., & Berkvens, J. (2010). Building a competency-based workplace curriculum around entrustable professional activities: the case of physician assistant training. *Medical Teacher*, *32*(10), E453–459. https://doi.org/10.3109/0142159x.2010.513719.

Nash, R. E., Chalmers, L., Brown, N., Jackson, S., & Peterson, G. (2015). An international review of the use of competency standards in undergraduate pharmacy education. *Pharmacy Education*, *15*(1), 131–141.

National Association of Boards of Pharmacy. (2017a). *North American Pharmacist Licensure Examination/ Multistate Pharmacy Jurisprudence Examination (NAPLEX®/MPJE®) 2017 Candidate Registration Bulletin*. Retrieved from https://nabp.pharmacy/wp-content/uploads/2017/07/NAPLEX_MPJE_Bulletin_07-06-17-to-TP.pdf.

National Association of Boards of Pharmacy. (2017b). *The Pharmacy Curriculum Outcomes Assessment (PCOA)*. Retrieved from https://nabp.pharmacy/programs/pcoa/.

Norcini, J., & Burch, V. (2007). Workplace-based assessment as an educational tool: AMEE guide no. 31. *Medical Teacher*, *29*(9), 855–871. https://doi.org/10.1080/01421590701775453.

Pearson, M. L., & Hubball, H. T. (2012). Curricular integration in pharmacy education. *American Journal of Pharmaceutical Education*, *76*(10), 204. https://doi.org/10.5688/ajpe7610204.

Pharmaceutical Society of Australia. (2010). *National competency standards framework for pharmacists in Australia*. Retrieved from https://www.psa.org.au/download/standards/competency-standards-complete.pdf.

Pharmacy Department, Faculty of Medicine, University of Zimbabwe. (1999). *Bachelor of pharmacy honours degree curriculum and regulations*. Zimbabwe.

Plaza, C. M., Draugalis, J. R., Slack, M. K., Skrepnek, G. H., & Sauer, K. A. (2007). Curriculum mapping in program assessment and evaluation. *American Journal of Pharmaceutical Education*, *71*(2), 20.

Ried, D. L., Doty, R. E., & Nemire, R. E. (2015). A psychometric evaluation of an advanced pharmacy practice experience clinical competency framework. *American Journal of Pharmaceutical Education*, *79*(2), 19. https://doi.org/10.5688/ajpe79219.

Skrabal, M. Z., Turner, P. D., Jones, R. M., Tilleman, J. A., & Coover, K. L. (2012). Portfolio use and practices in US colleges and schools of pharmacy. *American Journal of Pharmaceutical Education*, *76*(3), 46. https://doi.org/10.5688/ajpe76346.

Swing, S. R. (2007). The ACGME outcome project: retrospective and prospective. *Medical Teacher*, *29*(7), 648–654. https://doi.org/10.1080/01421590701392903.

Ten Cate, O. (2013). Nuts and bolts of entrustable professional activities. *Journal of Graduate Medical Education*, *5*(1), 157–158. https://doi.org/10.4300/jgme-d-12-00380.1.

Ten Cate, O., Chen, H. C., Hoff, R. G., Peters, H., Bok, H., & Van Der Schaaf, M. (2015). Curriculum development for the workplace using entrustable professional activities (EPAs): AMEE guide no. 99. *Medical Teacher*, *37*(11), 983–1002. https://doi.org/10.3109/0142159x.2015.1060308.

Ten Cate, O., & Scheele, F. (2007). Competency-based postgraduate training: can we bridge the gap between theory and clinical practice? *Academic Medicine*, *82*(6), 542–547. https://doi.org/10.1097/ACM.0b013e31805559c7.

Ten Cate, O., Snell, L., & Carraccio, C. (2010). Medical competence: the interplay between individual ability and the health care environment. *Medical Teacher*, *32*(8), 669–675. https://doi.org/10.3109/0142159x.2010.500897.

Ten Cate, O., Snell, L., Mann, K., & Vermunt, J. (2004). Orienting teaching toward the learning process. *Academic Medicine*, *79*(3), 219–228.

The American Nurses Association. (2013). *ANA leadership institute competency model*. Retrieved from https://learn.ananursingknowledge.org/template/ana/publications_pdf/leadershipInstitute_competency_model_brochure.pdf.

The Competency Development and Evaluation Group. (2007). *A competency framework for pharmacy practitioners: general level*. Retrieved from http://www.codeg.org/fileadmin/codeg/pdf/glf/GLF_Sept_2010.pdf.

The Competency Development and Evaluation Group. (2009). *Advanced to consultant level framework: a developmental framework for pharmacists progressing to advanced levels of practice*. Retrieved from http://www.codeg.org/fileadmin/codeg/pdf/ACLF.pdf.

The Council on Credentialing in Pharmacy. (2009). *Scope of contemporary pharmacy practice: roles, responsibilities, and functions of pharmacists and pharmacy technicians*. Retrieved from http://www.pharmacycredentialing.org/Contemporary_Pharmacy_Practice.pdf.

The Council on Credentialing in Pharmacy. (2010). *Credentialing in pharmacy: a resource paper*. Retrieved from http://www.pharmacycredentialing.org/Files/CCPWhitePaper2010.pdf.

The National Association of Pharmacy Regulatory Authorities. (2014). *The professional competencies for Canadian pharmacists at entry to practice*. Retrieved from http://napra.ca/Content_Files/Files/Comp_for_Cdn_PHARMACISTS_at_EntrytoPractice_March2014_b.pdf.

The Nursing and Midwifery Council. (2010). *Standards for competence for registered nurses*. Retrieved from https://www.nmc.org.uk/globalassets/sitedocuments/standards/nmc-standards-for-competence-for-registered-nurses.pdf.

The Pharmaceutical Society of Ireland. (2013). *Core competency framework for pharmacists*. Retrieved from http://www.thepsi.ie/gns/Pharmacy_Practice/core-competency-framework.aspx.

Wass, V., Van Der Vleuten, C., Shatzer, J., & Jones, R. (2001). Assessment of clinical competence. *Lancet*, *357*(9260), 945–949. https://doi.org/10.1016/s0140-6736(00)04221-5.

Whiddett, S., & Hollyforde, S. (2003). *A practical guide to competencies: how to enhance individual and organisational performance*. London: Chartered Institute of Personnel and Development Publishing.

Yip, H. K., Smales, R. J., Newsome, P. R., Chu, F. C., & Chow, T. W. (2001). Competency-based education in a clinical course in conservative dentistry. *British Dental Journal*, *191*(9), 517–522. https://doi.org/10.1038/sj.bdj.4801221a.

SECTION

SPECIAL ISSUES IN PHARMACY EDUCATION

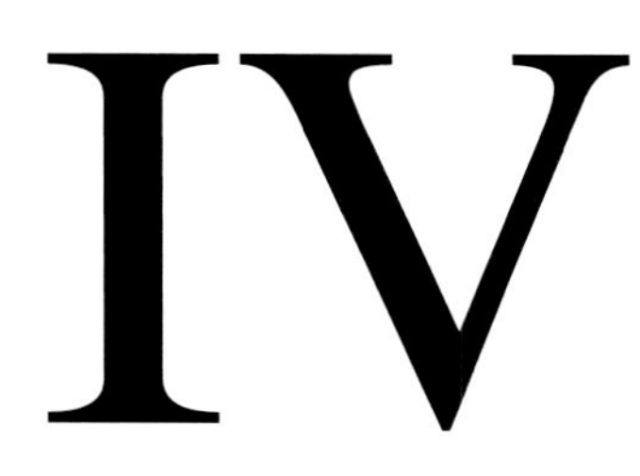

CHAPTER

CONTINUING PROFESSIONAL DEVELOPMENT AND SELF-LEARNING FOR PHARMACISTS

13

Nadir Kheir*, Kerry Wilbur[†]

University of Auckland, Auckland, New Zealand, [†]Faculty of Pharmaceutical Sciences, The University of British Columbia, Vancouver, BC, Canada

INTRODUCTION

Healthcare and its delivery have changed dramatically in the past decades due to many professional, technological, social, and environmental factors. Important forces driving this change are advances in biomedical knowledge and their application to the practice of medicine; changing expectations of patients and healthcare providers; incorporation of evidence-based medicine, and increasing accountability of healthcare practitioners towards their patients and to regulators, to mention a few (Bennett et al., 2000). These factors are accompanied by a realization of practitioners' need to keep up with the fast pace of change in order to provide care to patients that is appropriate, relevant, and evidence-based. Continuing medical education, or continuing education (CME and CE, respectively) and continuing professional development (CPD), are familiar concepts and frequently used in the different fields of the health professions. These "CME" and "CE" terms are widely used in the health professions and are considered organized learning experiences and activities in which healthcare professionals engage after they have completed entry-level academic education and training (Rouse, 2004).

LIFELONG LEARNING AND SELF-LEARNING

The concept of lifelong learning is not new. Lifelong learning (LLL) refers to education *through life as well as during childhood and adolescence* (Starke & Wade, 2005). Education in ancient Persia involved lifelong training, as it did in classical Greece, Rome, and ancient Western societies. Education in ancient Persia, for example, involved lifelong training that included knowledge of the sciences, moral virtues, and intellectual disciplines. Likewise, children and adolescents of the upper classes in Rome and Greece were diligent students, where schools endeavored to form harmonious personalities with balanced intellectual, aesthetic, and physical development (World Educational Forum, 2015)

Muslims were among the first to recommend the idea of lifelong education, exhorting Muslims to educate themselves "from the cradle to the grave," and it called for women and children to educate themselves in order to educate others in turn (Rouse, 2004). Historically, Persian science influenced

Pharmacy Education in the Twenty First Century and Beyond. https://doi.org/10.1016/B978-0-12-811909-9.00013-7

Greek philosophy and the first pre-Socratic thinkers settled in Asia Minor, under Persian rule. Thinkers such as Thales of Miletus and Heraclitus of Ephesus introduced Persian science into a liberal Greek society that willingly embraced these new sources.

The contemporary term "lifelong education" was popularized by the United Nations Educational, Scientific and Cultural Organization (UNESCO), which advocated basic concepts for all education policies in all countries of the world (Rouse, 2004). As a practice and a way of life, "learning for life" has been embraced globally and emphasizes continuing learning from childhood to adulthood. At its core, lifelong learning is a dynamic process that continues throughout the life of an individual. It entails the acquisition of knowledge that translates into one's ability, talent, and skills throughout life (Rouse, 2004). Three main dimensions of lifelong learning have been proposed by Dave (1976): expansion, innovation, and integration. Expansion defines lifelong learning as a process along with the situation and content. Innovation refers to the creative power of the learners in multiple and diverse learning situations. Integration unites the process of expansion and innovation through meaningful links (World Educational Forum, 2015).

In 2015, the World Educational Forum conducted in Korea advocated LLL for meeting the diverse and context-specific learning needs of all age groups, including the acquisition of basic literacy technical skills through both formal education and effective alternative pathways to learning.

The concept of self-learning (also autodidacticism or self-education) is education without the guidance of masters (such as instructors and professors) or institutions (such as colleges or schools). Various terms are used to describe self-education, including heutagogy, where a learner is at the center of his or her own learning (Chapnick, 2005).

CONTINUING PROFESSIONAL DEVELOPMENT AND CONTINUING EDUCATION: REFLECTIONS ON TERMS

A number of definitions of CPD exist. The Academy of Medical Royal Colleges in the United Kingdom defines it as "a continuing process, outside formal undergraduate and postgraduate training, that allows individual doctors to maintain and improve standards of medical practice through the development of knowledge, skills, attitudes and behavior" (Starke & Wade, 2005). The popularity of CPD in recent years reflects an emerging acceptance of a more complex and ambitious learning concept. Whereas CE and CME serve to update and reinforce knowledge, CPD is considered a model that addresses a myriad of interpersonal and professional skills (Merkur, Mossialos, Long, & McKee, 2008). As such, CPD presents a more self-directed and self-reflective approach, which is believed to better meet the educational needs of health professionals (Evans, Singleton, Nolan, & Bahrami, 2002). While traditional approaches to CE are not usually curricular in nature and do not optimally address all required competencies, CPD emphasizes the importance of practice-based learning and aims at ensuring that practitioners maintain their knowledge, skills, and competencies to practice throughout their careers in their specific area of practice (Peck, McCall, McLaren, & Rotem, 2000). CPD is therefore designed to meet specific goals and objectives of the individual practitioner and to, ultimately, improve the patient's health outcomes.

Self-learning (a more generic term that preceded the contemporary CPD term and embodies it) carries an element of autonomy, where the learner chooses the subject they will study, their studying material, and the study pace. This is an important requirement in professional development

Reflection
thinking about your practice
Planning
deciding how and when to learn
Action
recording what you learned
Evaluation
identifying the benefits of your learning

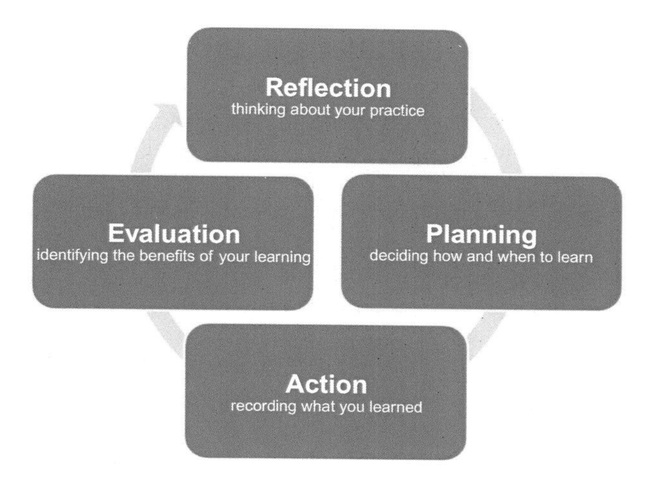

FIG. 1

The CPD cycle. Available in: General Pharmaceutical Council (GPhC): https://www.pharmacyregulation.org/regulate/article/keeping-record-continuing-update-and-record-your-cpd.

characterizing CPD, in which the learners identify their training needs and plan to close the knowledge and skill gaps through choosing the methods to close the existing gaps in their skills or knowledge. This is illustrated in Fig. 1.

Typically, a CPD cycle starts with reflecting on one's own practice and assessing learning needs. Following this, the learner develops specific learning goals and plans CPD activities to meet those goals. After completing the activities, the learner evaluates the outcomes regarding his or her performance. Documentation of needs and progress in learning is an integral aspect of CPD, and a personal portfolio is used for this purpose.

CPD AS AN ETHICAL REQUIREMENT

Learning in undergraduate and postgraduate training needs to be updated throughout a person's career to reflect changes in practice. Learning on the job is an important and indisputable part of the learning too, but it is not sufficient by itself (Gaga, Severin, & Stevenson, 2010). Attending seminars and meetings, reading journals and books, seeking expert advice, and getting information from web-based sources are some of the methods by which practitioners in current times learn and keep up to date. However, identifying sources for learning must be preceded by the desire (or need) for self-development. This desire reflects an ethical stance of the practitioner and a personal feeling of accountability and responsibility. Indeed, codes of ethics of different healthcare associations and professional bodies consistently place the maintaining of professional competency and knowledge as one of their main principles (American Pharmaceutical Association, 2007). The International Pharmaceutical Federation (FIP) has described lifelong maintenance of competency as a fundamental ethical requirement for all health professionals (FIP Statement of Professional Standards, 2002). Maintaining the standard of care through CPD does not only enhance job satisfaction and reduce wasteful staff turnover; it saves lives and improves the quality of people's lives (Gould, Kelly, Goldstone, & Maidwell, 2001).

CPD IN PHARMACY: GLOBAL PERSPECTIVE ON STATUS

The scope and implementation of CPD in pharmacy varies widely across countries and regions. It is still in a state of evolution and constant change reflected in the current diversity, from traditional provision of superficial and inconsistent offerings of CE sessions to full implementation of the most advanced and sophisticated CPD strategies. In a statement released by the FIP in 2002, CPD was defined as "the responsibility of individual pharmacists for systematic maintenance, development and broadening of knowledge, skills and attitudes, to ensure continuing competence as a professional, throughout their careers" (FIP Statement of Professional Standards, 2002). This definition emphasizes the cyclical nature of CPD and its main principles of structure and self-reliance. The FIP differentiates CPD from CE by stressing that CPD requires pharmacists to take personal responsibility for planning for their own development, meeting these needs, and subsequently evaluating their success in doing so. In contrast, CE refers to "pulses" of educational activities that could be components of a more overarching CPD program.

Regardless of geography, maintaining knowledge and skills to address emerging aspects of pharmaceutical care delivery and public health service responsibilities is challenging for pharmacists. CPD necessitates not only a learner's desire to learn but also access to resources to pursue identified self-learning needs. The principles of pharmaceutical care were initially embraced over 20 years ago in the United Kingdom, North America, Australia and New Zealand and, not coincidentally, this is where CPD may also be considered to have first developed and matured. Pharmacists recognized that to seize emerging opportunities and create new healthcare roles would require understanding and training beyond their initial pharmacy practice education. The World Health Organization, in the report of its consultative group on "Preparing the Future Pharmacist," included "lifelong learner" as one expectation of a "seven star pharmacist" (WHO, 1997). This is an essential credo for pharmacist role evolution and especially for those individuals aspiring to be patient-centered and assume greater involvement in management of patients' drug therapy. While the basic roles of the pharmacist in ensuring accurate dispensing of prescribed medicines and providing advice on responsible self-medication remain important elements of the service provided by pharmacists, pharmacists have also recognized that equally important roles are to advise other healthcare professionals on safe and rational use of medicines and to ensure that medicines are used safely and effectively by those to whom they are supplied. These roles contribute both to the welfare of the individual patient and to the overall improvement of public health (FIP, 2000). Pharmacists are also faced with continued influx of new medicine information that requires a new set of skills, such as appraisal of the literature and developing care plans. All these challenges make CPD as a tool for lifelong learning of paramount importance to pharmacists.

ACCREDITATION OF CPD

While initial professional development (CE and CPD) activities may be considered to have started in topical and unstructured fashions in many countries, educational programming rigor has now largely evolved. Various organizations worldwide (e.g., national pharmacy professional bodies, academic institutions) have now devised *accreditation standards* upon which CE and CPD activities should be developed and delivered. Professional development programmers seeking accreditation must submit documentation to the accrediting body demonstrating intended content that is scientifically robust and evidence-based, which may then be subject to external expert review. Program format and delivery must be described (e.g., independent study, live learner sessions or workshops, blended learning activities, conferences) and achievable participant learning outcomes expressed in clear and comprehensive language. Contributors (activity speakers or instructors) submit biographies confirming their content proficiencies and make conflict-of-interest disclosures as it pertains to the activity's sponsorship or paid association with any product/s included in the program content. Some accreditation guidelines (e.g., those of the Accreditation Council for Pharmacy Education (ACPE)) may even prohibit the use of brand, trade, or proprietary names in order to further exhibit the delivery of unbiased and evidence-based content (Accreditation Council for Pharmacy Education, 2017). Incorporation of participant learning assessment is often mandated through knowledge or skill measurement, reflective exercises, or authentic assessment whereby pharmacists are asked to perform tasks in real-world workplace settings to demonstrate achievement of learning outcomes. Accredited programming signals to the potential participant that measures have been taken to ensure the quality of the CPD program upon which they will embark.

The CPD accreditation process may also include an assignment of earned credit for participants. The number generally arises from a time-oriented formula whereby one hour of educational activity equates to one continuing educational unit (CEs or CEUs). Further computation of a program's CEU include the nature of the educational activities: (a) "live" or external activities (courses, seminars, meetings, conferences, audio and video presentations), (b) internal activities (practice-based activities, case conferences, grand rounds, journal clubs, teaching, consultation with peers and colleagues), and (c) "enduring" materials (print, CDROM, or web-based materials, possibly based on a curriculum, with testing or assessment). Currently, the majority of CPD programs worldwide ascribe to such "credit systems." As described earlier, CPD participants accumulate CEUs as required documentation for continuing professional registration (Peck, McLaren, & Rotem, 2000).

Increasingly, healthcare is moving toward interprofessional collaboration and interprofessional practice. Interprofessional collaboration in practice is a new paradigm and a new culture that is best learned through undergraduate education that uses interprofessional education (IPE) principles. Adoption strategies of IPE in CPD allows more interactions between learners and more integration of knowledge (Wadelin, Travlos, Janke, Zellmer, & Vlasses, 2017). CPD sessions and topics could be delivered through several platforms, including eLearning and face-to-face format in the shape of workshops. The latter mechanism allows for interactions between learners from diverse backgrounds, thus maximizing the benefits gained. Credentialing is becoming more critical for pharmacist practice activities.

MANDATING CPD

The debate is ongoing as to whether mandatory continuing education for retaining licensure to practice promotes professional growth or contributes to enhanced performance. Requirements for professional licensure and its renewal vary widely across countries. When pharmacist governing bodies require CPD documentation for relicensure, practitioners must attend more activities and events than they might otherwise do when no mandate is in place. This could also lead to taking courses on topics unrelated to specialty, or to need. Unfortunately, until CPD becomes a culture in practice and part of the practitioner's own personal routine, the phenomenon of taking courses for the sole reason of accumulating CE to meet licensure requirements shall continue. Like any good habit, lifelong learning and CPD need time to grow until they become second nature in the healthcare provider's personal agenda.

Decisions to mandate CPD should be preceded by basic foundational issues: for example, the development and use of a competency standards framework to guide professional development, educating practitioners on the skills of development of a professional practice profile, and the utilization of learning plans to guide the selection of relevant CPD activities. Before mandating CPD, regulators must ensure that practitioners have access to CE and other educational materials of the required quality. Unfortunately, there is always a risk that some, hopefully few, providers of CPD programs might use the need for CE points as a profit-generation exercise. Regulators must remain vigilant that this behavior does not take place through performance of audits, developing guidelines on best CPD practices and monitoring CPD providers' performance.

CPD/CE requirements within professions vary widely across countries. In the United States and Canada, jurisdictions of practice (i.e., provinces, territories), do not agree on requirements for CE and CPD as part of their processes for ensuring the competence of health professionals. In the European Union (EU), 17 of the member states require CPD for some sectors of healthcare providers, and many of the remaining have guidelines encouraging participation. The number of CE credit points expected varies widely, from a low in Slovenia of 10.7 points per year to a high in Bulgaria at 150 (Costa et al., 2010). Compulsory CPD programs in Austria, France, and Italy had few or no legal enforcement mechanisms. Austrian physicians are encouraged to comply with requirements because the likelihood of being subject to litigation increases without such compliance. Rather than implementing mandatory CME participation, Belgium and Norway encourage participation through financial incentives. In Belgium, nonhospital physicians receive yearly bonus payments and can ask higher fees per patient when they accumulate 20 CE credits per year (Garattini, De Campadri, & Casadei, 2010). General practitioners in Norway have no CPD requirements, but specialists will lose their specialization (and pay a 20% higher fee) if they fail to participate in specialty-specific CME courses.

Mandating CPD among pharmacists has been led by countries in which the practice of pharmacy is most developed. Worldwide, pharmacy registration authorities have clear requirements for initial registration as a pharmacist after graduation. These requirements may include examinations, successful completion of an internship after graduation, or meeting other requirements or a mixture of requirements. In 2014 at the 74th World Congress of Pharmacy and Pharmaceutical Sciences, the FIP released a document that contained data generated through a survey covering 66 countries and territories around the world (Cross, 2014). Regulation and licensing for most countries are controlled by either an independent agency or a government/ministry activity. The largest providers of CPD/CE are pharmacy professional bodies (90.6%) followed by universities (83.1%), employers (55.4%), and private providers (52.3%). The report also found that in 88% of the countries pharmacists are expected to provide some form of self-funding for their professional development, and that 77% of the countries reported contributions to CPD/CE by pharmaceutical companies. Half of the countries and territories surveyed by the FIP indicated that, after registration, there were no further regulatory or educational requirements to maintain registration, and most of the countries where CPD was mandated have continuing requirements in place (Cross, 2014). For example, in Japan, an online CPD provides a facility to maintain personal portfolios supported by professional standards and guidelines. In Namibia, CPD has a modular approach.

CHALLENGES AND BARRIERS TO THE IMPLEMENTATION OF CPD

CPD has become increasingly popular across countries, although its quality, content, and methods of implementation vary widely across the board. Governments and Ministries of Health are realizing that the availability of CPD programs within their structures is becoming an accreditation requirement and provides proof of quality. However; establishing CPD that is based on best practices is not an easy task. Some of the pitfalls of newly established CPD programs are lack of consistency in quality, lack or absence of clear objectives leading to provision of materials and activities that are not based on real need, absence of a strategy to assess impact, inability to gauge opinions and feedback of trainees, to name a few.

Several challenges and barriers facing the mandatory implementation of CPD have been reported. These include the shift of focus of learners to the CE points awarded rather than on the value and relevance of the CPD; absence of national CPD implementation plans; inconsistent use of the learning portfolio; ease of acquiring points for license renewal; lack of collaboration between stakeholders in education at the national level; and limited opportunities for practitioner engagement as speakers/lecturers in university educational activities (Cross, 2014).

However, and despite the inconsistent implementation methods of CPD programs around the world, there is agreement that embracing CPD as a tool for self-learning will put pharmacists in a learning mode on a day-to-day basis, and that ultimately CPD will become a culture for learning and a conscious choice that pharmacists, and other healthcare providers, will make.

ASSESSMENT OF CPD NEEDS

One of the most important requirements of any CE activity or CPD program is the relevance of its content to the real needs of trainees. In the past, and probably even currently in many locations, CE activities provided through CPD programs are selected at random with no evidence of need among practitioners. Accreditation bodies emphasize acquiring evidence that CE activities are based on needs assessment strategies. Structured needs assessment plays a central role in developing CE and CPD programs for healthcare professionals. Practitioners require learning experiences that address their real professional needs: hence the importance of utilizing a process mindful of the discrepancies between existing and desired proficiencies and the differences between needs, wants, and demands (Queeney, 1995). Although self-assessment of professional competence is often used to help thoughtful reflection on abilities before articulating training and educational needs, this approach has serious limitations. Healthcare professionals at all levels of training and experience have difficulty with accurate self-assessment (Gamble, 2014; Hodges, Regehr, & Martin, 2001). Self-evaluation and self-assessment of competency require knowledge of what constitutes best practice to allow comparison between "what is" and "what should be" (Ekbatani & Pierson, 2000). Without that benchmark, inflation of confidence or satisfaction with poor performance would be the natural outcomes. The difficulty in self-assessment is compounded when it is used in assessing poorly defined concepts, like clinical skills, which creates problems with reliability and validity (Fotheringham, 2010). This situation has led to a search for other strategies either to complement or replace self-assessment. Among them is triangulation. Triangulation as a research concept was first articulated by Campbell and Fiske when they suggested the application of a multimethod procedure to assess the validity of measures and traits in the psychological fields (Campbell, 2005). Patton subsequently described four types of triangulation: (1) methods triangulation using different data collection methods; (2) triangulation of sources, drawing on different data sources using the same method; (3) analyst triangulation, using multiple analysts to review findings; and (4) theory/perspective triangulation using multiple lenses to interpret the data (Patton, 2002). Using "observers" to identify training needs, complemented by self-assessment of needs (through well-structured surveys and/or qualitative research such as focus groups) represents a triangulation approach. However, the use of a triangulation approach could yield discrepancies between self and observed needs. Developing CPD content based on observer's assessment alone could be perceived as a paternalistic act that compromises the practitioner's autonomy and right of self-rule. Therefore, it may be that simple source triangulation strategies might not be sufficient or practical as a strategy in determining educational content of CPD programs or curricula. It may be that the accuracy of self-assessments can be improved through the use of strategies like rubrics (Motycka, Rose, Ried, & Brazeau, 2010). However, the use of multiple strategies concurrently to assess training needs still remains the most accurate method.

CPD PROGRAM ASSESSMENT

From idea to execution, CPD programming requires significant investment of time and human and financial resources. Prior to delivery of any specific CPD activity (that was picked based on needs assessment), teams are assembled to develop content and choose instructional methods, identify presenters and speakers, prepare and submit accreditation documents, coordinate promotion and registration, and arrange venues and materials. A set of other tasks is completed after the delivery of the activity. These include, but are not limited to, assessment of knowledge gained, analyzing the demographics of the participants, and gauging the opinions and comments of participants on the activity (including what went well and what didn't). However, the real challenge is assessing the impact of the CPD activities on the individual learner and, subsequently, on the performance in practice. This assessment merits purposeful evaluation. Although no data is currently available for pharmacy, in physician-oriented CPD literature, only minimal evidence of the effect on patient outcomes has been reported. Kirkpatrick's framework for determining the effectiveness of training programs is a model that studies have used to help measure CPD outcomes (Kirkpatrick, 1994). Four levels are described, including (1) participant reaction (i.e., this level measures how trainees reacted to the training, and this could be achieved by simply asking them through a self-administered questionnaire); (2) degree of learning (i.e., what trainees had gained in respect to improvement in their knowledge, and this could simply be achieved through a pre-post quiz based on a preset of learning objectives); (3) transfer of learning to work behavior (i.e., how far trainees have changed their behavior, based on the training they received, and specifically how trainees apply or intend to apply the information they gained); and finally (4) results, or in other words reflection on patient outcomes.

While Kirkpatrick's framework is widely used, there are many issues that warrant consideration. First, the framework as it stands is time consuming and requires trained personnel to apply. Second, it is often extremely difficult to apply levels 3 and 4 for the sole purpose of evaluating training. Impact of training on patient outcomes requires full coordination and collaboration with high-level management, which might not be practical in most situations.

Increases in participant knowledge and practice skills following CME have been objectively and reliably determined, but measured behavior change and patient benefits are often negligible (Cervero & Gaines, 2015). Features of CPD programming the support knowledge acquisition and transfer to change provider performance and patient health outcomes include those that are interactive, use varied instructional methods, and involve repeated exposures to the same or related material (Cervero & Gaines, 2015). Purposeful consideration of such elements of design and evaluation should be adopted by both established and emerging CPD programs. Additionally, much further research is warranted on how distance-based CPD activity impacts learning, provider behavior and patient outcomes, as it must be acknowledged that many motivated place-bound pharmacists throughout the world still do not have opportunities to access live events.

CONCLUSION

Continuing professional development is now considered an ethical requirement in healthcare. One of WHO's features of a Seven-Star Pharmacist is one who is a lifelong learner. It is an obligation towards the patients, and pharmacy professional bodies and regulators are therefore increasingly mandating CPD among their practitioners. However, until CPD becomes a professional culture and part of the pharmacists' personal agenda, accumulating CE points for the sake of meeting the legal requirements for relicensure will continue.

REFERENCES

Accreditation Council for Pharmacy Education (ACPE). (2017). www.acpe-accredit.org/.

American Pharmaceutical Association AP. 2007. Oath of the Pharmacist. Available from: http://www.pharmacist.com/oath-pharmacist.

Bennett, N. L., Davis, D. A., Easterling, W. E. J., Friedmann, P., Green, J. S., Koeppen, B. M., et al. (2000). Continuing medical education: A new vision of the professional development of physicians. *Academic Medicine*, *75*(12), 1167–1172.

Campbell, M. E. (2005). *Investigating self-assessment accuracy from the heuristics and biases perspective (Ph.D.)*. Ann Arbor: University of Toronto (Canada).

Cervero, R. M., & Gaines, J. K. (2015). The impact of CME on physician performance and patient health outcomes: An updated synthesis of systematic reviews. *Journal of Continuing Education in the Health Professions*, *35*(2), 131–138.

Chapnick, S. M. J. (2005). *Renaissance eLearning: Creating dramatic and unconventional learning experiences*. John Weily.

Costa, A. F. V., Aparicio, W., Gatzemeier, J. W., Leer, B., Hossfeld, D., & Continuing, K. (2010). medical education in Europe: Towards a harmonized system. *European Journal of Cancer*, *46*(13), 2340–2343.

Cross, C. T. T. (2014). *Continuing professional development/continuing education in pharmacy: Global report*. The Hague, The Netherlands: International Pharmaceutical Federation.

Dave, R. H. (1976). In R. H. Dave (Ed.), *Foundations of lifelong education* (1st ed). Elsevier.

Ekbatani, G., & Pierson, H. (Eds.), (2000). *Learner directed assessment in ESL* (pp. ix–xiii). New Jersey: Lawerance Erlbaum Associates.

Evans, A. A. S., Singleton, C., Nolan, P., & Bahrami, J. (2002). The effectiveness of personal education plans in continuing professional development: An evaluation. *Medical Teacher*, *24*(1), 79–84.

FIP. 2000 First statement of policy on good pharmacy education practice.
FIP. 2002 FIP statement of professional standards continuing professional development 24/12/2016. pp. 1–4. Available from: https://www.fip.org/www/uploads/database_file.php?id=221&table_id=.
Fotheringham, D. (2010). Triangulation for the assessment of clinical nursing skills: a review of theory, use and methodology. *International Journal of Nursing Studies*, *47*(3), 386–391.
Gaga, M., Severin, T., & Stevenson, R. (2010). Continuing medical education across Europe: The role of EBAP and the ERS in facing the challenges of life-long learning. *The European Respiratory Journal*, *35*(4), 721–722.
Gamble, K. N. (2014). *Revealing and dealing with the "messy stuff": The role of needs assessment in identifying, negotiating and planning for complex district learning needs [PhD]*. New Brunswick: Rutgers, The State University of New Jersey.
Garattini, L. G. S., De Campadri, P., & Casadei, G. (2010). Continuing medical education in six European countries: A comparative analysis. *Health Policy*, *94*(3), 246–254.
Gould, D., Kelly, D., Goldstone, L., & Maidwell, A. (2001). The changing training needs of clinical nurse managers: exploring issues for continuing professional development. *Journal of Advanced Nursing*, *34*(1), 7–17.
Hodges, B., Regehr, G., & Martin, D. (2001). Difficulties in recognizing one's own incompetence: novice physicians who are unskilled and unaware of it. *Academic Medicine: Journal of the Association of American Medical Colleges*, *76*(10 Suppl), S87–S89.
Kirkpatrick, D. L. (1994). *Evaluating training programs: The four levels*. San Francisco: Berrett-Koehler.
Merkur, S., Mossialos, E., Long, M., & McKee, M. (2008). Physician revalidation in Europe. *Clinical Medicine, Journal of the Royal College of Physicians of London*, *8*(4), 371–376.
Motycka, C. A. P., Rose, R. L. P., Ried, L. D. P., & Brazeau, G. P. (2010). Self-assessment in pharmacy and health science education and professional practice. *American Journal of Pharmaceutical Education*, *74*(5), 1–7.
Patton, M. (2002). *Training and educational needs were similar between the pharmacists and observers* (3rd ed.). Sage Publications.
Peck, C., McCall, M., McLaren, B., & Rotem, T. (2000). Appendix C: International comparison of continuing education and continuing professional development. *BMJ*, *320*, 432–435. Available from [Internet]: http://www.bmj.com/content/320/7232/432.full.
Peck, C. M. M., McLaren, B., & Rotem, T. (2000). Continuing medical education and continuing professional development: International comparisons. *BMJ*, *320*(7232), 432–435.
Queeney, D. S. (1995). Assessing needs in continuing education. An essential tool for quality improvement. *The Jossey-Bass Higher and Adult Education Series* (1st ed.). San Francisco, CA: Jossey-Bass.
Rouse, M. J. (2004). Continuing professional development in pharmacy. *Journal of the American Pharmacists Association*, *44*(4), 517–520.
Starke, I., & Wade, W. (2005). Continuing professional development—supporting the delivery of quality healthcare. *Annals of the Academy of Medicine, Singapore*, *34*(11), 714–716.
Wadelin, J. W., Travlos, D. V., Janke, K. K., Zellmer, W. A., & Vlasses, P. H. (2017). Current and future opportunities and challenges in continuing pharmacy education. *American Journal of Pharmaceutical Education*, *81*(3), 44.
WHO. 1997. The role of the pharmacist in the health care system. Preparing the future pharmacist: Curricular development. Consultative Report. Vancouver, Canada: World Health Organization. Report No.: WHO/PHARM/97/599.
World Educational Forum WE. 2015. Lifelong learning. Korea.

FURTHER READING

Faur, E. H. F., Kaddoura, A., Lopez, H., Petrovesky, A., Rahnema, M., & Ward, F. (1972). *Learning to be: A world of education today and tomorrow*. UNESCO.

CHAPTER

CAPACITY BUILDING IN PHARMACY EDUCATION

14

Claire Anderson*, Arijana Meštrović[†,‡,§]

**University of Nottingham, Nottingham, United Kingdom,* [†]*Near East University, Nicosia, Cyprus,* [‡]*University of Split, Split, Croatia,* [§]*Pharma Expert—Consultancy and Education, Zagreb, Croatia*

BUILDING ACADEMIC CAPACITY

Countries need to have a strong academic sector to be able to develop their own intellectual resources, promote innovation and knowledge, and optimize their capacity for social and economic development. The phrase "building capacity" is a widely used educational term and it refers to any effort being made to improve the abilities, skills, and expertise of educators and of those being educated. It can include human capacity building as well as institutional capacity building—for example, buildings, equipment, and infrastructure.

A well-prepared pharmacy workforce is essential for future safe and effective medicine access and use. The capacity to provide pharmaceutical services, cost-effective healthcare, research, innovations in technology, and pharmaceutical industry in each country is dependent upon having a competent, adaptable, and capable workforce, and a similarly integrated academic workforce to train and support sufficient numbers of new registrant pharmacists and other support staff, at both entry to practice and advanced levels. We have a global health workforce crisis (WHO, 2016). There is incredible variability across countries. The world is a long way from universal health coverage. Pharmacy is recognized as a key health workforce by the United Nations (UN), Organisation for Economic Co-operation and Development (OECD), International Labor Organization (ILO), and other NGOs.

The FIP*Ed* Workforce Development Goals (WDGs) were launched in Nanjing in 2016 (FIP, 2017). Workforce Development Goal number one is "academic capacity" and calls for all countries and FIP member organizations to engage in higher-education development policies and encourage leaders in pharmaceutical science and clinical practice to:

- Support supply-side workforce development agendas. The rationale and drivers for this goal are to increase the capacity to provide a competent pharmaceutical workforce by developing initial education and training programs that are fit for purpose, according to national health resource needs (clinical practice, pharmaceutical science areas, and stakeholders across all cadres).
- Develop new and innovative ways to attract young pharmacists into all areas of pharmaceutical practice and science (e.g., encourage young pharmacists to consider careers in clinical academia, as preceptors/trainers, in industrial pharmacy, regulatory sciences, research, nuclear and veterinary pharmacy, among others).

Pharmacy Education in the Twenty First Century and Beyond. https://doi.org/10.1016/B978-0-12-811909-9.00014-9

- Include the ability to meet minimum national standards of facilities, educators, and student support in order to ensure access to quality education for all students and practitioners.
- Enhance interprofessional education and collaboration with key stakeholders, including governments, national and international pharmacy/pharmaceutical organizations, and patient advocacy groups to achieve sustainable solutions for capacity development.
- Include experiential education in the curricula, as well as teacher-practitioners to assure translation of science to practice and backwards.
- Enforce more attention to training, career development, and capacity building of the clinical academic educator workforce needs, which must, importantly, include research capacity enhancement.

The health priorities of the UN post-2015 Sustainable Development Goals, which include ending AIDS, tuberculosis, and malaria; achieving drastic reductions in maternal mortality; ending preventable deaths of newborns and children under 5; reducing premature mortality from noncommunicable diseases; promoting mental health; and addressing chronic diseases, will all remain aspirational unless the health workforce including the pharmacy workforce is transformed (WHO, 2016).

The 2013 FIP*Ed* education report (FIP, 2013) suggests that pharmacy education, in both capacity and infrastructure, varies considerably between countries, territories, and World Health Organization (WHO) regions, and generally correlates with country-level economic development indicators. Those countries and territories with lower economic indicators tend to have the least academic capacity and produce fewer pharmacists.

SOCIAL ACCOUNTABILITY

Educational systems, and specifically universities, are not currently held accountable for the professionals they develop. A global independent Commission on the Education of Health Professionals for the 21st Century (Frenk et al., 2010) concluded that “all health professionals in all countries should be educated to mobilise knowledge and to engage in critical reasoning and ethical conduct so that they are competent to participate in patient and population-centred health systems as members of locally responsive and globally connected teams.” The Commission reviewed the global status of postsecondary health professional education in health. The Commission adopted a global outlook, focusing on the health needs of populations, recognizing the increasing demand for integrated health professionals’ education and leadership, and took a systems approach to educational reform, considering health professionals’ education itself as a system that overlaps with the health system it attempts to serve.

The report from the Lancet Commission on Medical Education for the 21st Century states that a renaissance of a new professionalism that is patient-centered and team-based has been much discussed but has lacked the leadership, incentives, and power to deliver on its promise; they concluded that changes were needed because of fragmented, outdated, and static curricula that produce ill-equipped graduates. The Commission argued for major reform across the entire health professional education system, to produce competency-led curricula for the future. The problems that are systemic across the health professions, including pharmacy, were identified as: mismatch of competencies to patient and population needs; poor teamwork; persistent gender stratification of professional status; narrow technical focus without broader contextual understanding; episodic encounters rather than continuous care; predominant hospital orientation at the expense of primary care; quantitative and qualitative imbalances in the professional labor market; and weak leadership to improve health-system performance. The commission also condemned the tribalism of the health professionals, who are largely working in professional silos instead of calling for professions to work together.

There is increasing evidence that coverage and numbers of health professionals have a direct effect on health outcomes (Zulfiqar, 2010). The Lancet Commission, while acknowledging that reforms are particularly challenging in poor countries, stated how difficult it is for any country rich or poor to implement educational reform and develop competencies that are responsive to health needs, overcome professional silos, harness IT, enhance critical thinking, and strengthen professional identity and values.

The transition to integrated patient-oriented pharmacy services in the developed world has been a factor of health system planning and investment in academic and practice orientation and quality assurance over many years. Developed countries have led competency-based pharmacy curricula, which have been a product of these tertiary healthcare environments. In contrast, within developing countries the population's access to health services is reduced and healthcare provision is the primary aim of the healthcare system. Expansion was indicated by an increase in the number of pharmacy schools or increases in enrollments at existing schools or increased numbers of entrants to the profession. However, this expansion presented many concerns regarding quality of teaching, the number of available pharmacy-trained faculty, and the academic standard of applicants. In addition, alignment of pharmacy curricula with pharmacy practice was considered important for job satisfaction and hence retention of pharmacists.

There is a global shortage of pharmacist academics and of practice-based supervisors/preceptors/educators to train student pharmacists and interns in practice. One response to shortages of pharmacists at the beginning of this century was a planned expansion of the number of pharmacy graduates, which occurred or was recommended in the United Kingdom, the United States, Australia, Canada, Ireland and Malaysia; this led to rapid expansion of pharmacy schools and of the numbers of students admitted into existing courses.

There is an increasing trend in some countries towards doctor of pharmacy (PharmD) level education. Thailand, Pakistan, India, Bangladesh, many African countries, and parts of the Middle East are changing their entry-level qualification to a PharmD. PharmD courses are characterized by a considerable number of precepted clerkships with measurable outcomes. Many of these countries do not yet have a trained and available workforce practicing clinical pharmacy who are competent to act as preceptors (Anderson & Futter, 2009).

As the pharmacy curriculum has evolved to become more clinical, some countries have employed more clinical academics who may be working in practice but also spending some time teaching and sometimes doing research. However, in some countries, including many developing countries, all academics have been required to have PhDs and be active in both research and teaching. There is a dilemma, though, exemplified in the current UK situation: as the curriculum has become more clinical and more integrated, many leading universities have appointed academics to teaching-only contracts and fewer people are coming into academia via more traditional routes, leading to there being too few people to be the future full professors and associate professors in clinical pharmacy, social pharmacy, and pharmacy practice. There is also a potential issue that, as the curriculum has become more clinical, fewer of the pharmaceutical scientists are no longer pharmacists as they have been in the past.

Universities and policymakers need to think of new ways to attract pharmacists into academic roles. In many countries, there is a need to create clear career pathways and training schemes to address the academic workforce in general, and a practitioner-academic workforce in particular.

An understanding of pharmacy education and its significant influencing factors are essential for planning human resources for health and for achieving universal access to medicines and medicine expertise. Collaboration with key partners, including governments and national and international pharmacy organizations, is crucial to achieving sustainable solutions to the challenges surrounding pharmacy education.

Opinion leaders and governments in developed countries are calling for pharmacy education to take the lead in medicine optimization and public health, to build accountability for medication therapy outcomes, and to develop curricula to prepare pharmacy students for specialized areas such as personalized medicine, independent prescribing, and team-based patient care, especially in settings where tertiary pharmacy education has not been in place previously (Hassali, 2011). It is critically important that pharmacy degree courses prepare future pharmacists for the wide range of career pathways that are needed to better meet health system needs. Many countries are moving from curricula that focus on knowledge and skills to curricula that will develop pharmacists who will "think, act, and do things in a way that shows they are truly patient-centred pharmacists" (Noble, Shaw, Nissen, Coombes, & O'Brien, 2011; Rennie et al., 2011). There is an increasing focus on values and behaviors in the UK following the findings of the Francis Inquiry into serious failings of care at the Mid Staffordshire hospital, where many patients died unnecessarily. The failure of the healthcare system in this example has led to many national recommendations including enhancing education, training, and support (Francis, 2013). There is also a desire to prepare flexible graduates for a varied and unknown future, but pharmacy educators may not be moving quickly enough toward these goals (Carter, 2011; DiPiro, 2011).

The role of pharmacists in these environments is still evolving, but trends toward a focus on access to medicines, including availability, affordability, and acceptability, are emerging. In a number of countries—for example, India, South Africa and Mexico—pharmacists are also widely employed in the pharmaceutical industry and students are prepared for careers in the industry. In Brazil pharmacists are widely employed in primary-care clinics and in the UK in general practice.

Globally, pharmacy practice, science, and education are undergoing unprecedented changes. Expanded roles for pharmacists, as providers of healthcare services and as scientists, are increasingly recognized and valued. Pharmacists worldwide are serving as the medicine experts in the collaborative healthcare team and are providing critical information to other health providers on the benefits, risks, and potential adverse interactions between therapeutic agents for communicable diseases such as malaria, TB, HIV/AIDS and noncommunicable diseases such as diabetes, hypertension, and cancer. Countering these achievements, many countries still face critical shortages of pharmacists, pharmaceutical scientists, and pharmaceutical support personnel. Although there have been calls for changes in preservice education, better approaches are needed in continuing education for the existing health workforce, and for training pharmacists to supervise a lower cadre of assistants.

INTRODUCTION OR EXPANSION OF PRACTICE EXPERIENCE IN THE CURRICULUM; NEED FOR PRECEPTORS/PRACTITIONER EDUCATORS

There is a need to define, measure, build, and monitor the academic capacity required to produce the workforce necessary for safe and effective medicine discovery, manufacture, distribution, and use. At the Nanjing workshop on WDG 1—Academic capacity, a number of priorities were developed:

(1) defining "fit for purpose" during a time of great change in healthcare and education,
(2) recruiting and training classroom and practice-based instructors for new and nontraditional pharmacy roles,

(3) academic collaborations with practice, industry, and interprofessional stakeholders,
(4) practice-based definitions of pharmacists, pharmacy technicians, and other support cadres, and
(5) the need to include students in discussions of academic capacity.

Workshop participants agreed that, while local needs may vary, academic capacity was an important global issue. Diagnostic models and benchmarking tools are needed to help countries estimate the number of and specific competencies for pharmacy-related academics. Additionally, pharmacy leaders must develop skills in advocacy in order to demonstrate to educational, healthcare, and financial policymakers the value of investing in the pharmacy-related academic workforce. This investment is critical for the future of safe and effective medicine development, access, and use.

Barriers identified include the wide range of degree offerings (diploma, BPharm, MPharm, PharmD) globally and potential misunderstandings about these, a lack of shared academic terminology, a lack of skill in distance-based education models that could be critical in achieving capacity, mistrust associated with a historical brain drain from lower-middle income countries, local legal constraints in education, and a disconnect between academic advancement expectations (teaching, research, service) and outcomes.

While previous work regarding counting and describing pharmacy-related academics has been initiated (FIP, 2013), the outputs of this work has not been complete nor has it been used widely to drive policy. Diagnostic models and benchmarking tools are needed to enable these numbers and competencies to motivate global action as well as to be useful in needs-based educational models. WDG1 provides an opportunity to develop the passive and active surveillance systems required to produce the pharmacy-related workforce necessary for safe and effective medicine discovery, manufacture, distribution, and use worldwide.

BUILDING CAPACITY: KNOWLEDGE, SKILLS, ATTITUDES, AND VALUES DEVELOPMENT OF EDUCATORS

Developing or enhancing pedagogy and andragogy skills, including new teaching methods and philosophies (active learning, problem-based learning, team-based learning, "flipped classroom," OSCEs, etc.) is one of the most important indicators for quality of teaching. There is no doubt that academics in pharmacy are knowledgeable in their area of expertise and teaching, but it is not always required for them to demonstrate teaching and assessment skills on the highest-quality level when in the classroom. Also, in many schools in the world, the only assessment required to evaluate teaching skills and attitudes of academic staff is the student's evaluation and satisfaction. There are many tools developed to evaluate pedagogy skills and an interactive approach to teaching (Eady & Lockyer, 2013). Andragogy is another discipline that should be introduced to the faculty members and quality management to meet the learners' needs is recommended.

Adults learn in many ways, especially if they already have their own practice experience. Students, as adult learners, are becoming more independent and have developed different learning styles (Kaufman, 2003). They value meaningful learning that shows perspectives to be applied in their future or current practice and integrates their everyday life situations. New generations especially value debates and problem-centered approaches; they like to learn in small groups, not always individually. It is important that the learning climate surrounds learners in a creative atmosphere, where learners feel safe and comfortable in sharing their experience and knowledge. Learning methods also vary in communication style, especially in discussions and the habit of asking questions. Students in some cultures do not feel comfortable speaking openly and asking for explanations when they need it (Jubraj, 2009).

If it is possible, it is always good to involve learners in explaining their own needs and expectations, participating at least in some parts of creating the curricular content and identifying resources for learning. If the learner is an active contributor to the educational process, learning flow can be more natural and better accepted by the learners.

Teachers need to have mechanisms to assess learners' current level of knowledge and understanding and to implement them in the learning process. In many ways, the teacher needs to be the role model to achieve the desired impact on students, and especially on adult learners. As people often teach the way they were taught, medical educators should model these educational principles with their students and junior doctors. This will help the next generation of teachers and learners to become more effective and should lead to better care for patients.

In teaching design it is important to recognize different aspects of teaching to address all perceptive segments of learning such as: behavioral, cognitive, developmental, and psychoanalytic approaches to develop judgment skills and the decision-making process (Romanelli, Bird, & Ryan, 2009).

This leads to another important aspect of academic capacity: How to use new educational technologies (e.g., online education, distance education, high-fidelity simulation) in teaching?

Simulations and virtual patients, on-line courses and webinars, interactive assessment, and feedback are having a greater role in teaching and learning methodologies in pharmacy. It is already well known that e-learning in pharmacy education effectively increases knowledge and is a highly acceptable format both for pharmacy students and healthcare professionals. There is still very limited evidence that e-learning effectively improves skills or developing attitudes in the profession. It is still early to say whether e-learning will be effective at increasing knowledge in the long term. The most common methodologies are online modules, enhanced by an audio component. Multimedia vignettes, virtual patients, or workshop activities with a blended or hybrid approach can use both traditional (face-to-face) and virtual methods. Academic capacity should be building those skills and methodologies to meet the needs of the learners of the 21st century (Salter, SKaria, Sanfilippo, & Clifford, 2014).

One very important aspect of teaching is also developing or enhancing assessment and feedback skills. This includes assessment of achievement of the range of needed competencies by all students, especially in helping students to develop self-directed lifelong learning skills and to assume a greater responsibility for their own learning in the future.

It is important not to forget about developing and enhancing research skills of educators, to stay up-to-date in the field and to contribute to scientifically valuable data and resources. Research should be part of educators' continuing professional development, as they must mentor students to develop research skills and publish in the pharmacy field. It is an essential requirement for academic advancement, but not always well supported in educators' capacity building program. Research skills should be developed during the undergraduate period and applied during all aspects of pharmacy practice and education (Fuji & Galt, 2009).

Motivation and dedication for teaching is visible in teachers' performance. Developing the attitudes and values of educators is extremely important in their capacity building and competency development. Expanding and enhancing cocurricular activities, service learning, community engagement, and similar activities can help in this regard. Seeing the patients can be a very strong motivator to teach and transfer knowledge to the students and healthcare professionals who are facing routine and low levels of motivation in their own professional development. Attitudes and values can be built based on an ethical approach in teaching, addressing open ethical questions and debating different solutions of presented case studies (Meštrović & Rouse, 2015).

Mentoring junior educators is also a skill that needs to be developed, as it is required in everyday activities of academic staff. This is a special aspect of teaching, in leading by example and providing assertive feedback to the less-experienced colleague. It is also important to include administration and management skills, which include time and change management, planning, stress management, financial basic skills, and teamwork.

QUALITY ASSURANCE OF PROFESSIONAL DEVELOPMENT PROGRAMS FOR EDUCATORS

Assessing and improving the quality of education is especially important for educators in their own lifelong learning cycle. Using the recently accepted concept of pillars and foundations of educational quality in pharmacy, it is possible to choose the best educational activity and to design activities that will develop desired skills and knowledge for academic teachers and preceptors (International Pharmaceutical Federation, 2014).

The educational activity needs to be provided in this specific context, so educators can be empowered to educate others. Most appropriate courses are even called "learning for teaching" or "educating the educators" to be recognized by this specific target audience. The structure and process of educational activity can be designed to promote quality in preparation and delivery. Skilled and experienced presenters and interactive teaching methods would open the possibility to be a part of the educational process and experience it from the learner's perspective. Outcomes should be well defined and targeted to develop competencies and improve performance in teaching and educational activity preparations. But the most important part of the quality assessment should be impact, not only because of participants' development, but also to raise the awareness that teachers can really have an impact on the learners' skills and attitudes. Impact is not always easy to measure, as it is usually a long-term result of learning activity, but it must be taken into consideration also in evaluation of learning.

Measuring the learning outcomes and impact of competency-based pharmacy education is probably easiest if competency assessment is provided before and after educational activity. It could be a self-assessment or peer assessment method, but if the development of knowledge, skills, attitudes, and values is visible, it can be considered to be competency-based education.

Therefore, it is important that such educational activities are based on three fundamental aspects: science, practice, and ethics. Science will provide a firm and needed background of evidence-based facts and will assure the quality of the content and outcomes. Practice aspects will be visible in the structure and process of educational activity, using interactive methods, case studies, debates, problem-solving approaches and providing of practical solutions. Ethical aspects will trigger the behavioral change, including development of new attitudes and values, hopefully to be included and transferred during future teaching activities of the participants (International Pharmaceutical Federation, 2014).

TOOLS AND RESOURCES TO SUPPORT EDUCATORS IN THEIR PROFESSIONAL DEVELOPMENT, INCLUDING NETWORKS AND RESOURCE-SHARING SITES (PHARMACADEMY, UNITWIN, FIP'S CENTRES OF EXCELLENCE, ETC.)

FIP Education (or FIP*Ed)* is bringing together all of the International Pharmaceutical Federation's education actions, strengthening their projects and partnerships with the WHO and with the United Nations Educational, Scientific and Cultural Organization (UNESCO). FIP*Ed* is comprised of the Academic Institutional Membership (AIM), the Pharmacy Education Development Team, and the Academic Section (see www.fip.org/education). FIP*Ed* is working to stimulate transformational change in pharmacy education and engender the development of science and practice, toward meeting present and future societal and workforce needs around the world. They are advocating for the use of needs-based strategies where pharmacy education is socially accountable, where practice and science are evidence-based and practitioners have the required competencies to provide the needed services to their communities.

PHARMACADEMY

Many other tools are available to support the academic community at http://pharmacademy.org. PharmAcademy is a platform supported by FIP*Ed* where academics from around the world can download, use, and share resources to improve teaching and learning. Enhanced pharmacy education creates better pharmacists, but creating high-quality student learning resources takes time and money. Sharing educational resources makes sense so students can benefit and learn more, especially in a global profession such as pharmacy where teaching needs are often similar. Sharing and collaborating creates and strengthens partnerships based on goodwill and a shared commitment to educational excellence. The platform is a place to share, discover, acquire, and repurpose resources for pharmacy education. It also encourages the collaborative creation of new content. PharmAcademy is available to educators in pharmacy schools around the world, hosting quality-assured educational resources and providing a trustworthy source of relevant and current material. Being multitiered, it allows various access levels for a broad range of users. The success of PharmAcademy depends on academics contributing resources they have developed to share via the database.

THE UNESCO UNITWIN PROGRAM

In August 2010, at the 70th International FIP World Congress, FIP and UNESCO launched a global University Twinning and Networking Programme. The Global Pharmacy Education Development network is a UNESCO-sponsored initiative hosted under the UNITWIN scheme. This UNITWIN collaboration is the first ever in the field of higher education for health professionals and the first for global pharmacy education. The UNESCO UNITWIN program seeks to advance research, training, and program development in higher education by building university networks and encouraging interuniversity cooperation worldwide. In bringing together pharmacy schools from all regions of the world with UNESCO and FIP, the UNITWIN Network in Global Pharmacy Education Development (G-PhEd) will enable synchronized and powerful development in pharmacy and pharmaceutical sciences education and improve communication for scientific innovation, healthcare outcomes, and ultimately the attainment of the Millennium Development Goals (MDGs). The FIP-UNESCO University Twinning Network for Pharmacists has been formally approved by UNESCO. The initial focus has been on bringing together a number of African pharmacy schools to work together to facilitate the sharing of ideas, skills, resources, and good practice, including staff exchange for skills and capacity building. The Centre provides a forum for discussion and debate on trends and developments in pharmacy education, facilitated by network partners, including NGOs and professional agencies, and coordinated by the founding partners.

FIP UNESCO-UNITWIN CENTRE OF EXCELLENCE

Africa was chosen to establish the first FIP UNESCO-UNITWIN Centre of Excellence because the region is in great need of a pharmacy workforce and lacks educational resources for universities. A recent meeting of the five founding partner countries of a FIP*Ed* UNITWIN African Centre of Excellence—Ghana, Namibia, Nigeria, Uganda, and Zambia—was held in Lusaka, Zambia to determine the future activities of the Centre of Excellence. Five domains for the Centre of Excellence were determined (communication, capability, quality, innovation, and clinical). Each founding partner agreed to take the lead in one of these domains and coordinate projects or activities within them. The founding partners developed and agreed to a communications strategy and will contribute to advocacy, local network building, and communications to ensure the wider success of the Centre of Excellence. Proposed projects of the Centre include a survey of African colleges and schools of pharmacy to establish a database of academic capacity and expertise to facilitate intraregional sharing of expertise through a visiting academic program. Another project is the development of a "Lab-box" of basic laboratory equipment to improve students' ability to undertake laboratory experiments to support their learning of basic science concepts. The Centre of Excellence will invite additional countries to become part of the center to expand its activities and provide a broader base of communication and support in the African region. Centre of Excellence activities will also seek to promote gender equality and empowerment for women academics and scientists in collaborative research and policy development.

OVERCOMING CHALLENGES

Many challenges remain and succession planning is important to build the academics of the future. What will the 21st century academics look like? Will they be the same as previously and do they have to do it all? Is research alone or teaching alone enough? The PharmD remains an entry-level qualification and is not sufficient to pursue a research-focused career in academia. However, PharmD or MPharm level qualifications may be appropriate for teaching focused staff. Research and scholarship remain important and should stay part of the expectations of an academic position. However, other factors need to be taken into account, in other subjects: for example, law and business academic staff are appointed based on the skills they bring from their professions. It is needed to include this aspect for future pharmacy academics. At many UK universities, promotions are largely based on the teaching only, with less of a focus on research. We also need to provide new pathways for clinical academics. The University of Nottingham has recently developed the role of research practitioner, where young practitioners have been employed to do a PhD, teach, and maintain their practice. We hope that these junior practitioners will then have the opportunity to develop into clinical practice academics. The

National Institute of Health Research in England has opened up their clinical fellowships, lecturers, professors, and so on to pharmacists wishing to pursue a clinical academic career. Other countries also need to look at promotion routes/tenure tracks for clinical academics; otherwise they tend to leave for practice positions.

The American College of Clinical Pharmacy (ACCP) states that clinical pharmacy practice academics in the United States should possess PharmD from an Accreditation Council for Pharmacy Education accredited institution, have completed a postgraduate year one (PGY1) residency, or possess at least 3 years of direct patient care experience. Those who practice in identified areas of pharmacotherapy specialization, as identified by the American Society of Health-System Pharmacists postgraduate year two (PGY2) residency guidelines, should have completed a PGY2 residency in that area of specialty practice. Alternatively, faculty should have completed a minimum of a PGY1 residency and 1 additional year of practice, with at least 50% of time spent in their area of specialization, which is documented in a portfolio, or 4 years of direct patient care in their area of specialization, which is documented in a portfolio. Fellowship training or a graduate degree (e.g., PhD) should be required for research-intensive positions. All academics should obtain structured teaching experience during or after postgraduate training, preferably through a formal teaching certificate program or through activities documented in a teaching portfolio (Engle et al., 2014).

CONCLUSION

It is essential that there be a well-prepared pharmacy workforce for future safe and effective medicine access and use. The capacity to provide clinical pharmaceutical services, cost-effective healthcare, research, and innovations in technology and pharmaceutical industry in each country is dependent upon having a competent, adaptable and capable workforce. In order to provide appropriate training of an academic workforce, it is essential to train and support sufficient numbers of new registrant pharmacists and other support staff at both entry to practice and advanced levels. There is very little existing data on academic capacity in pharmacy globally, and it is imperative that pharmacy member organizations, regulatory bodies, heath departments, educational institutions, and other stakeholders start to collect and review this data alongside other workforce data. A whole systems approach over a long period of time is needed for countries to bring about the changes required. Evaluation needs to be coproduced and developed with all stakeholders. A mixed methods approach needs to be employed, using a range of established evaluative techniques designed to assess process, outcomes, and impacts. It is also necessary to focus on key quantitative variables around supply of graduates, employability, and analysis of competencies and measures of stakeholder satisfaction. It will be important to explore effectiveness of partnerships, both qualitatively and through use of tools like social network analysis. Curriculum change can be analyzed through standard curriculum evaluation methodologies, for example with the FIP benchmarks as a key reference point for pharmacy students.

REFERENCES

Anderson, C., & Futter, B. (2009). PharmD or needs based education: Which comes first? *American Journal of Pharmaceutical Education*, *73*(5), 92.

Carter, R. A. (2011). The new American pharmacist. *American Journal of Pharmaceutical Education*, *75*(9), 172.

DiPiro, J. T. (2011). Preparing our students for the many opportunities in pharmacy. *American Journal of Pharmaceutical Education*, *75*(9), 170.

Eady, M. J., & Lockyer, L. (2013). Tools for learning: Technology and teaching strategies. In *Learning to teach in the Primary School*. Australia: Queensland University of Technology. 71 p.

Engle, J. P., Erstad, B. L., Anderson, D. C., Jr., Bucklin, M. H., Chan, A., Donaldson, A. R., et al. (2014). Minimum qualifications for clinical pharmacy practice faculty. *Pharmacotherapy*, *34*(5), e38–e44. Available at https://www.accp.com/docs/positions/commentaries/EducAffrs13Commentary_FINAL.pdf.

FIP*Ed*. 2013. Global Education Report. FIP, The Hague. Available at http://www.fip.org/files/fip/FIPEd_Global_Education_Report_2013.pdf.

Francis, RQC (2013) Final report of the independent Inquiry into care provided by mid Staffordshire NHS Foundation Trust (on-line). Available at http://www.midstaffsinquiry.com/pressrelease.html.

Frenk, J., Chen, L., Bhutta, Z. A., Cohen, J., Crisp, N., Evans, T., et al. (2010). Health professionals for a new century: transforming education to strengthen health systems in an interdependent world. *The Lancet*, *376* (9756), 1923–1958.

Fuji, K. T., & Galt, K. A. (2009). Research skills training for the Doctor of Pharmacy in US Schools of Pharmacy: A descriptive study. *Indian Journal of Physiology and Pharmacology*, *17*(2), 115–121.

Hassali, M. A. (2011). Challenges and future directions for public health pharmacy education in developing countries. *American Journal of Pharmaceutical Education*, *75*(10), 195.

International Pharmaceutical Federation, (Ed.), (2014). *Quality assurance of pharmacy education: The FIP global framework* (2nd ed). The Hague: International Pharmaceutical Federation.

International Pharmaceutical Federation (FIP). (2017). *Transforming pharmacy and pharmaceutical sciences education in the context of workforce development*. The Hague: International Pharmaceutical Federation. Available at http://fip.org/files/fip/PharmacyEducation/2017/FIP_Nanjing_Report.pdf.

Jubraj, B. (2009). Developing a culture of self-directed workplace learning in pharmacy. *The Pharmaceutical Journal*, *275*, 48–52.

Kaufman, D. M. (2003). ABC of learning and teaching in medicine: Applying education theory in practice. *BMJ*, *326*, 213–216.

Meštrović, A., & Rouse, M. (2015). Pillars and foundations of quality for continuing education in pharmacy. *American Journal of Pharmaceutical Education*, *79*(3), 45.

Noble, C., Shaw, P. N., Nissen, L., Coombes, I., & O'Brien, M. (2011). Curriculum for uncertainty: Certainty may not be the answer. *American Journal of Pharmaceutical Education*, *75*(1), 13a.

Rennie, T. W., Haoses-Gorases, L., Lates, J., Mabirizi, D., Nyarang'o, P., & Sagwa, E. (2011). Sustaining Namibia: Improving the nation's health through sustainable pharmacy competency. *International Journal of Pharmaceutics*, *27*(1), 21–24.

Romanelli, F., Bird, E., & Ryan, M. (2009). Learning styles: A review of theory, application, and best practices. *American Journal of Pharmaceutical Education*, *73*(1), 9.

Salter, S., Karia, A., Sanfilippo, F., & Clifford, R. (2014). Effectiveness of E-learning in pharmacy education. *American Journal of Pharmaceutical Education*, *78*, 83.

WHO. (2016). *Global Strategy on human resources for health. Workforce 2030*. Geneva: WHO. Available at http://who.int/hrh/resources/pub_globstrathrh-2030/en/.

FURTHER READING

Bhutta, Z. A., Chen, L., Cohen, J., Crisp, N., Evans, T., Fineberg, H., et al. (2010). Education of health professionals for the 21st century: A global independent Commission. *Lancet*, *375*, 1137–1138.

CHAPTER

QUALITY AND ACCREDITATION IN PHARMACY EDUCATION

15

Ahmed Ibrahim Fathelrahman*,[a], Michael J. Rouse[†]

**College of Pharmacy, Taif University, Taif, Saudi Arabia, [†]Accreditation Council for Pharmacy Education (ACPE), Chicago, IL, United States*

INTRODUCTION

OVERVIEW

By reading this chapter the readers will appreciate basic concepts related to the quality and accreditation of pharmacy programs and be able to answer a group of questions such as;

- In general terms what is the meaning of quality, accreditation and certification?
- What are the philosophies behind accreditation?
- Are there differences and/or relationships between accreditation and certification?
- Does accreditation really indicate quality of education or improve the quality of education provided by the accredited colleges?
- What are the important bodies responsible for the academic accreditation of pharmacy education worldwide?
- Are there differences between accrediting bodies in the requirements for accreditation?
- Mapping accreditation standards of several accreditation bodies (ACPE, CCAPP, APC) against FIP's Global QA Framework.
- What important advice can be provided to a college planning for accreditation?

Quality is a universal issue, sought everywhere and involved in almost all fields of science, professions, and human activities. The culture and concepts of quality are very important for the pharmacy profession in particular, and quality is classically built in various pharmacy-related practices, such as manufacturing of medicines and pharmaceutical products, quality control analyses and assays for medicines and pharmaceutical products, preparation of some products in community pharmacies such as topical use preparations (e.g., ointments and creams), and other activities related to inventory control and drug supply management. Even in the modern era, the mission of pharmacy practice is described as

[a]Part of the chapter was written while the author was working with College of Pharmacy, Qassim University, Buraydah, Saudi Arabia.

Pharmacy Education in the Twenty First Century and Beyond. https://doi.org/10.1016/B978-0-12-811909-9.00015-0

contributing to health improvement and helping patients to make best use of their medicines, which is a philosophy built on a concept of quality (International Pharmaceutical Federation, 2012).

The concept of quality which was developed primarily in the industry environment was subjected to changes over decades starting from the notion of *quality control*, which focuses mainly on the inspection of the final product to check for its compliance with predetermined criteria, to the notion of *quality assurance*, which is based on monitoring quality during manufacturing processes at certain check points to provide confidence that quality will be fulfilled in the final product, to the notion of *total quality management*, which aims at building quality via controlling all factors that may determine the quality of the final product, including the financial and human resources, systems and policies, and leadership. These developments and changes in quality concept aimed at achieving more control of quality of the intended products. However, such changes reflect the dilemma that humanity faces while looking for quality. This means that every time people discover that what has already been established by way of concepts and criteria in order to achieve quality is found to be not enough to satisfy the quality-related needs, and that some amendments are needed. If we ask ourselves why people look for quality:

1. Some would say to achieve a low rate of errors in manufacturing or provision of services. In the context of pharmacy education, quality results in producing competent pharmacy graduates who commit lower rates of mistakes while practicing (e.g., fewer dispensing errors and fewer mistakes in pharmacotherapeutic and pharmaceutical care recommendations).
2. Some would say to improve customers' satisfaction by producing products or services that meet their expectations (e.g., a healthcare provider is satisfied with a drug information service and a patient is satisfied with a counseling session provided by a pharmacist).
3. Some would say to improve safety and reduce risk, which is another result of reducing errors and mistakes (e.g., reducing the drug-related mortality and reducing the health-related negative consequences associated with medication errors or using low-quality medications).
4. Some would say to optimize the use of the limited resources (i.e., serving a maximum number of patients using the minimum amount of resources including money, time, and facilities). This would lead us to an important conclusion: an important measure of quality should always be focusing on the final product (e.g., reducing deaths from diseases in hospitals, protecting the community from illness, reducing the rate of drug-related problems, increasing patients' quality of life, and increasing customers' satisfaction), although it is important to build quality through different steps and processes.

THE FIP GLOBAL FRAMEWORK FOR QUALITY ASSURANCE OF PHARMACY EDUCATION

In 2007, FIP in collaboration with WHO and UNESCO developed a global framework for quality assurance of pharmacy education. The framework was adopted by the FIP officially in September 2008 and a second edition was published in 2014.

The FIP Global Framework for Quality Assurance of Pharmacy Education included four main sections (International Pharmaceutical Federation, 2014):

Section A: Prerequisites for quality assurance in pharmacy education
Section B: Quality criteria and quality indicators for pharmacy education
Section C: The quality assurance agency
Section D: Glossary

According to the FIP Global Framework for Quality Assurance of Pharmacy Education:

1. Section A "describes the prerequisites and foundational elements that need to be in place or agreed in order to design, develop and implement an optimal quality assurance system for pharmacy education. It discusses the key players (stakeholders) who have an interest in quality education, and how they should be involved. It explores different approaches to quality assurance and continuous quality improvement." Fig. 1 describes the FIP Education Needs-Based Education Model.
2. Section B "discusses in more detail the criteria (areas) that must be addressed to assure quality under broad headings of context, structure, process, outcomes, and impact of pharmacy education (five "pillars" of quality), and science, practice, and ethics (three "foundations" of quality)" (Fig. 2).

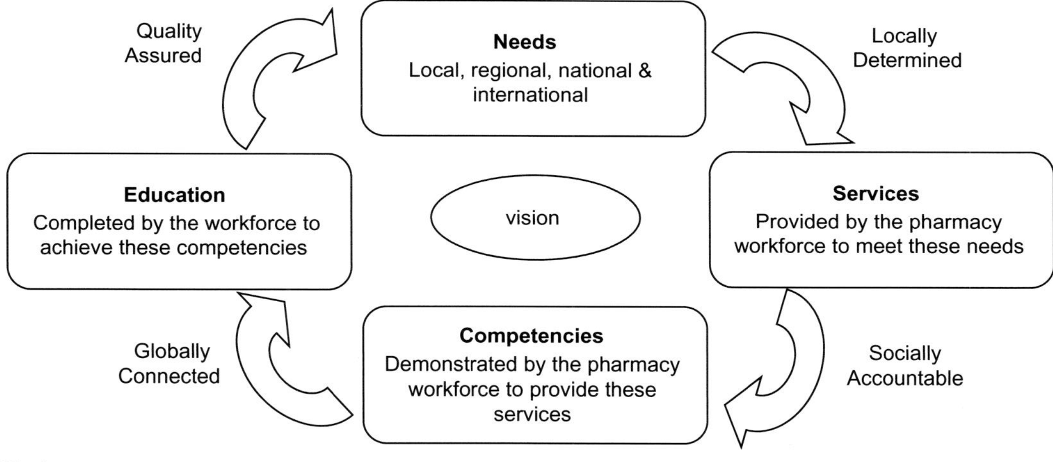

FIG. 1

FIP education needs-based education model (International Pharmaceutical Federation, 2014) used with permission from FIP.

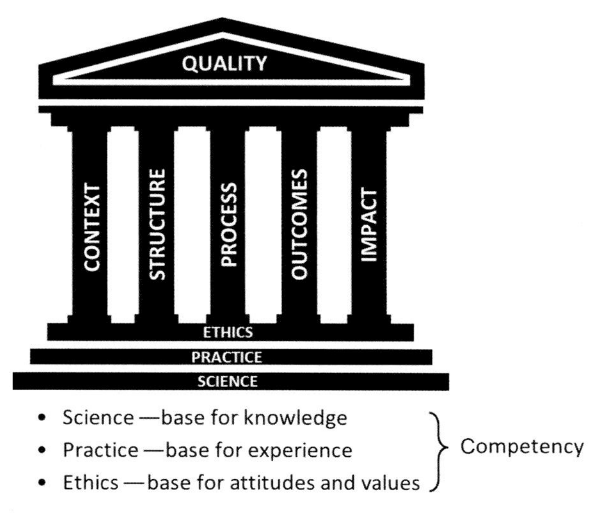

FIG. 2

The pillars and foundations of quality (International Pharmaceutical Federation, 2014; Meštrović & Rouse, 2015) used with permission from FIP and the American Journal of Pharmaceutical Education.

3. Section C "identifies the key elements or aspects of structure, governance, policies, and procedures that should be considered when establishing or restructuring a quality assurance agency/ organization/council or committee."
4. Section D represents a description of the general context in which important terms were used in the document by the authors.

IN GENERAL TERMS WHAT IS THE MEANING OF QUALITY, ACCREDITATION, AND CERTIFICATION?

Van Kemenade, Pupius, and Hardjono (2008) wrote about "more value to defining quality" and they said, "Former ways of thinking about quality are not sufficient any more to explain what is happening." About the meaning of quality of education, Van Kemenade et al. (2008) wrote "But what is quality of education? There is probably no answer to that question as there is no simple answer to the question: "What is life?" Van Kemenade et al. (2008) continued: "One of the most cited articles on quality in higher education was written by Harvey and Green (1993) under the title 'Defining quality.' Harvey and Green stated that quality is a slippery concept." According to Van Kemenade et al. (2008) those who wrote about quality and have tried to define it approached this from different perspectives and tend to define it based on multiple components, which indicates that quality is not a simple concept. Prisacariu and Shah (2016) argued that the "literature shows that it is still difficult to find agreement on a single definition of the concept. University leaders and quality assurance professionals define quality in many different ways." Prisacariu and Shah (2016) said, "Quality is a slippery and vague concept for which it is still difficult to find agreement on a single definition, regardless of its increasing popularity in higher education policy and practice." They mentioned also, "Rather, the definition is a matter of negotiation between the different parties involved. Hence, instead of trying to impose a global interpretation on the word, different definitions of quality have been used depending on the circumstances."

Harvey and Williams (2010) argued that "Quality in educational programmes has been variously conceptualised as meeting specified standards, being fit for purpose or as transformative. Melrose suggested a link between different concepts of quality and the paradigms of curriculum evaluation that influence the evaluative operations of academics. Readers were enabled to critically review their own evaluative practice against these descriptions and interpretations."

Promoting a culture of quality in the institution is essential to achieve quality and a quality journey is based on setting up the requirements/standards and having a good documentation of procedures, processes, and activities. Dellana and Hauser (1999) found an association between total quality management and organizational culture.

On the other hand, accreditation is "the process by which a (non-)governmental or private body evaluates the quality of a higher education institution (i.e., institutional accreditation) as a whole or of a specific educational program (i.e., programmatic accreditation) in order to formally recognize it as having met certain predetermined minimal criteria or standards" (Vlasceanu, Grunberg, & Parlea, 2007).

According to the FIP Global Framework for Quality Assurance of Pharmacy Education, accreditation means "the process whereby a statutory body, association or agency grants public recognition to an organization, site or program that meets certain established qualifications or standards, as determined through initial and periodic peer-review based evaluations" (International Pharmaceutical Federation, 2014).

The Council for Higher Education Accreditation (CHEA, USA) defines accreditation as "a process of external quality review created and used by higher education to scrutinize colleges, universities and programs for quality assurance and quality improvement."

According to the Canadian Council for Accreditation of Pharmacy Programs (CCAPP) "Accreditation is the public recognition accorded to a program that meets established educational standards through initial and periodic evaluation. Accreditation concerns itself with both quality assurance and program enhancement. It applies to programs and is to be distinguished from certification or licensure, which applies to individuals." It is clear from the CCAPP definition of accreditation that certification and licensure are different and they are used only linked to the individual practitioners' practice, including pharmacists, and do not indicate recognition of educational programs.

Harvey (2003) defines accreditation as "the establishment or re-statement of the status, legitimacy or appropriateness of an institution, program (i.e., composite of modules) or module of study.

McDavid and Huse (2015) define accreditation as a mechanism whereby an educational program of an educational institution is evaluated by a third party (accrediting body) against predetermined criteria, whereas they define certification as a process by which a person masters certain skills and competencies in a field as assessed by an external body (usually a professional society in the specialty). On the other hand, McDavid and Huse (2015) define licensure as an approval from a state or national legal governmental body to practice the profession with presence of penalties for those practicing without license. In some situations, the criteria for licensing are the same as certification and are based on professional societies' standards.

WHAT ARE THE PHILOSOPHIES BEHIND ACCREDITATION?

THE NATURE OF ACCREDITATION

In general, the term accreditation can be viewed as a mechanism for the achievement and the recognition of quality of an accredited academic program. It does not guarantee quality and it is not supposed to be the only way to achieve and sustain quality. This is like the fact that provision of healthcare services to the patients and the community does not guarantee health and wellness and it is not the only way to get them, but it is one mechanism used by those who are looking for health after losing it. A logical question might be raised: "Does a particular healthcare service provided to a patient or a group of patients actually contribute to an improvement or gain in health?" In a real situation, the answer may sometimes be "Yes" and sometimes "No." We wanted to find an answer to a similar question regarding accreditation: "Does a particular accreditation exercise undertaken by a pharmacy college actually contribute to an improvement or gain in quality?" The reader may find an answer to this question in Section "Does Accreditation Really Indicate Quality of Education or Improve the Quality of Education Provided by the Accredited Colleges?" of this chapter. Gaston (2014), while trying to answer the question "Is accreditation the best possible form of quality assurance for US higher education?" wrote, "We can transpose the well-known statement by Winston Churchill regarding democracy in describing accreditation as the worst form of quality assurance, except for all those other forms that have been tried from time to time." This is Gaston's philosophy and others may agree or disagree with him. As one mechanism concerned with quality, accreditation uses methods and has purposes that overlap with audit, quality assessment, and external examination (Harvey, 2003).

THE RATIONALE FOR ACCREDITATION

Some institutions seek accreditation to be recognized and receive credit from others (i.e., an accrediting body) regarding what is achieved. This can be used for marketing purpose to increase the demand for the accredited institution.

In the United States, not all academic programs look for accreditation. It is sought mainly by disciplines that qualify students for licensure, such as pharmacy, nursing, and engineering (i.e., the graduates who cannot practice without getting licensure must study at accredited programs) and the institutions looking to obtain federal funds, such as student aid (Gaston, 2014). Therefore, currently all established schools of pharmacy in the United States are accredited or in the process of applying. Eaton (2012) identified four roles for accreditation in the United States: assuring quality, enabling students to get access to federal and state funds, engendering private sector confidence, and allowing students to easily transfer courses and programs among colleges and universities.

GOVERNMENT VERSUS PRIVATE PLAYERS

In the United States, accreditation is not directly controlled by government. It is a self-regulated process of recognition of institutional viability by nongovernmental voluntary associations despite the presence of a government link via eligibility for federal funding (Harvey, 2003). However, in some countries, accreditation (especially national accreditation) might be a government requirement to get permission to operate under the umbrella of the Ministry of Higher Education. Achieving such accreditation means fulfilling minimum requirements of quality in the provided education. In Europe, for example, accreditation is controlled by national entities—either government departments or government-initiated agencies (Harvey, 2003). Accreditation is normally divided into two main categories: institutional and programmatic. This chapter focuses mainly on the programmatic accreditation. Institutional accreditation is a "license" for the institution to operate and it indicates the presence of minimum quality standards, such as qualifications of staff, research activities, student intake, and learning resources at the institution as a whole (Harvey, 2003).

ACCREDITATION AND INSTITUTIONAL VALUES

According to Gaston (2014), accreditation in the United States "has always reflected the values and priorities of those it accredits." Gaston (2014) concludes "accreditors therefore can usually be counted on to respect institutional autonomy: the right (within some constraints) of an institution or program to define its mission, to organize itself in pursuit of that mission, and to enjoy in that pursuit a healthy measure of self-determination, from the boardroom to the classroom."

Since accreditation is a mechanism of quality action and quality cannot be established unless it becomes an embedded culture in the academic institution, it should be established based on a core set of traditional academic values and beliefs (Eaton, 2012). According to Eaton, the US accreditation is based on five concepts:

1. Higher education institutions have primary responsibility for academic quality; colleges and universities are the leaders and the key sources of authority in academic matters.
2. Institutional mission is central to judgments of academic quality.
3. Institutional autonomy is essential to sustaining and enhancing academic quality.
4. Academic freedom flourishes in an environment of academic leadership of institutions.
5. The higher education enterprise and our society thrive on decentralization and diversity of institutional purpose and mission.

ARE THERE DIFFERENCES AND/OR RELATIONSHIPS BETWEEN ACCREDITATION AND CERTIFICATION?

It is clear from the previous section that certification is commonly applied to individuals who seek permission to practice, whereas accreditation is applied to the institutions and institutional programs to provide evidence that they are following certain quality criteria making them eligible for recognition. Table 1 describes the differences between accreditation, licensure, and certification. The two terms licensure and certification, however, are used interchangeably, sometimes inappropriately, to indicate the same thing.

Although many accreditation and practice regulatory bodies worldwide use the term certification to describe only individuals' credentials, the term is used by the US Accreditation Council for Pharmacy Education (ACPE) to describe the ACPE recognition of pharmacy degree programs outside the United States, instead of using "international accreditation." This is to differentiate it from the accreditation of the US national pharmacy programs.

Table 1 The Differences Between Certification, Licensure, and Accreditation

	Certification	Licensure	Accreditation
Scope	A process that is generally applicable to individuals[a]	A process that is applicable to individuals	A mechanism applicable to institutions and programs
Attribute	A credential to indicate eligibility for practice	Indicate eligibility for practice	Should indicate quality; compliance with a set of standards
Purpose	May qualify for licensure	Compulsory for practice	May be compulsory or voluntary; depends on the country's regulatory requirements
Offered by	A professional national or international society in the specialty	A state or national legal governmental body	An accrediting body can be a private nonprofit organization (NGO) or government

[a]*Certification is used by ACPE to describe the ACPE recognition of international pharmacy degree programs (outside the United States).*

Although they are basically different, accreditation, certification, and licensure sometimes are related. According to Harvey (2003), "in many professional areas, graduation from an appropriately accredited academic program is a preliminary step and full professional certification, and thus a licence to practice, follows only after some period of work experience." This means graduating from an accredited program may lead automatically to receiving a professional certification and such certification leads to receiving a licensure for practicing.

For the rest of the chapter, we are only going to use the term accreditation, as certification is a process that is generally applicable to individuals and refers to something else that is not included in the scope of this chapter. Certification, as it has been used by the ACPE, refers to the recognition of pharmacy degree programs outside the United States, and it can be treated in the same way as accreditation. However, readers will notice that some literature presented in some sections from this chapter uses the terminology "certification" to describe ISO-certification which is sought by some healthcare institutions and this can be considered as another mechanism for quality achievement and assessment.

WHAT IS ISO CERTIFICATION?

The ISO 9000 series, originally introduced in 1987, was created by the International Organization for Standardization (ISO) and over decades became a popular mechanism for quality management systems (QMS: a set of policies, processes, and procedures required for planning and execution in the core business area of an organization). ISO 9001 lists requirements an organization must maintain in their quality system for ISO 9001:2008 certification (i.e., ISO 9001-2008 is the only ISO standard that requires certification), while the other standards in the 9000 family provide guidelines and information. However, it is a common mistake that ISO 9001:2008 certification is described as "ISO 9000 certification" (9000 Store, 2017a). Slightly lower than half (43%) of the organizations seeking ISO 9001:2008 certification are service providers for various reasons, among which is to improve customer satisfaction and for market needs (9000 Store, 2017b). ISO 9001:2008 is focused on meeting customer expectations and delivering customer satisfaction via achieving consistent results and continually improving the process, and evaluating whether an organization's quality management system is appropriate and effective, while also forcing the organization to identify and implement improvements (9000 Store, 2017c).

DOES ACCREDITATION REALLY INDICATE QUALITY OF EDUCATION OR IMPROVE THE QUALITY OF EDUCATION PROVIDED BY THE ACCREDITED COLLEGES?

The literature documenting the impact of accreditation on pharmacy education and the link between them is limited. However, some evidence can be generated from studies conducted from other higher education fields. The literature on the impact of accreditation of healthcare institutions on the quality of care is another source of information that can be used to extrapolate the evidence.

SOME EVIDENCE FROM HEALTHCARE INSTITUTIONS (STUDIES ARE ARRANGED IN CHRONOLOGICAL ORDER)

The perceived impact of national accreditation of Lebanese hospitals on quality of care was assessed among nurses (El-Jardali, Jamal, Dimassi, Ammar, & Tchaghchaghian, 2008). The study revealed a positive perception among the nurses about the role of accreditation on the improvement of care. Respondents perceived improved teamwork and productivity in hospitals after accreditation. The study revealed differences in the impact of accreditation by hospital size. Medium-sized hospitals were more responsive to quality needs such as establishing policies and procedures and establishing new services (i.e., quality management). Hospital staff was more involved in accreditation in small-sized hospitals, which assisted hospitals to improve their quality. The researchers conclude "according to Lebanese nurses, hospital accreditation is a good tool for improving quality of care." It is important to note here that accreditation has been described by the researchers as a tool. The study proves a positive impact for accreditation on quality of care, but does not indicate an impact on the actual patient outcomes.

Thirty recently accredited (within 1 year) nongovernmental organizations' health units in Egypt matched with 30 units not programmed for accreditation were evaluated by a study conducted by Al Tehewy, Salem, Habil, and El Okda (2009). The study evaluated the providers' and the patients' satisfaction in the accredited health units compared to those in the nonaccredited ones. The satisfaction of the patients in the accredited health units was significantly higher with regards to cleanliness, waiting area, waiting time, and unit staff, and with regards to the overall satisfaction. The providers of the healthcare in the accredited health units expressed higher overall satisfaction, although no significant differences were found in the detailed evaluation items. Greater compliance with certain patient care standards was evident in the accredited health units; examples included the availability of clinical guidelines and an emergency drug list. Accredited health units showed better records of patient visits and greater compliance to infection control and safety standards.

The quality management in 89 hospitals from six European countries (Belgium, Czech Republic, France, Ireland, Poland, Spain, and the UK) was evaluated to identify systematic differences between accredited, ISO certified and neither accredited nor certified hospitals (Shaw, Groene, Mora, & Sunol, 2010). Accredited hospitals scored higher on the quality and safety standards: management, patient safety, clinical organization, clinical practice, environment and global scores compared with ISO certified or neither accredited nor certified hospitals. Analysis confirmed statistically significant differences comparing mean scores by type of hospital (accredited, ISO certified, and neither), but variations between accredited and certified hospitals were not substantially high. Two-factorial ANOVA analysis revealed an interaction between type of hospital and country. It appears that the effect of the country on the mean scores is greater than the contribution of hospital type (i.e., accredited, ISO certified, and neither).

Shaw et al. (2014) assessed the effect of ISO 9001 certification and accreditation on quality management in 4 clinical services in 73 hospitals from 7 European countries. The measures for quality management included the following items: (1) SER: specialized expertise and responsibility, which reflects clinical leadership and dissemination of clinical guidelines; (2) EBOP: evidence-based organization of pathways, which refers to critical elements in evidence-based clinical management; (3) PSS: patient safety strategies, which measure the use of commonly recommended safety procedures, such as hand hygiene, patient identification, and reporting of adverse events; (4) CR: clinical review, which reflects professional participation in the measurement of clinical practice against formal guidelines. SER, EBOP, PSS, and CR were treated as dependent variables and the measure of external assessment status (i.e. accreditation and certification) was treated as independent variable. Among findings was that both accreditation and certification are positively associated with clinical leadership, systems for patient safety, and clinical review, but not with clinical practice. Both of the two mechanisms promote structures and processes, which support patient safety and clinical organization but have limited impact on the provision of evidence-based patient care.

A mixed-method approach involving surveying 669 staff, documentary analyses, and semistructured interviews with 12 senior managers from 3 accredited public hospitals in Saudi Arabia was used to evaluate the impact of national accreditation on quality of care (Almasabi & Thomas, 2016). More than half of the respondents agreed that hospital accreditation has a positive impact on leadership, strategic planning, assessment of patient needs and expectations, using data and information on quality and records keeping and on the quality of care provided to patients. Accreditation allowed the hospitals to better use their internal resources. The documentary analyses indicated no significant improvement in terms of mortality rate; the infection rate had increased significantly in two hospitals and decreased in one hospital; and length of stay was significantly higher in one hospital and lower in another. However, substantial proportions of the respondents perceived a positive impact for accreditation on mortality rate, infection rate, and length of stay. A majority of respondents to the open-ended question declared that accreditation was focused on paperwork rather than on patient care. The researchers concluded that the study reported some improvement in procedure but no evidence of effect on quality outcomes was found.

SOME EVIDENCE FROM ACADEMIC INSTITUTIONS (STUDIES ARE ARRANGED IN CHRONOLOGICAL ORDER)

Coria, Deluca, and Martinez (2010) evaluated the impact of academic accreditation with special focus on curricular changes in pharmacy (19 degrees), biochemistry (19 degrees), and agriculture (30 degrees) undergraduate programs in Argentina. The accreditation process, which was implemented by the National Commission for University Evaluation and Accreditation (CONEAU), was compulsory. Respondents described the impact of the accreditation process on the quality of programs to be positive due to its contribution to curricular changes, getting more financial resources for upgrading infrastructure and equipment, and improving the program's information management. The authors concluded that "The accreditation processes had a significant impact on programmes since they allowed universities to implement the necessary changes in curricula, which for several reasons, could not be done before."

The experience of a medical college in Saudi Arabia with academic accreditation was reported by Al Mohaimeed, Midhet, Barrimah, and Saleh (2012). It was a mixed qualitative-quantitative study conducted in Qassim University College of Medicine after an accreditation process led by The Saudi National Commission for Academic Accreditation and Assessment (NCAAA). The accreditation exercise had a positive impact on various aspects, among which were reformulating the students' learning outcomes to match professional practice and regulation requirements, quality standards of education, curriculum planning and modifications to accommodate changes in national and international requirements in medical education, regular curriculum review and improvement, increasing the diversity of teaching and learning methods, and increasing the availability and access to educational resources.

Dattey, Westerheijden, and Hofman (2014) evaluated the differential impacts of accreditation during two cycles of assessments for accreditation between public and private universities in Ghana. Evaluators' reports revealed no statistically significant differences (i.e., improvement or deterioration) between the two cycles of assessments for both public and private institutions. Public universities achieved better aggregated assessment scores representing the two cycles, indicating greater improvements. Private universities were more likely than the public to implement suggestions for improvement by the evaluators. The authors explained the latter finding by concluding that the private universities more than the public had to struggle with coercive (complying with legislation), mimetic (copying the ways of their mentors), and normative (accepting the norms as established by the mentor institutions and the accreditation procedure) isomorphic pressures.

Hou et al. (2015) presented a case study of the impact of three programs' accreditors on higher education institutions in Taiwan, namely the Higher Education Evaluation & Accreditation Council of Taiwan (HEEACT), which is a nongovernmental quality assurance agency; Association to Advance Collegiate Schools of Business International (AACSB), which is a private US quality assurance agency; and Institute of Engineering Education Taiwan (IEET), which is a private Taiwanese quality assurance agency. The authors evaluated the impact of accreditation on Taiwanese universities with special focus on what has been described by prominent Australian scholar, Simon Marginson, as a *glonacal* education phenomenon, which means education institutes need to effectively respond to the global, national, and local needs and requirements. Analysis revealed that the three accreditation systems did have a great impact on learning outcomes-based teaching, self-enhancement mechanisms and internationalization in Taiwan's higher education institutions. However, the increased time and efforts by staff and faculty have created a resistance to all three program accreditations. The *glonacal* quality assurance system helped institutions setting up a self-enhancement quality mechanism and provided them with an opportunity to have more autonomy to develop their own features by choosing a suitable accreditation activity.

Sin, Tavares, and Amaral (2017) studied the impact of program accreditation on Portuguese higher education provision. Analyses proved that program accreditation has had great impact, reducing the number of programs (by 40% out of 5262 programs offered in the academic year 2009/2010 with a higher proportion of private sector programs discontinuing), increasing the number of PhD holders among teaching staff, and raising institutional awareness of quality.

CONCLUSIONS ON THE EVIDENCE OF THE EFFECT OF ACCREDITATION

Most of the evidence from the healthcare and academic institutions indicate that accreditation enhances the procedures, the processes, and the outputs; keeps the providers alert and enthusiastic for providing better services, and may enhance the satisfaction of the customers and the providers. However, no evidence is available on the presence of a positive effect of accreditation on the actual outcomes of the healthcare services or the academic programs.

WHAT ARE THE IMPORTANT BODIES RESPONSIBLE FOR THE ACADEMIC ACCREDITATION OF PHARMACY EDUCATION WORLDWIDE?

The International Network for Quality Assurance Agencies in Higher Education (INQAAHE) is a worldwide association of over 200 organizations active in the theory and practice of quality assurance in higher education. INQAAHE works closely with national bodies such as the Council for Higher Education Accreditation (CHEA, USA) and academicians to control educational quality in around 140 countries and acts to develop and promote standards of professional practice in quality assurance (QA). In 2003, the INQAAHE established Guidelines of Good Practice in Quality Assurance (commonly referred to as GGP) to promote professional practices among quality agencies. The GGP was revised in 2006 and 2014–2015 and published in its current version in 2016. The purpose of the GGP is to promote good practice for internal and/or external quality assurance. Specific goals include:

1. Creating a framework to guide the creation of new External Quality Assurance Agencies (EQAAs).
2. Providing criteria for use in the self and external evaluation of EQAAs.
3. Promoting professional development among EQAAs and their staff.
4. Promoting public accountability of EQAAs.

According to INQAAHE, a quality agency described as an External Quality Assurance Agency (EQAA) is a recognized, credible organization, trusted by the higher education institutions and the public. It has adequate mechanisms to prevent conflicts of interest in the decisions it makes and its staff has the needed skills to carry out the functions associated with external QA. The EQAA has the needed resources to carry out its mission.

The US Department of Education (USDE) establishes criteria for recognition of institutional and programmatic accreditors to assure that federal funding is provided to quality assured organizations (Gaston, 2014). CHEA is the top-level private organization in the United States that cares about the accreditation of higher education institutions (Eaton, 2012). It is a nonprofit national organization. It provides advocacy and recognizes higher education accrediting organizations that meet the CHEA standards in the United States (Gaston, 2014). However, this recognition is voluntary for the accreditation organization. CHEA is a member of INQAAHE.

The Accreditation Council for Pharmacy Education (ACPE, USA), the Canadian Council for Accreditation of Pharmacy Programs (CCAPP) and the Australian Pharmacy Council (APC) are examples of accreditation organizations (i.e., EQAAs) that work nationally and internationally to recognize pharmacy programs.

ARE THERE DIFFERENCES BETWEEN ACCREDITING BODIES IN THE REQUIREMENTS FOR ACCREDITATION?

Internationally active accrediting bodies have established certain requirements for accreditation of pharmacy programs. Such requirements are described as criteria in the case of ACPE and as standards in the case of CCAPP and APC. Most of the requirements are articulated in three main domains:

1. Curriculum: including teaching and learning strategies, learning outcomes, and required graduates' competencies, assessment of student learning, and curricular effectiveness.
2. Administration and systems: including management, planning, policies, leadership, mission and vision, collaboration within and outside the organization.
3. Resources: including human and financial resources and the available facilities.

However, different accreditation bodies state certain items much more explicitly than others and include some items implicitly under others.

Since quality requirements of pharmacy education depend on the local, regional, national, and international community's needs as described by the FIP Education Needs-Based Education Model (Fig. 1), accrediting bodies adopted criteria/standards for the international pharmacy programs that differ from those of the local/national programs. Accrediting bodies differentiated between the local and the international requirements in different ways. The ACPE replaced the term accreditation, which they used only to indicate their recognition of Doctor of Pharmacy (PharmD) degree programs using US standards, with the term "certification" to indicate their recognition of the international programs and accordingly adopted different criteria (note: the PharmD program in Lebanese American University, Lebanon, is the only pharmacy program outside the US ACPE accredited using US PharmD standards). The CCAPP, although describing their recognition of both local and international programs as "accreditation," adopted different sets of standards. APC also adopted the same descriptive term "accreditation" and used the same set of standards for both the local and the international programs; however, they considered some standards only applicable for the local (Australian) programs and accordingly the only possible accreditation status of the international programs is "accreditation with condition." Certification status in the case of ACPE is either certification or provisional certification. Provisional certification may be awarded to a program that has factors that compromise compliance with the Certification Quality Criteria, but that has initiated appropriate plans to address such factors, and meets all ACPE's requirements for such recognition. Accreditation status in the case of CCAPP is either accreditation (i.e., full), conditional accreditation (meaning there are some areas that need to be improved), or provisional accreditation (for those programs that have not graduated students yet). However, the CCAPP Board has agreed to use the term accreditation rather than full accreditation, etc. Accreditation will be for a defined period of time. If there are things to fix, the length of the accreditation awarded will be shorter.

As of 2017, programs of seven international pharmacy schools are certified by ACPE, five international pharmacy schools are accredited by CCAPP, and a program of one international pharmacy school is accredited (with condition) by the APC. Table 2 summarizes the differences between ACPE, CCAPP, and APC.

Table 2 The Differences Between ACPE, CCAPP, and APC

	ACPE	CCAPP	APC
Descriptive term of recognition	Accreditation for the US[a] versus certification for the international programs	Accreditation for the local and international accreditation for international programs	Accreditation for both the local and international programs
Requirements	Described as criteria for certification of international programs and standards for accreditation of local programs	Described as standards/ different for accreditation of international programs compared to local programs	Described as standards/ some are not applicable for international programs compared to local programs
Accreditation status	Certification or provisional certification for international programs; accreditation for US[a] programs	Full accreditation, conditional accreditation or provisional accreditation	Only accredited with conditions for international programs and accreditation for local programs

Continued

Table 2 The Differences Between ACPE, CCAPP, and APC—cont'd

	ACPE	CCAPP	APC
Recognized international pharmacy degree programs	**1.** Jagadguru Sri Shivarathreeswara (JSS) University College of Pharmacy, Mysuru and Ooty, India **2.** The University of Jordan (UJ) School of Pharmacy—Amman, Jordan **3.** Near East University Faculty of Pharmacy—Nicosia, Northern Cyprus **4.** King Faisal University College of Clinical Pharmacy—Al Ahsa, KSA **5.** King Saud University College of Pharmacy—Riyadh, KSA **6.** Qassim University College of Pharmacy—Al Qassim, KSA **7.** Al Ain University of Science and Technology College of Pharmacy—Al Ain and Abu Dhabi, United Arab Emirates (UAE) Source: ACPE (2017)	**1.** Beirut Arab University, Lebanon (Conditional International Accreditation Status 2015–2017) **2.** King Abdulaziz University—Jeddah, KSA (International Accreditation Status 2017–2023) **3.** King Faisal University—Al Ahsa, KSA (Conditional International Accreditation Status 2014–2017) **4.** King Saud University—Riyadh, KSA (Provisional International Accreditation Status 2014—June 2017) **5.** Qatar University—Doha, Qatar (Full Accreditation Status 2014–2018) Source: CCAPP (2017a, 2017b)	*Monash University*, Malaysia (Accredited with Conditions) Source: APC (2017)

[a] *The PharmD program in Lebanese American University, Lebanon is the only pharmacy program outside the US accredited using US PharmD standards.*

MAPPING ACCREDITATION STANDARDS OF SEVERAL ACCREDITATION BODIES (ACPE, CCAPP, APC) AGAINST FIP'S GLOBAL QA FRAMEWORK

Table 3 shows the mapping of accreditation standards of ACPE (2016), CCAPP (2017a, 2017b), and APC (2012) against FIP's Global QA Framework indicators (International Pharmaceutical Federation, 2014). ACPE, CCAPP, and APC were invited to review and edit the draft mapping produced by the authors. Some changes, but not all changes, proposed by the accreditors were accepted. A standard or criterion was considered matching a FIP indicator whenever there is some similarity in the principal focus and or scope of the compared items. However, it is important to notice that:

1. Similarity between an accreditation standard/criterion and an FIP indicator in some situation is partial and not full.

2. Mapping is based on the main standards (in case of CCAPP and APC) and criteria (in case of ACPE) of the accreditor. However, in certain situations the relationship between an accreditor's standard/criteria and a FIP indicator might not be very clear without reading the substandard/subcriteria or reading the guidance/best practice that elaborates more on the standard/criteria. So, the absence of a relationship in Table 3 does not indicate total absence of an actual relationship as the purpose of the mapping is the general comparison.
3. The categorization of the standards/criteria (e.g., under sections in the case of ACPE and parts and subparts ranked with alphabetical numbering in the case of CCAPP) is not similar among the accreditation bodies but comparable.
4. Some items might be stated earlier in the criteria of one accreditor and stated later in the criteria of another accreditor, so they are not similarly arranged.
5. The FIP indicators are very detailed (71 indicators) whereas ACPE, CCAPP and APC criteria might be generally stated (26 criteria for ACPE, 24 standards for CCAPP, and 36 standards for APC). However, some accreditors provide a breakdown on their criteria/standards into substandards in separate documents.
6. Variations among accreditors and between their criteria and the FIP indicators sometimes are due to:

a. The same ideas being emphasized in different resources (accreditor criteria or FIP indicators) but using different wordings and descriptions. For example, FIP stated that "Learning objectives of courses are appropriate to achieve the desired competencies" (indicator 21), whereas APC stated "pharmacy program produces graduates who have the graduate attributes of the university and the knowledge, skills and attitudes necessary to commence supervised practice as an intern pharmacist" (standard 25), which describes competencies using different wordings (i.e., knowledge, skills, and attitudes).

b. The same descriptions are used by different accreditors or the FIP in different contexts to highlight different ideas. For example, the involvement of "stakeholders" is mentioned by the FIP (indicator 4) and ACPE (criterion 1) in the development of the school's mission, goals, and values and mentioned by ACPE with regards to strategic planning (criterion 3) and mentioned by the APC regarding the "review of curriculum content, delivery and evaluation and student assessment methods" (standard 18).

c. Some ideas are described by the particular accreditor partially, stressing specific quality needs, while other accreditors described the idea in a broader scope. For example, the FIP quality indicator number 19 "collaborative relationships and partnerships," which is described by the FIP using general terms, was covered by APC in the context of experiential learning (standard 7) and with regards to review of curriculum content, delivery, and evaluation and student (standard 18).

d. Some standards/criteria of an accreditor may represent a breakdown of a generally stated standard/criterion of the other accreditor.

Table 4 describes the accreditation standards of ACPE, CCAPP, and APC that were not matched well with FIP's Global QA Framework indicators.

Table 3 Mapping Accreditation Standards of Several Accreditation Bodies (ACPE, 2016; APC, 2012; and CCAPP, 2017a, 2017b) Against FIP's Global QA Framework

	FIP Global Framework Quality Indicator	ACPE Criteria	CCAPP Standards	APC Standards
Quality indicators related to Context				
1	The mission and goals of the school reflect and consider the national environment, needs, and priorities	*Criterion No. 1*: *Mission, Goals, and Values* The school operates under a defined mission, which is compatible with the mission of the university and is developed with broad input from school stakeholders. The mission, goals, and values reflect a commitment to continuous quality improvement in education, research, scholarship, and community service, and to being socially accountable in its activities	*Standard 10*: The Faculty has a vision and mission aligned with that of the University in education, practice, research, and other scholarly activities	*Standard 4*: The School of Pharmacy has an operational plan that is aligned to deliver the objectives of the university's strategic plan and which specifies the School's mission, objectives, and key performance indicators/targets against which performance and achievements are regularly measured *Guidance*[a] "In developing its operational plan, the School of Pharmacy should consult with both internal and external stakeholders who have a legitimate interest in the program, such as academic staff, members of the profession, professional organizations and the community, students, and relevant government and healthcare entities"
2	The mission and goals of the school are aligned with the profession-wide vision for pharmacy practice and education	*Criterion No. 2*: *Professional, Ethical and Harmonious Environment* The school values and provides an environment that promotes professional and ethical behavior, effective	*Standard 2*: The Faculty provides an environment and culture that promotes professional behavior and harmonious relationships among students, and between students and faculty members,	

Table 3 Mapping Accreditation Standards of Several Accreditation Bodies (ACPE, 2016; APC, 2012; and CCAPP, 2017a, 2017b) Against FIP's Global QA Framework—cont'd

	FIP Global Framework Quality Indicator	ACPE Criteria	CCAPP Standards	APC Standards
		communication, and harmonious and productive relationships among administrators, academic and other staff, preceptors, and students	administrators, preceptors, and staff	
3	The mission and goals of the school are aligned with the mission and goals of the university (if applicable)	*Criterion No. 1*: *Mission, Goals, and Values*	*Standard 10*: The Faculty has a vision and mission aligned with that of the University in education, practice, research, and other scholarly activities	*Standard 4*: The School of Pharmacy has an operational plan that is aligned to deliver the objectives of the university's strategic plan and that specifies the School's mission, objectives, and key performance indicators/targets against which performance and achievements are regularly measured
4	The mission, goals, and values of the school are developed with input from key stakeholders (internal and external)	*Criterion No. 1*: *Mission, Goals, and Values*	*Standard 14*: The Faculty has a current strategic plan that is systematically reviewed and updated to facilitate the achievement of the Faculty's mission, vision, goals, and objectives. *Criterion 14.1* The planning process provides for broad-based input from faculty members, students, practitioners, alumni, and other key stakeholders or constituent groups[a]	*Standard 4*: The School of Pharmacy has an operational plan that is aligned to deliver the objectives of the university's strategic plan and that specifies the School's mission, objectives, and key performance indicators/targets against which performance and achievements are regularly measured *Guidance*[a] "In developing its operational plan, the School of Pharmacy should consult with both internal and

Continued

Table 3 Mapping Accreditation Standards of Several Accreditation Bodies (ACPE, 2016; APC, 2012; and CCAPP, 2017a, 2017b) Against FIP's Global QA Framework—cont'd

	FIP Global Framework Quality Indicator	ACPE Criteria	CCAPP Standards	APC Standards
				external stakeholders who have a legitimate interest in the program, such as academic staff, members of the profession, professional organizations and the community, students, and relevant government and healthcare entities"
5	The education program is designed and delivered based on national and professional needs and priorities	*Criterion No. 1*: *Mission, Goals, and Values*	*Criterion 1.1*: Educational outcomes and entry-to-practice competencies are based, at a minimum, on a recognized national body's current description of the ethical, legal and professional responsibilities of a pharmacist in the nation where the professional program is based[a]	
6	Changes in science, practice, and regulation influence the content, design, and delivery of the program	*Criterion No. 8*: *Competencies of Graduates* The school clearly identifies and publishes the competencies that graduates must achieve to address current and future national medication and health-related needs and policies	*Criterion 1.2*: The curriculum educational framework and any subsequent changes are documented and evaluated against the entry-to-practice competencies and edcucation competencies[a]	*Standard 20*: The curriculum of the pharmacy program demonstrates congruency with contemporary pharmaceutical sciences, pharmacotherapeutics and pharmacy practice and the pharmacy learning domains
7	Curricular changes are visible, consensus based, and aligned with changes impacting the pharmacy profession	*Criterion No. 8* *Criterion No. 9*: *Design and Development of the Curriculum* The school, through a defined process, uses	*Standard 17*: A governance structure within the faculty directs and supports the design, development, implementation,	

Table 3 Mapping Accreditation Standards of Several Accreditation Bodies (ACPE, 2016; APC, 2012; and CCAPP, 2017a, 2017b) Against FIP's Global QA Framework—cont'd

	FIP Global Framework Quality Indicator	ACPE Criteria	CCAPP Standards	APC Standards
		the desired graduate competencies to design and develop the curricular philosophy, structure, content, and instructional methods	formative assessment, and review of a curriculum that satisfies the educational outcomes required for the professional program in pharmacy. *Criterion 17.2*: Regular systematic review of the curricular structure, content, process, and outcomes are conducted[a]	
8	The educational program provides national and international perspectives on the topics being taught.			
9	The school implements strategies and programs to broaden the scientific and professional horizons of students.	*Criterion No. 11*: *Curricular Foundation in the Sciences* The curricular content provides students with the necessary foundation in the biomedical, pharmaceutical, social/behavioral/administrative and clinical sciences to achieve the desired graduate competencies. The science foundation courses are appropriately sequenced, and the desired knowledge and skills are introduced, reinforced, and advanced progressively throughout the curriculum	*Standard No. 4*: The curriculum includes foundational content in: biomedical, pharmaceutical, behavioral, social, and administrative pharmacy sciences; clinical sciences including clinical practice skills and practice experiences	

Continued

Table 3 Mapping Accreditation Standards of Several Accreditation Bodies (ACPE, 2016; APC, 2012; and CCAPP, 2017a, 2017b) Against FIP's Global QA Framework—cont'd

	FIP Global Framework Quality Indicator	ACPE Criteria	CCAPP Standards	APC Standards
10	The school provides and/or supports the delivery of educational programs to its graduates and other pharmacy professionals in the form of CE and CPD activities to inform and influence pharmacy practice			
11	The school's commitment to the generation, dissemination, and application of new knowledge is evident and demonstrated by productive research, publications, and other scholarly activities	*Criterion No. 1*: *Mission, Goals, and Values* *Criterion No. 19*: *Academic and Other Staff Resources—Quantitative* The school has a sufficient number of qualified full-time academic staff, other staff, and preceptors to effectively deliver and evaluate the degree program, while providing adequate time for academic staff development, research and other scholarly activities, student advising, service, and, where applicable, pharmacy practice. *Criterion No. 20*: *Academic Staff Resources—Qualitative* The composition of the academic staff, including contributions from collaborative relationships and preceptors,	*Criterion 8.2*: The university demonstrates a commitment to research and other scholarly activities through appropriate infrastructure, in order to create an environment of scholarship for faculty members and students[a]	*Standard 14*: The School of Pharmacy actively promotes and supports research and scholarship

Table 3 Mapping Accreditation Standards of Several Accreditation Bodies (ACPE, 2016; APC, 2012; and CCAPP, 2017a, 2017b) Against FIP's Global QA Framework—cont'd

	FIP Global Framework Quality Indicator	ACPE Criteria	CCAPP Standards	APC Standards
		encompasses the biomedical, pharmaceutical, social/behavioral/administrative, and clinical science disciplines, and meets the needs of the education, research, and service elements of the mission of the school		
12	The school embraces the obligation to be socially accountable and strives to address national and community needs through its educational, research and service activities	*Criterion No. 1*: *Mission, Goals, and Values*	*Standard 9*: The Faculty has University support for affiliations, collaborations, and partnerships (internal and external to the University) necessary to advance the education, research, clinical practices, and service mission of the Faculty	
13	The school provides and supports projects and activities that bring about positive changes in society	*Criterion No. 1*: *Mission, Goals, and Values*		
Quality indicators related to structure				
14	The director of the school has appropriate qualifications and experience in pharmacy education to provide strong and visible leadership and ensure the quality of the professional degree program	*Criterion No. 7*: *Organizational Structure and Governance of the School* The dean of the school and other administrative leaders are qualified, have defined lines of responsibility and authority, and function in an organizational structure that assures	*Standard 13*: The Faculty, under the leadership of a Dean/Director, fulfills its mandate in its professional program, research and scholarly mission	*Standard 5*: The School of Pharmacy has a designated leader with requisite profession-specific experience and expertise who is responsible for the provision of professional and academic leadership, engagement and advocacy for the School and the

Continued

Table 3 Mapping Accreditation Standards of Several Accreditation Bodies (ACPE, 2016; APC, 2012; and CCAPP, 2017a, 2017b) Against FIP's Global QA Framework—cont'd

	FIP Global Framework Quality Indicator	ACPE Criteria	CCAPP Standards	APC Standards
		the optimal use and development of academic and nonacademic staff resources. The governance documents of the school (such as bylaws and policies) describe the organizational structure, the decision-making process, responsibility for human, physical, technological, educational, and financial resources, and the functions and responsibilities of committees and meetings of academic staff		profession within and beyond the institution
15	Members of the school administration have defined lines of authority and responsibility	*Criterion No. 7: Organizational Structure and Governance of the School*	*Standard 12*: The Faculty is organized in a manner that facilitates the accomplishment of its mission and progress towards its vision	*Standard 2*: The School of Pharmacy is a clearly defined operational entity within the organizational, corporate, and academic governance structures, and has systems of academic and administrative responsibility and accountability within the university *Standard 6*: The School of Pharmacy has designated authority and autonomy within the university to design, develop, deliver, and evaluate their pharmacy program

Table 3 Mapping Accreditation Standards of Several Accreditation Bodies (ACPE, 2016; APC, 2012; and CCAPP, 2017a, 2017b) Against FIP's Global QA Framework—cont'd

	FIP Global Framework Quality Indicator	ACPE Criteria	CCAPP Standards	APC Standards
16	Members of the school's administration foster organizational unit development and collegiality, and appropriately allocate resources	*Criterion No. 7*: *Organizational Structure and Governance of the School*		*Standard 2*: The School of Pharmacy is a clearly defined operational entity within the organizational, corporate, and academic governance structures, and has systems of academic and administrative responsibility and accountability within the university
17	Time, facilities and resources are well managed	*Criterion No. 7*: *Organizational Structure and Governance of the School*	*Standard 21*: The Faculty has adequate financial resources so that continuing operation of the professional programs and other elements of the Faculty mission are fulfilled	*Standard 9*: The School of Pharmacy has general and specialized teaching facilities, learning resources, and equipment of appropriate type, size, and quantity for the effective delivery of the pharmacy program *Standards 10*: The School of Pharmacy has a planned approach for the review of facilities, resources, and support infrastructure to accord with significant program changes and to inform future needs and facilitate the requisite forward planning *Standard 36*: The School of Pharmacy has a documented risk management plan for assuring continuity of program delivery

Continued

Table 3 Mapping Accreditation Standards of Several Accreditation Bodies (ACPE, 2016; APC, 2012; and CCAPP, 2017a, 2017b) Against FIP's Global QA Framework—cont'd

	FIP Global Framework Quality Indicator	ACPE Criteria	CCAPP Standards	APC Standards
18	Committees are established to identify and address key components of the mission and goals	*Criterion No. 7*: *Organizational Structure and Governance of the School*	*Standard 12*: The Faculty is organized in a manner that facilitates the accomplishment of its mission and progress towards its vision	*Standard 3*: The university governance structures facilitate appropriate representation of the School of Pharmacy on decision-making committees within the university and establish the functions/roles, authority, and reporting relationships of the committees at a School, faculty and/or university level
19	The school develops collaborative relationships and partnerships with stakeholders (internal and external)	*Criterion No. 3*: *Strategic Planning and Continuous Quality Improvement* The school has a systematic process of planning, implementation, and monitoring to support the achievement and advancement of its mission and values. Strategic planning involves input from the stakeholders of the school. Administrators identify and allocate the necessary resources to implement and achieve desired improvements *Criterion No. 5*: *School and University Internal Relationships*: The school and its leadership are defined within the university structure. The university and school policies and procedures clearly define	*Criterion 14.1*: The planning prcess provides for broad-based input from faculty members, students, practitioners, alumni, and other key stakeholders or constituent groups[a]	*Standard 7*: The School of Pharmacy has active and ongoing partnerships or associations with relevant professional, government, health, indigenous and community agencies through which matters of mutual interest are progressed. formal relationships exist with healthcare providers, practitioners, and services to facilitate access to appropriate experiential placements *Standard 18*: Review of curriculum content, delivery, and evaluation and student assessment methods is undertaken through broad stakeholder engagement and use of a consultative and collaborative approach

Table 3 Mapping Accreditation Standards of Several Accreditation Bodies (ACPE, 2016; APC, 2012; and CCAPP, 2017a, 2017b) Against FIP's Global QA Framework—cont'd

	FIP Global Framework Quality Indicator	ACPE Criteria	CCAPP Standards	APC Standards
		respective authority and responsibility. The school contributes to the activities and governance of the university. The school works effectively with other units within the university. The university and school leadership collaborate to secure adequate human, physical, technological, educational, and financial resources to maintain and advance the program *Criterion No. 6*: *External Collaborative Relationships* To support and advance its mission, the school establishes and maintains, with the support of the university, collaborative relationships with organizations and entities outside the university that work in education, research, and other scholarly activity, industry, practice, and community service		
20	The school evaluates the outcomes and impact of collaborative relationships and partnerships	*Criterion No. 3*: Strategic Planning and Continuous Quality Improvement *Criterion No. 4*: *Assessment of Achievement of Mission and Goals* The school establishes	*Standard 15*: The Faculty establishes and maintains systems that measure and evaluate the extent to which the mission, vision, goals, and objectives are achieved	*Standard 4*: The School of Pharmacy has an operational plan that is aligned to deliver the objectives of the University's strategic plan and that specifies the School's mission, objectives, and key

Continued

Table 3 Mapping Accreditation Standards of Several Accreditation Bodies (ACPE, 2016; APC, 2012; and CCAPP, 2017a, 2017b) Against FIP's Global QA Framework—cont'd

	FIP Global Framework Quality Indicator	ACPE Criteria	CCAPP Standards	APC Standards
		and uses measures to evaluate the achievement of the mission and goals. Assessment data are used to identify opportunities for quality improvement and shape future goals and planning. Assessment involves input from stakeholders of the school		performance indicators/targets against which performance and achievements are regularly measured
21	Learning objectives of courses are appropriate to achieve the desired competencies	*Criterion No. 9: Design and Development of the Curriculum* The school, through a defined process, uses the desired graduate competencies to design and develop the curricular philosophy, structure, content, and instructional methods	*Standard 15*: The Faculty establishes and maintains systems that measure and evaluate the extent to which the mission, vision, goals, and objectives are achieved	*Standard 25*: The pharmacy program produces graduates who have the graduate attributes of the university and the knowledge, skills, and attitudes necessary to commence supervised practice as an intern pharmacist
22	Curricular content is well aligned with the official (legal) scope of practice of pharmacists	*Criterion No. 12: Simulation and Practice Experiences* The curriculum provides educational experiences in actual and simulated pharmacy practice settings to develop and demonstrate achievement of the desired competencies, under academic staff responsibility and practitioner guidance. The practice experiences and simulations integrate, apply, reinforce, and advance the knowledge, skills, attitudes, and values developed throughout the curriculum		*Standard 25*: The pharmacy program produces graduates who have the graduate attributes of the university and the knowledge, skills, and attitudes necessary to commence supervised practice as an intern pharmacist

Table 3 Mapping Accreditation Standards of Several Accreditation Bodies (ACPE, 2016; APC, 2012; and CCAPP, 2017a, 2017b) Against FIP's Global QA Framework—cont'd

	FIP Global Framework Quality Indicator	ACPE Criteria	CCAPP Standards	APC Standards
23	The curriculum provides a thorough foundation (knowledge base) in the biomedical, pharmaceutical, social, behavioral, administrative, and clinical sciences	*Criterion No. 11*: *Curricular Foundation in the Sciences*	*Standard 4*: The curriculum includes foundational content in: biomedical, pharmaceutical, behavioral, social, and administrative pharmacy sciences; clinical sciences including clinical practice skills; and practice experiences	*Standard 20*: The curriculum of the pharmacy program demonstrates congruency with contemporary pharmaceutical sciences, pharmacotherapeutics and pharmacy practice, and the pharmacy learning domains
24	Educational activities are based on science, practice, and ethics to address all competency areas (knowledge, skills, attitudes, values)	*Criterion No. 2*: *Professional, Ethical and Harmonious Environment* *Criterion No. 11*: *Curricular Foundation in the Sciences*	*Standard 2*: The Faculty provides an environment and culture that promotes professional behavior and harmonious relationships among students, and between students and faculty members, administrators, preceptors, and staff *Standard 5*: Practice experiences are of adequate intensity, breadth, structure, duration, and variety so as to achieve educational outcomes. Practice experiences are acquired in high-quality practice settings in a variety of care sectors, involving patients with a variety of healthcare service needs. Experiences integrate, reinforce, and advance the knowledge, skills, attitudes, and values developed through the other components of the professional program	*Standard 20*: The curriculum of the pharmacy program demonstrates congruency with contemporary pharmaceutical sciences, pharmacotherapeutics and pharmacy practice and the pharmacy learning domains *Standard 22*: The School of Pharmacy has clearly defined experiential learning outcomes embedded within the curriculum, provides students with learning opportunities in hospital and community practice settings to meet those outcomes, and applies assessment methods for assuring those outcomes are met

Continued

Table 3 Mapping Accreditation Standards of Several Accreditation Bodies (ACPE, 2016; APC, 2012; and CCAPP, 2017a, 2017b) Against FIP's Global QA Framework—cont'd

	FIP Global Framework Quality Indicator	ACPE Criteria	CCAPP Standards	APC Standards
25	The school has a sufficient number of qualified full-time academic (including pharmacy trained) and other staff to effectively deliver and evaluate the professional degree program	*Criterion No. 19*: *Academic and Other Staff Resources—Quantitative* *Criterion No. 20*: *Academic Staff Resources—Qualitative*	*Standard 19*: The Faculty has sufficient human resources, including appropriately qualified faculty members, support and administrative staff, and preceptors to effectively deliver and evaluate the professional program	*Standard 11*: The School of Pharmacy has an academic staff complement that ensures an appropriate level of expertise in the pharmaceutical sciences, pharmacotherapeutics, and pharmacy practice to: • Effectively develop, deliver and evaluate the pharmacy program; • provide for timely access and interaction with students as individuals or small groups; and • achieve a balance between teaching, administration, research/scholarship and clinical/professional practice by the academic staff *Standard 15*: The School of Pharmacy has sufficient type and number of administrative and professional staff to support the educational program, the operation of the School, and the effective management of resources

Table 3 Mapping Accreditation Standards of Several Accreditation Bodies (ACPE, 2016; APC, 2012; and CCAPP, 2017a, 2017b) Against FIP's Global QA Framework—cont'd

	FIP Global Framework Quality Indicator	ACPE Criteria	CCAPP Standards	APC Standards
26	The school identifies trained pharmacist preceptors who have the expertise, experience, and commitment to facilitate learning and evaluate the achievement of required competencies by students	*Criterion No. 20*: *Academic Staff Resources—Qualitative*	*Standard 19*: The Faculty has sufficient human resources, including appropriately qualified faculty members, support and administrative staff, and preceptors to effectively deliver and evaluate the professional program	*Standard 11*: The School of Pharmacy has an academic staff complement that ensures an appropriate level of expertise in the pharmaceutical sciences, pharmacotherapeutics, and pharmacy practice to: • Effectively develop, deliver, and evaluate the pharmacy program; • provide for timely access and interaction with students as individuals or small groups; and • achieve a balance between teaching, administration, research/ scholarship, and clinical/ professional practice by the academic staff *Standard 23*: The School of Pharmacy coordinates, monitors and regularly reviews the quality and performance of the experiential learning elements of the program

Continued

Table 3 Mapping Accreditation Standards of Several Accreditation Bodies (ACPE, 2016; APC, 2012; and CCAPP, 2017a, 2017b) Against FIP's Global QA Framework—cont'd

	FIP Global Framework Quality Indicator	ACPE Criteria	CCAPP Standards	APC Standards
27	The school has established and implemented criteria for the selection of an adequate number and mix of pharmacy practice facilities and sites for students' experiential education	*Criterion No. 25*: *Pharmacy Practice Sites and Preceptors* The school has an adequate number, balance, and mix of practice sites and preceptors in community, hospital, and other settings to support the curricular pharmacy practice experiences, taking into account any national regulations or expectations. The school has criteria to ensure that sites and preceptors are of high quality and committed to advancing practice in their respective settings. The school uses the established criteria to approve sites and preceptors prior to students undertaking their practice experience at the site. The school has an effective system for communicating with sites and preceptors, and evaluating the site, preceptor, and students' experiences and outcomes	*Standard 20*: The Faculty selects practice sites where student learning and skills development are adequately managed, supported, and supervised. Practice sites meet relevant regulatory requirements	*Standard 7*: The School of Pharmacy has active and ongoing partnerships or associations with relevant professional, government, health, indigenous, and community agencies through which matters of mutual interest are progressed, formal relationships exist with healthcare providers, practitioners, and services to facilitate access to appropriate experiential placements *Standard 9*: The School of Pharmacy has general and specialized teaching facilities, learning resources, and equipment of appropriate type, size, and quantity for the effective delivery of the pharmacy program *Standard 22*: The School of Pharmacy has clearly defined experiential learning outcomes embedded within the curriculum, provides students with learning opportunities in hospital and community practice settings to meet those outcomes, and applies assessment methods for assuring those outcomes are met

Table 3 Mapping Accreditation Standards of Several Accreditation Bodies (ACPE, 2016; APC, 2012; and CCAPP, 2017a, 2017b) Against FIP's Global QA Framework—cont'd

	FIP Global Framework Quality Indicator	ACPE Criteria	CCAPP Standards	APC Standards
				Standard 23: The School of Pharmacy coordinates, monitors, and regularly reviews the quality and performance of the experiential learning elements of the program
28	The physical facilities are safe, well maintained, and adequately equipped for teaching, learning, and research	*Criterion No. 23*: *Physical Facilities* The school has adequate physical facilities to achieve its mission. The facilities provide a comfortable, well-equipped, and safe environment for administration, teaching, learning, and research, and enable effective interaction between administrators, academic and other staff, and students. Facilities and resources for different groups of students, academic and other staff assure comparable experiences and opportunities, and comparable educational outcomes for all students	*Standard 22*: Physical facilities and infrastructure of the Faculty and those at other University sites where students and faculty members are located are adequate and appropriately equipped to achieve the stated mission	*Standard 9*: The School of Pharmacy has general and specialized teaching facilities, learning resources, and equipment of appropriate type, size, and quantity for the effective delivery of the pharmacy program *Standards 10*: The School of Pharmacy has a planned approach for the review of facilities, resources, and support infrastructure to accord with significant program changes and to inform future needs and facilitate the requisite forward planning *Standard 14*: The School of Pharmacy actively promotes and supports research and scholarship *Standard 36*: The School of Pharmacy has a documented risk management plan for assuring continuity of program delivery

Continued

Table 3 Mapping Accreditation Standards of Several Accreditation Bodies (ACPE, 2016; APC, 2012; and CCAPP, 2017a, 2017b) Against FIP's Global QA Framework—cont'd

	FIP Global Framework Quality Indicator	ACPE Criteria	CCAPP Standards	APC Standards
29	The school has a broad base of financial support to provide a stable environment for the delivery and ongoing development and growth of the program	*Criterion No. 26*: *Financial Resources* The school has the financial resources necessary to provide the human, physical, technological, and educational resources needed to accomplish its mission. The budget of the school is planned, developed, and managed according to university policies and sound management practices	*Standard 21*: The Faculty has adequate financial resources so that continuing operation of the professional programs and other elements of the Faculty mission are fulfilled	*Standard 8*: There are clearly defined mechanisms by which the Head of School can secure and be accountable for the financial resources necessary to ensure the effective operation of the School and its pharmacy program *Standard 36*: The School of Pharmacy has a documented risk management plan for assuring continuity of program delivery
30	The school ensures access for all academic staff, preceptors, and students to a comprehensive library and other learning/educational resources, including electronic and web-based resources	*Criterion No. 24*: *Library and Educational Resources* The academic staff and students have access to library, learning and educational resources that are sufficient to support the degree program, research and other scholarly activities according to the mission and goals of the school	*Standard 24*: The Faculty ensures access for all faculty members, preceptors and students to library and information resources that are sufficient in quantity and quality to support all educational and scholarly activities in accordance with the Faculty's mission and goals	*Standard 9*: The School of Pharmacy has general and specialized teaching facilities, learning resources, and equipment of appropriate type, size, and quantity for the effective delivery of the pharmacy program
31	The school's physical facilities include simulated pharmacy practice settings where the school organizes active learning and performance assessment supervised by preceptors and/or academic staff with appropriate pharmacy practice experience	*Criterion No. 12*: *Simulation and Practice Experiences*		

Table 3 Mapping Accreditation Standards of Several Accreditation Bodies (ACPE, 2016; APC, 2012; and CCAPP, 2017a, 2017b) Against FIP's Global QA Framework—cont'd

	FIP Global Framework Quality Indicator	ACPE Criteria	CCAPP Standards	APC Standards
Quality indicators related to Process				
32	The strategic plan is developed based on an examination of the current environment, assessing strengths, weaknesses, opportunities, and threats relevant to the school	*Criterion No. 3*: *Strategic Planning and Continuous Quality Improvement*	*Standard 14*: The Faculty has a current strategic plan that is systematically reviewed and updated to facilitate the achievement of the Faculty's mission, vision, goals, and objectives. Plans and planning processes have the support and cooperation of the University administration	*Standard 4*: The School of Pharmacy has an operational plan which is aligned to deliver the objectives of the university's strategic plan and which specifies the School's mission, objectives and key performance indicators/targets against which performance and achievements are regularly measured
33	The strategic plan is developed and adopted with input from key stakeholders (internal and external)	*Criterion No. 3*: *Strategic Planning and Continuous Quality Improvement*		
34	Enrollment of students is transparent and well organized	*Criterion No. 14*: *Student Services* The school and/or university provides student services, including recruitment, admission, orientation, career counseling, records maintenance, and access to healthcare services. The school and/or university provides tutoring, advising by academic staff, and remediation for students experiencing academic difficulty *Criterion No. 15*: *Program Information* The school produces a complete and accurate description of the	*Standard 16*: The Faculty utilizes published criteria, policy, and procedures to admit students to the professional program in pharmacy	*Standard 28*: The School of Pharmacy has clearly documented and regularly reviewed eligibility or admission criteria and policies that are applied consistently, equitably, and fairly *Standard 29*: Potential students receive information on: • the accreditation status of the course; • student groups for whom defined affirmative action policies exist • specific academic entry requirements and arrangements

Continued

Table 3 Mapping Accreditation Standards of Several Accreditation Bodies (ACPE, 2016; APC, 2012; and CCAPP, 2017a, 2017b) Against FIP's Global QA Framework—cont'd

	FIP Global Framework Quality Indicator	ACPE Criteria	CCAPP Standards	APC Standards
		academic requirements and student services and makes this information available to students and prospective students *Criterion No. 17: Enrollment Management* The school plans, manages, and aligns the number of students enrolled with available resources, and local and national needs and policies		by which advanced standing may be granted; • English language proficiency requirements; • criteria to be met for right of entry to experiential placement sites; and • PBA registration standards (e.g., criminal history and English language skills) *Standard 30*: The School of Pharmacy ensures that students seeking admission who have not completed their secondary education in English, or earlier prerequisite tertiary studies in English, have demonstrated English language of a proficiency to undertake the program
35	Enrollment of students is aligned with the resources of the school and university	*Criterion No. 17: Enrollment Management*		*Standard 28*: The School of Pharmacy has clearly documented and regularly reviewed eligibility or admission criteria and policies that are applied consistently, equitably, and fairly
36	Enrollment of students is aligned with the national needs	*Criterion No. 17: Enrollment Management*		

Table 3 Mapping Accreditation Standards of Several Accreditation Bodies (ACPE, 2016; APC, 2012; and CCAPP, 2017a, 2017b) Against FIP's Global QA Framework—cont'd

	FIP Global Framework Quality Indicator	ACPE Criteria	CCAPP Standards	APC Standards
37	Academic policies and procedures are defined and available for all students and prospective students	*Criterion No. 16*: *Academic Policies and Procedures* The school publishes policies, procedures, and criteria related to admissions, academic progression, graduation, academic probation, remediation, missed course work, or credit, dismissal, readmission, and rights to due process. These documents are made available to academic staff, students, and prospective students. The school regularly assesses student admission and progression criteria, policies, and procedures based on how successfully graduates attain the desired competencies		*Standard 24*: The School of Pharmacy has clearly documented procedures for management of experiential placements that safeguard students and healthcare consumers *Standard 27*: The School of Pharmacy has policies and procedural controls that involve external assessment or moderation to assure integrity, reliability, fairness, and transparency in the assessment of students *Standard 28*: The School of Pharmacy has clearly documented and regularly reviewed eligibility or admission criteria and policies that are applied consistently, equitably, and fairly *Standard 29*: Potential students receive information on: • the accreditation status of the course; • student groups for whom defined affirmative action policies exist; • specific academic entry requirements and arrangements by which advanced standing may be granted;

Continued

Table 3 Mapping Accreditation Standards of Several Accreditation Bodies (ACPE, 2016; APC, 2012; and CCAPP, 2017a, 2017b) Against FIP's Global QA Framework—cont'd

	FIP Global Framework Quality Indicator	ACPE Criteria	CCAPP Standards	APC Standards
				• English language proficiency requirements; • criteria to be met for right of entry to experiential placement sites; and • PBA registration standards (e.g., criminal history and English language skills) *Standard 31*: Enrolling students are provided with an orientation to the School/University and its facilities, and information about: • program objectives, structure and delivery; • policies and procedures relevant to academic assessment and progression, student obligations, conduct and access to resources/facilities; and • available student support services
38	Comprehensive student services are available to all students, assuring individual attention, guidance, and support	*Criterion No. 14*: *Student Services*	*Standard 18*: Students are supported and have a positive, safe, inclusive, nondiscriminatory, inspiring experience while enrolled in the	*Standard 31*: Enrolling students are provided with an orientation to the School/university and its facilities, and information about:

Table 3 Mapping Accreditation Standards of Several Accreditation Bodies (ACPE, 2016; APC, 2012; and CCAPP, 2017a, 2017b) Against FIP's Global QA Framework—cont'd

	FIP Global Framework Quality Indicator	ACPE Criteria	CCAPP Standards	APC Standards
			professional program of pharmacy *Standard 23*: The Faculty provides space for student activities and organizations	• program objectives, structure and delivery; • policies and procedures relevant to academic assessment and progression, student obligations, conduct and access to resources/ facilities; and • available student support services *Standard 32*: The School of Pharmacy has processes in place for the early identification of students in need of support or remediation *Standard 33*: Students have access to relevant remedial and counseling support services, including appropriate English language support, to assist their successful progression through the pharmacy program and the School of Pharmacy has measures in place to ensure progression through the program is continued

Continued

Table 3 Mapping Accreditation Standards of Several Accreditation Bodies (ACPE, 2016; APC, 2012; and CCAPP, 2017a, 2017b) Against FIP's Global QA Framework—cont'd

	FIP Global Framework Quality Indicator	ACPE Criteria	CCAPP Standards	APC Standards
39	The school considers student perspectives and includes student representation on appropriate committees, including curriculum and assessment and evaluation activities	*Criterion No. 18: Student Representation, Perspectives, and Grievances* The school has clearly defined structures and mechanisms that provide a forum for student dialogue, facilitate student representation and input to the administrative leaders of the school, and foster the development of student leadership and professionalism. The administrative leaders of the school consider student input and respond within an appropriate time to problems and issues of concern. The school has a policy to be followed in the event of a formal student grievance related to the program or school	*Standard 18*: Students are supported and have a positive, safe, inclusive, nondiscriminatory, inspiring experience while enrolled in the professional program of pharmacy	*Standard 34*: The School of Pharmacy actively promotes the engagement and involvement of students in the governance and curriculum management processes of the School
40	Curricular revision ensures the overall integrity of the curriculum, avoiding curricular overload, redundancy, dilution of focus, and insufficient depth of coverage for essential components of the curriculum	*Criterion No. 9: Design and Development of the Curriculum* *Criterion No. 13: Assessment of Student Learning and Curricular Improvement* Assessment methods for student learning are valid and reliable to evaluate the desired curricular outcomes. Objective and subjective assessment data are used to	*Standard 17*: A governance structure within the Faculty directs and supports the design, development, implementation, formative assessment, and review of a curriculum that satisfies the educational outcomes required for the professional program in pharmacy	*Standard 17*: The School of Pharmacy has responsibility and authority for curriculum design and evaluation and has established mechanisms for doing so *Standard 18*: Review of curriculum content, delivery, and evaluation and student assessment methods is undertaken through broad stakeholder

Table 3 Mapping Accreditation Standards of Several Accreditation Bodies (ACPE, 2016; APC, 2012; and CCAPP, 2017a, 2017b) Against FIP's Global QA Framework—cont'd

	FIP Global Framework Quality Indicator	ACPE Criteria	CCAPP Standards	APC Standards
		evaluate and improve individual and collective student learning. The school analyzes, interprets, and uses these data to determine the level of attainment of the desired competencies and to continuously improve the content, organization, and delivery of the curriculum		engagement and use of a consultative and collaborative approach *Standard 20*: The curriculum of the pharmacy program demonstrates congruency with contemporary pharmaceutical sciences, pharmacotherapeutics, and pharmacy practice and the pharmacy learning domains
41	Students are actively encouraged and supported to assume responsibility for their own learning, including the self-identification of learning needs and gaps	*Criterion No. 10*: *Teaching and Learning Methods* The curricular teaching and learning methods ensure that students can develop the necessary knowledge, skills, attitudes, and values to enter practice (or the next stage of education and training) and be self-directed, lifelong learners		*Standard 21*: The School applies a variety of teaching and learning approaches to stimulate student engagement and to enhance student learning *Standard 34*: The School of Pharmacy actively promotes the engagement and involvement of students in the governance and curriculum management processes of the School
42	Educational content appropriately and adequately addresses traditional, contemporary, and future practice	*Criterion No. 8*: *Competencies of Graduates* The school clearly identifies and publishes the competencies that graduates must achieve to address current and future national medication and health-related needs and policies		*Standard 20*: The curriculum of the pharmacy program demonstrates congruency with contemporary pharmaceutical sciences, pharmacotherapeutics, and pharmacy practice and the pharmacy learning domains

Continued

Table 3 Mapping Accreditation Standards of Several Accreditation Bodies (ACPE, 2016; APC, 2012; and CCAPP, 2017a, 2017b) Against FIP's Global QA Framework—cont'd

	FIP Global Framework Quality Indicator	ACPE Criteria	CCAPP Standards	APC Standards
43	Curricular content and teaching methodologies prepare students for practice in a variety of practice settings			*Standard 19*: Cultural competence and cultural sensitivity are fostered through embedded curriculum content that enables students to develop an appreciation and respect for cultural diversity, and specifically addresses the health and wellbeing of Aboriginal and Torres Strait Islander people in Australia and Māori in New Zealand *Standard 22*: The School of Pharmacy has clearly defined experiential learning outcomes embedded within the curriculum, provides students with learning opportunities in hospital and community practice settings to meet those outcomes, and applies assessment methods for assuring those outcomes are met
44	Teaching and learning methodologies account for and cater to diverse learners, including different learning styles and preferences of students	*Criterion No. 10*: *Teaching and Learning Methods*	*Standard 7*: The Faculty utilizes a variety of teaching, learning and assessment methodologies to produce graduates who meet the required educational outcomes	*Standard 21*: The School applies a variety of teaching and learning approaches to stimulate student engagement and to enhance student learning

Table 3 Mapping Accreditation Standards of Several Accreditation Bodies (ACPE, 2016; APC, 2012; and CCAPP, 2017a, 2017b) Against FIP's Global QA Framework—cont'd

	FIP Global Framework Quality Indicator	ACPE Criteria	CCAPP Standards	APC Standards
45	Materials and resources are provided to the students (or cited) to enhance understanding and application of the educational material in practice	*Criterion No. 24*: *Library and Educational Resources*		*Standard 9*: The School of Pharmacy has general and specialized teaching facilities, learning resources, and equipment of appropriate type, size, and quantity for the effective delivery of the pharmacy program
46	The program provides opportunities for interprofessional education and activities		*Standard 3*: The professional degree program in pharmacy has a minimum of four academic years, or the equivalent number of hours or credits, including a series of core courses, practice experiences and interprofessional experiences that support educational outcomes *Standard 6*: The curriculum includes required intra- and interprofessional learning experiences, offered throughout the professional program, to broaden understanding of roles and competencies of pharmacists and other health professionals, including pharmacist support staff such as clerks, assistant or technician where those roles exist	
47	The program offers a broad range of elective subjects			

Continued

Table 3 Mapping Accreditation Standards of Several Accreditation Bodies (ACPE, 2016; APC, 2012; and CCAPP, 2017a, 2017b) Against FIP's Global QA Framework—cont'd

	FIP Global Framework Quality Indicator	ACPE Criteria	CCAPP Standards	APC Standards
48	Curricular contents is evidence-based, balanced, objective, and unbiased			
49	The educational activities use active learning strategies and exercises and promote and develop problem solving and critical thinking skills			
50	The school has effective measures and processes to evaluate the achievement of each stated learning objective and competency development goal by all graduates	*Criterion No. 13: Assessment of Student Learning and Curricular Improvement* Assessment methods for student learning are valid and reliable to evaluate the desired curricular outcomes. Objective and subjective assessment data are used to evaluate and improve individual and collective student learning. The school analyzes, interprets, and uses these data to determine the level of attainment of the desired competencies and to continuously improve the content, organization, and delivery of the curriculum	*Standard 15*: The Faculty establishes and maintains systems that measure and evaluate the extent to which the mission, vision, goals, and objectives are achieved	*Standard 17*: The School of Pharmacy has responsibility and authority for curriculum design and evaluation and has established mechanisms for doing so *Standard 26*: The School of Pharmacy uses a range of assessment methods that are appropriate to the outcomes of the program. *Standard 27*: The School of Pharmacy has policies and procedural controls that involve external assessment or moderation to assure integrity, reliability, fairness, and transparency in the assessment of students
51	Student assessment criteria and methodologies are defined and implemented, serving as a basis for future curricular improvement	*Criterion No. 13: Assessment of Student Learning and Curricular Improvement*		*Standard 17*: The School of Pharmacy has responsibility and authority for curriculum design and evaluation and has established mechanisms for doing

Table 3 Mapping Accreditation Standards of Several Accreditation Bodies (ACPE, 2016; APC, 2012; and CCAPP, 2017a, 2017b) Against FIP's Global QA Framework—cont'd

	FIP Global Framework Quality Indicator	ACPE Criteria	CCAPP Standards	APC Standards
				so *Standard 18*: Review of curriculum content, delivery, and evaluation and student assessment methods is undertaken through broad stakeholder engagement and use of a consultative and collaborative approach *Standard 26*: The School of Pharmacy uses a range of assessment methods that are appropriate to the outcomes of the program *Standard 27*: The School of Pharmacy has policies and procedural controls that involve external assessment or moderation to assure integrity, reliability, fairness, and transparency in the assessment of students
52	The evaluation process for academic and other staff involves self-assessment and includes appropriate input from peers, supervisors, and students	*Criterion No. 22*: *Performance Evaluation of the Academic and Other Staff* The school regularly evaluates the productivity, scholarship, and performance of its academic and other staff. The criteria for promotion (and tenure, if applicable) are articulated clearly to academic staff and consistently applied		*Standard 12*: The School of Pharmacy clearly defines and regularly reviews the reciprocal responsibilities that exist between the School and part-time or sessional contributors to the program *Standard 16*: All staff are regularly provided with feedback on their performance through formal performance planning, development and review processes

Continued

Table 3 Mapping Accreditation Standards of Several Accreditation Bodies (ACPE, 2016; APC, 2012; and CCAPP, 2017a, 2017b) Against FIP's Global QA Framework—cont'd

	FIP Global Framework Quality Indicator	ACPE Criteria	CCAPP Standards	APC Standards
				and are encouraged and supported to undertake professional development activities relevant to their roles within the School of Pharmacy
Quality indicators related to Outcomes				
53	Learning outcomes are competency-based, specific, and measurable	*Criterion No. 8: Competencies of Graduates* The school clearly identifies and publishes the competencies that graduates must achieve to address current and future national medication and health-related needs and policies *Criterion No. 9: Design and Development of the Curriculum* The school, through a defined process, uses the desired graduate competencies to design and develop the curricular philosophy, structure, content, and instructional methods	*Standard 1*: The professional program in pharmacy is based on an organized educational framework that facilitates development of graduates with competencies to meet the entry-level scope of practice	*Standard 25*: The pharmacy program produces graduates who have the graduate attributes of the university and the knowledge, skills, and attitudes necessary to commence supervised practice as an intern pharmacist
54	Validated measures are used to evaluate the extent to which the desired outcomes of the professional degree program (including assessment of student learning and evaluation of the effectiveness of the curriculum) are being achieved	*Criterion No. 4: Assessment of Achievement of Mission and Goals* *Criterion No. 13: Assessment of Student Learning and Curricular Improvement* Assessment methods for student learning are valid and reliable to evaluate the desired		*Standard 26*: The School of Pharmacy uses a range of assessment methods that are appropriate to the outcomes of the program *Standard 27*: The School of Pharmacy has policies and procedural controls that involve external assessment or

Table 3 Mapping Accreditation Standards of Several Accreditation Bodies (ACPE, 2016; APC, 2012; and CCAPP, 2017a, 2017b) Against FIP's Global QA Framework—cont'd

	FIP Global Framework Quality Indicator	ACPE Criteria	CCAPP Standards	APC Standards
		curricular outcomes. Objective and subjective assessment data are used to evaluate and improve individual and collective student learning. The school analyzes, interprets, and uses these data to determine the level of attainment of the desired competencies and to continuously improve the content, organization, and delivery of the curriculum		moderation to assure integrity, reliability, fairness and transparency in the assessment of students
55	Evaluation of learning outcomes includes all competencies (knowledge, skills, attitudes, and values)	*Criterion No. 13*: *Assessment of Student Learning and Curricular Improvement*		*Standard 26*: The School of Pharmacy uses a range of assessment methods that are appropriate to the outcomes of the program
56	Competencies to be achieved by graduates are clearly stated by the school	*Criterion No. 8*: *Competencies of Graduates* The school clearly identifies and publishes the competencies that graduates must achieve to address current and future national medication and health-related needs and policies		*Standard 31*: Enrolling students are provided with an orientation to the School/University and its facilities, and information about: • program objectives, structure, and delivery; • policies and procedures relevant to academic assessment and progression, student obligations, conduct, and access to resources/ facilities; and • available student support services

Continued

Table 3 Mapping Accreditation Standards of Several Accreditation Bodies (ACPE, 2016; APC, 2012; and CCAPP, 2017a, 2017b) Against FIP's Global QA Framework—cont'd

	FIP Global Framework Quality Indicator	ACPE Criteria	CCAPP Standards	APC Standards
57	Competencies to be achieved by graduates aligned with national and global needs and trends	*Criterion No. 8*: *Competencies of Graduates*		*Standard 19*: Cultural competence and cultural sensitivity are fostered through embedded curriculum content that enables students to develop an appreciation and respect for cultural diversity, and specifically addresses the health and wellbeing of Aboriginal and Torres Strait islander people in Australia and Māori in new Zealand *Standard 25*: The pharmacy program produces graduates who have the graduate attributes of the University and the knowledge, skills, and attitudes necessary to commence supervised practice as an intern pharmacist
58	Students develop new knowledge and skills to improve patient and population health	*Criterion No. 8*: *Competencies of Graduates*		*Standard 25*: The pharmacy program produces graduates who have the graduate attributes of the University and the knowledge, skills and attitudes necessary to commence supervised practice as an intern pharmacist
59	Students adopt an ethical approach to develop their self-awareness, attitudes, and values	*Criterion No. 2*: *Professional, Ethical, and Harmonious Environment*	*Standard 2*: The Faculty provides an environment and culture that promotes professional behavior	

Table 3 Mapping Accreditation Standards of Several Accreditation Bodies (ACPE, 2016; APC, 2012; and CCAPP, 2017a, 2017b) Against FIP's Global QA Framework—cont'd

	FIP Global Framework Quality Indicator	ACPE Criteria	CCAPP Standards	APC Standards
			and harmonious relationships among students, and between students and faculty members, administrators, preceptors, and staff	
60	The school assesses student professionalism, behavior, and attitudes	*Criterion No. 13*: *Assessment of Student Learning and Curricular Improvement*		*Standard 26*: The School of Pharmacy uses a range of assessment methods that are appropriate to the outcomes of the program
61	Through the research, publications, and other scholarly activities of its academic staff and students, the school contributes to the generation, dissemination, and application of new knowledge	*Criterion No. 1*: *Mission, Goals, and Values*	*Standard 8*: The Faculty is located in a University within an academic health sciences network or has a close relationship with a network of healthcare facilities that have an academic mission toward research and other scholarly activities	*Standard 14*: The School of Pharmacy actively promotes and supports research and scholarship
62	The school supports initiatives and projects that serve the health-related needs of the population and advance pharmacy practice models in community pharmacy and hospital settings	*Criterion No. 1*: *Mission, Goals, and Values*		
63	The school with the support of the university, establishes productive and effective collaborations and networks with other schools, universities, the	*Criterion No. 6*: *External Collaborative Relationships*	*Standard 9*: The Faculty has University support for affiliations, collaborations, and partnerships (internal and external to the University) necessary to advance the	*Standard 7*: The School of Pharmacy has active and ongoing partnerships or associations with relevant professional, government, health, indigenous and

Continued

Table 3 Mapping Accreditation Standards of Several Accreditation Bodies (ACPE, 2016; APC, 2012; and CCAPP, 2017a, 2017b) Against FIP's Global QA Framework—cont'd

	FIP Global Framework Quality Indicator	ACPE Criteria	CCAPP Standards	APC Standards
	pharmacy practice community, the pharmaceutical industry, national and international organizations, the government, and other appropriate partners		education, research, clinical practices, and service missions of the Faculty	community agencies through which matters of mutual interest are progressed. Formal relationships exist with healthcare providers, practitioners, and services to facilitate access to appropriate experiential placements
Quality indicators for Impact				
64	Learning leads to behavior and performance changes by graduates			
65	The school's students and graduates feel honor and pride in belonging to the international pharmacy community and are aware that they are a direct reflection on the profession			
66	New projects, services, or activities are visible in pharmacy practice as the result of the impact of students' and graduates' knowledge, skills, and motivation			
67	Advocacy and impact on the development of the profession is achieved through the leadership of the school, its academic staff, and graduates who are agents of change			

Table 3 Mapping Accreditation Standards of Several Accreditation Bodies (ACPE, 2016; APC, 2012; and CCAPP, 2017a, 2017b) Against FIP's Global QA Framework—cont'd

	FIP Global Framework Quality Indicator	ACPE Criteria	CCAPP Standards	APC Standards
68	Innovations and changes that address or solve national and/or international healthcare-related needs and priorities are achieved	*Criterion No. 1: Mission, Goals, and Values*		
69	Ethical aspects, such as building the self-image of pharmacists, enhancing professional autonomy and personal development, are visible as a result of the program			
70	The school has developed and adopted an "Oath of a pharmacist," to be taken by students before they enter practice			
71	Pharmacy students and new pharmacy graduates promise, in public, before their mentors and peers, to follow the highest standards of professional practice and ethics and commit to lifelong learning to maintain and enhance their competence			

ACPE, CCAPP, and APC were invited to review and edit the draft mapping produced by the authors. Some changes, but not all changes, proposed by the accreditors were accepted.

[a]For CCAPP, standards are broken down into criteria and sometimes the relevance of a standard with a FIP indicator can't be understood without mentioning the particular relevant criteria. The same is true for APC: the relevance of certain standards with a FIP indicator is explained by mentioning the guidances that provide detailed breakdowns of the standards.

Table 4 Accreditation Standards of Several Accreditation Bodies (ACPE, CCAPP, APC) not Well Matched With FIP's Global QA Framework

	ACPE Criteria	CCAPP Standards	APC Standards
1	*Criterion No. 21*: Continuing Professional Development of the Academic and Other Staff The school promotes, facilitates, and supports the training and ongoing development of its academic and other staff and preceptors, commensurate with their programmatic responsibilities *Under SECTION 5: STAFF RESOURCES*	*Standard 11*: The professional degree in pharmacy program is housed in a unit that is equivalent to a Faculty, College, or School *Under part II Governance and Program Management*: *B. Faculty Organization and Leadership*	*Standard 1 (Australia)*: The university in which the School of Pharmacy operates holds current registration with the tertiary education Quality and Standards Agency (teQSA) as a higher education provider in the Australian university category OR *Standard 1 (new Zealand)*: The School of Pharmacy's qualifications are approved by universities' New Zealand quality assurance body, the Committee on university Academic Programmes (CuAP), listed on the new Zealand Qualifications framework (nZQf), and eligible for funding through the tertiary education Commission (teC) *Under 1. Standards for Governance, Structure and Administration, 1.1 Governance*
2			*Standard 13*: The School of Pharmacy actively encourages contribution to program delivery in Australia by Aboriginal and Torres Strait Islander people, and in New Zealand by Māori *Under 2. Standards for Resource Allocation and Management, 2.3 Human Resources*
3			*Standard 35*: The School of Pharmacy has a demonstrable and continuous quality improvement program and is responsive to both internal and external feedback and review *Under 5. Standards for Quality and Risk Management, 5.1 Quality Management*

WHAT IMPORTANT ADVICE CAN BE PROVIDED TO A COLLEGE PLANNING FOR ACCREDITATION?

Institutions that are applying for accreditation or continuation of accreditation will typically be required to undertake a self-assessment against the accreditation standards (sometimes referred to as a "self-study"), submit a self-study report (SSR), and undergo an on-site evaluation visit by a team of trained evaluators. The following section provides guidance and advice to assist institutions in the planning and execution of the self-study, development of the SSR, and preparation for the on-site visit.

PLANNING FOR A SELF-STUDY

- Start the planning well in advance

A comprehensive self-study and the development of a quality SSR take time, especially if it is the first time that an institution has gone through an accreditation process. Do not underestimate the time that it will take. There is a large amount of information, data, and documentation to be collected, analyzed, and interpreted. Adequate time should be allowed for development and review of multiple iterations (drafts) of the SSR. The timeline should include opportunities for input and feedback from all key stakeholders, as well as internal quality control of the SSR prior to its finalization. Anticipate that some stakeholders will not meet required deadlines for submission; build such a contingency into the schedule. Accreditation agencies usually operate with defined accreditation schedules (cycles) and timelines, which do not allow much, if any, flexibility. Submission delays of a few weeks may force the process into the next accreditation cycle, resulting in significant delays in achieving accreditation. Typically, a self-study would take a minimum of 8–10 months; some institutions start as early as 18–24 months before the on-site evaluation. A self-study can be conducted in parallel or in conjunction with strategic planning.

The self-study is usually managed by a steering committee and subcommittees. Some accreditation agencies recommend that the self-study steering committee not be chaired by the dean/head of school/institution. Institutions sometimes have individuals with specific responsibility for quality assurance/accreditation and such individuals frequently chair the self-study steering committee. Subcommittees typically work on a number of accreditation standards that are related and combined in one section of the standards. The work and deliverables, respective responsibilities, and meeting schedule for the steering committee and subcommittees should be agreed upon in advance, building in some flexibility for contingencies as noted previously.

- Identify and involve all key stakeholders

Importantly, the SSR should not be written by an individual or a small, select group. The self-study should be a truly inclusive and representative process. While full agreement may not be reached in all areas, the process—including enough time for meaningful debate—should allow for consensus to be reached. If consensus cannot be reached in any area, the different perspectives can be provided for the information of the team, which should come to its own conclusion. There are many different stakeholders—internal and external—who have an interest (or "stake") in the quality of the institution and its educational program(s). Internal stakeholders include members of the academic, technical/support, and administrative staff; students; graduates/alumni; and administrators of the institution.

External stakeholders include preceptors, employers/practitioners, regulators, and professional associations. Ideally, a broad range of stakeholders, including students, should be included on all self-study committees, especially the subcommittees working on self-assessment against the standards. If necessary, students can be excluded from specific discussions, rather than excluding them from the entire work of a subcommittee. All members of the academic staff should either serve on one of the committees or at least be provided with the opportunity to provide input and feedback on the draft(s) of the SSR. In addition to providing direct input via membership on committees, the institution's external stakeholders should also be invited and given opportunities to provide input throughout the process, review drafts, and provide feedback and suggestions for improvement.

- Early identification of areas of noncompliance and opportunities for quality improvement

Allowing ample time for a self-study affords the institution the opportunity for early identification of areas of noncompliance and/or areas for quality improvement. In both of these areas, the institution can then develop an appropriate plan that will achieve the desired outcome, secure the necessary resources and permissions (if applicable), assign the responsible/accountable persons, implement the plan, and start to compile evidence that the plan is working before the evaluation team arrives. Progress with the implementation of the plan and any data/evidence already compiled can be included in the SSR or presented to the team during the on-site evaluation visit. This commitment to quality and quality improvement is what accreditation agencies like to see, as opposed to institutions being in "denial" of areas needing improvement and the evaluation team having to identify them during the visit.

THE SELF-STUDY REPORT

- Quantitative and qualitative analysis

The SSR should present a comprehensive (yet concise) quantitative and qualitative assessment of the quality of the institution and its program(s) using the standards as the point of reference. In essence, the self-study and SSR are a self-assessment of *strengths*, *weaknesses*, *opportunities*, and *threats*: i.e., a SWOT analysis. Areas of the program that are noteworthy, innovative, or exceed the expectation of the standard should also be included.

The key is to be transparent, candid, and honest. Institutions that are committed to quality and continuous quality improvement (CQI) have nothing to lose by identifying and disclosing any areas needing improvement. Many accreditation agencies that see *quality advancement* as a part of their mission will—when invited by the institution—be very happy to provide advice and guidance to institutions on how to address areas of noncompliance, improve quality, or otherwise strengthen the institution and its program(s).

- Address all "Pillars" of educational quality (International Pharmaceutical Federation, 2014) but focus on outcomes and impact

While quality is dependent on good *structure* and *process*, and they should be self-assessed in the SSR, accreditation agencies should now be focusing more on the *outcomes* and *impact* of an institution and its program(s) and, accordingly, should be looking more for evidence of these "pillars" to demonstrate compliance with standards. Accreditors may revert to a more thorough evaluation of *structure* and *process* to identify deficiencies when the desired *outcomes* and *impact* are not being achieved. It is, however, also important for evaluators to understand the *context* in which the education is delivered. Helping evaluators to understand the *context,* as it relates to any unique aspects of the institution's environment, mission, vision, goals, culture, values, etc., is also important in the SSR and later during the on-site visit.

- Follow requirements and guidelines of the agency

Many agencies have a required or suggested template for the SSR; this should be followed as closely as possible and specified page or word limits adhered to. Page and word limits give an indication of the level of detail expected by the agency; hence, the length of the SSR should also not be significantly less than the suggested/required page limit, as this would tend to indicate that inadequate detail has been provided. Additionally, accreditation agencies require submission of specific data and documentation, either in the SSR or for review during the on-site visit. If, for any reason, requested data or documentation cannot be provided or is not applicable, a clear explanation should be provided.

- What? So what? What next?

Answering these three questions throughout the SSR is the key to a quality report:

- The *What* should provide a brief, objective, factual description of the situation at the institution and its program(s)—the *strengths*, *weaknesses*, *opportunities* and *threats*. All statements that are intended to demonstrate compliance with a standard should be supported by clear evidence in the form of data and/or documentation.
- The *So What* should provide a subjective analysis of the situation. It's more reflective, focusing on the meaning and implications of the situation (SWOT) to the quality of the institution and its program(s) in terms of appropriately addressing *context*, *structure*, *process*, *outcomes* and *impact*—the five pillars of educational quality described in FIP's Global Framework for Quality Assurance of Pharmacy Education (International Pharmaceutical Federation, 2014). If changes have recently been made, the impact of the change should be assessed and discussed.
- The *What Next* should provide a detailed description of the institution's *plan* (as opposed to "what the institution plans to do") to address the area of noncompliance or desired quality improvement. The plan should be SMART—*specific*, *measurable*, *achievable*, *relevant*, and *timed*. The stage of implementation and progress with the plan should be described and any evidence to demonstrate that the plan is likely to achieve the desired outcome should be submitted.

These three questions illustrate well how the "CQI loop" should be closed when it comes to assessment data. Institutions can sometimes expend a huge amount of effort collecting and reporting on assessment data (the *What*), but then fail to adequately analyze and interpret the data and the implications for the quality of the program (the *So What*), and don't develop specific interventions and strategies to achieve the needed impact (the *What Next*).

- Self-assessment of compliance

Accreditation agencies will invariably require institutions to self-assess their performance/compliance against the standards. The self-assessment must be realistic and evidence-based. Evidence should also be provided to demonstrate that compliance will be maintained in the future.

- Appendices

Appendices are an important element of the SSR. They typically include required data and documentation as well as additional (voluntary) data and documentation that an institution wishes to submit as extra evidence of compliance, innovations, or quality improvement initiatives. Appendices should, in the main, *support* the main text in the SSR, not *substitute* for it. Appendices should be used judiciously, so as not to overload evaluators, and should be well organized and formatted so that the needed information or data is easy to find and assimilate. Where only a part(s) of a document is/are important/relevant, it/they should be extracted or clearly identified. Appendices should be numbered and indexed appropriately, and if the SSR is electronic (e.g., in PDF format), the appendices should ideally be bookmarked and/or hyperlinked.

- Quality control of the report

Good quality control (QC) of the SSR is essential, ensuring accuracy of spelling and grammar and consistency of style and format (font, font-size, line spacing, tabbing, pagination, etc.). Tables and figures should be clear and easy to interpret; explanatory text should be provided when necessary. Digital links to external sources (e.g., URLs) should be checked to ensure that they are still valid and not access-controlled. Incorrect spellings, poor grammar, inconsistent formatting, and contradictory data or statements can be a major distraction for evaluators, something that is not in the best interests of the institution. This is particularly important when a report is submitted in a language that is not the first language of the authors. The steering committee as a whole should also ensure consistency of information and data (including in tables) between the different sections of the SSR which may have been written by different people; inconsistencies are a "red flag" for evaluators.

A vital aspect of the QC process should be to ensure that the three key questions identified above have been addressed in each component of the SSR.

A useful quality assurance strategy is to ask someone who is not directly connected to the institution to provide an independent and objective review of the final draft. The SSR should be clear and understandable to someone who has no or little prior knowledge of the institution. Such a person can provide valuable feedback to improve the completeness and clarity of the final product.

PREPARING FOR AN ON-SITE VISIT

- Plan all aspects of the visit carefully

All aspects of the visit should be carefully planned in collaboration with the accreditation agency. Planning for an on-site visit should start well in advance. Arrangements for travel (including visas, if applicable) and accommodation for the team should be finalized as far in advance as possible, and confirmations of the arrangements sent to the agency. The visit schedule is typically busy and somewhat rigid; days are long for the members of the on-site evaluation team ("team"). It is important that the schedule is agreed in advance and communicated with adequate notice to everyone affected by the schedule. The visit should be planned for when students are on campus and, if applicable, at practice sites.

The schedule must be efficiently managed and delays, changes, and disruptions kept to a minimum. The institution should not arrange additional (unscheduled) events. Some flexibility, however, should be built into the schedule to allow for contingencies and breaks, and experienced team members can usually adjust for unforeseen scenarios.

The team should be provided with a secure, private room(s) for meetings with committees and individuals, and their own discussions. It is helpful if the room has secure Internet access, light refreshments, and some administrative support on hand if needed (e.g., for printing, photocopying, access to documents).

- Inform key stakeholders

The members of the team will meet with committees and various individuals during the visit. People who meet with the team should be aware of the visit and its purpose, the findings and conclusions from the self-study, and the types of questions that could be asked of them. As with the text of the SSR, answers and statements given to the team should be honest, candid, and objective. Team members will triangulate what is written in the SSR with responses to questions, and very likely will "see through" prepared answers that do not accurately represent the situation at the institution. Interviews and other activities/assessments conducted during the on-site visit should validate the findings and conclusions presented in the SSR; inconsistencies are another "red flag" for evaluators.

- The on-site visit

Typical sessions/meetings during an on-site visit could include: introductory meeting with the dean; document review; tour of campus and physical facilities (laboratories, lecture theaters, library, etc.); meetings with committees (Self-Study, Executive/Leadership, Curriculum, Assessment, etc.); Student Services staff; students; individual interviews with members of the academic staff; visits to practice/experiential sites; preceptors; experiential staff/coordinators; graduates; and exit interviews with the dean and institutional administrators.

Photographs may be allowed by the accreditation agency but, if so, should be kept to a minimum. If sessions are conducted in a language other than the primary language of the country, the services of an independent translator may be necessary.

CHAPTER SUMMARY AND CONCLUSION

The concept of quality that was developed primarily in the industry environment was subjected to changes over decades, starting from the notion of quality control, to the notion of quality assurance, to the notion of total quality management. Since quality cannot be established unless it becomes an embedded culture in the academic institution, it should be established based on a core set of traditional academic values and beliefs. Accreditation can be viewed as a mechanism for the achievement and the recognition of quality of an accredited academic program. It does not guarantee quality and it is not supposed to be the only way to achieve and sustain quality.

Except for ACPE, certification is commonly applied to individuals who seek a permission to practice, whereas accreditation is applied to the institutions and institutional programs to provide evidence that they are following certain quality criteria making them eligible for recognition.

Although they are basically different, accreditation, certification, and licensure sometimes are related. Graduating from an accredited program may lead automatically to receiving a professional certification and such certification leads to receiving a licensure for practicing.

As of 2017, programs of seven international pharmacy schools are certified by ACPE, five international pharmacy schools are accredited by CCAPP, and a program of one international pharmacy school is accredited (with condition) by the APC.

Some institutions seek accreditation to be recognized and receive credit from others (i.e., an accrediting body) regarding what is achieved. In the United States, not all academic programs look for accreditation and accreditation is not directly controlled by government. It is sought mainly by disciplines that qualify students for licensure such as pharmacy, nursing, and engineering (i.e., the graduates who cannot practice unless getting licensure must study at accredited programs) and the institutions looking to obtain federal funds, such as student aid. Currently all established schools of pharmacy in the United States are accredited or in the process of applying. On the other hand, in many countries, accreditation is compulsory and controlled by a governmental agency.

Most of the evidence indicates that accreditation enhances procedures, processes, and outputs, but no evidence is available on its positive effect on the actual outcomes of the healthcare services or the academic programs.

ACKNOWLEDGMENTS

The authors of this chapter would like to acknowledge the invaluable assistance from Dr. Peter H. Vlasses, the Executive Director Accreditation Council for Pharmacy Education (ACPE), who has made useful comments and corrections in the manuscript, and Dr. K. Wayne Hindmarsh, the Executive Director Canadian Council for Accreditation of Pharmacy Programs (CCAPP) and Dr. Bronwyn Clark, Chief Executive Officer Australian Pharmacy Council (APC), who reviewed the mapping section and made useful corrections. The assistance of Kate Spencer, Senior Pharmacist, Accreditation, the APC and Glenys Wilkinson, Executive Director Professional Services, the APC in reviewing the mapping section is also highly appreciated.

REFERENCES

9000 Store. (2017a). ISO 9000 series of quality standards. http://the9000store.com/what-are-iso-9000-standards/ (accessed 20 October 2017).

9000 Store. (2017b). Who is ISO? (International Organization for Standardization). http://the9000store.com/articles/who-is-iso/ (accessed 20 October 2017).

9000 Store. (2017c). ISO 9001: What is it? Who needs certification and why? http://the9000store.com/what-are-iso-9000-standards/what-is-iso-9001/ (accessed 20 October 2017).

ACPE. (2016). International quality criteria for certification of professional degree programs in pharmacy. International Services Program, Accreditation Council for Pharmacy Education.

ACPE. (2017). Accreditation Council for Pharmacy Education Directory of Programs with Certification Status. Retrieved 10 October 2017, from https://www.google.com.sa/url?sa=t&source=web&rct=j&url=https://www.acpe-accredit.org/pdf/DirectoryCertifiedPrograms.pdf&ved=0ahUKEwiij6WEw-XWAhXqHpoKHXCcAFYQFggwMAE&usg=AOvVaw2eDn1akldLS34vhiPfzXTv.

Al Mohaimeed, A., Midhet, F., Barrimah, I., & Saleh, M. N. (2012). Academic accreditation process: Experience of a medical college in Saudi Arabia. *International Journal of Health Sciences, Qassim University*, *6*(1), 23–29.

Al Tehewy, M., Salem, B., Habil, I., & El Okda, S. (2009). Evaluation of accreditation program in non-governmental organizations' health units in Egypt: Short-term outcomes. *International Journal of Quality in Health care*, *21*(3), 183–189.

Almasabi, M., & Thomas, S. (2016). The impact of Saudi hospital accreditation on quality of care: A mixed methods study. *The International Journal of Health Planning and Management*. https://doi.org/10.1002/hpm.2373.

APC. (2012). *Accreditation standards for pharmacy programs in Australia and New Zealand*. Australian Pharmacy Council Ltd.

APC. (2017). Accredited providers. Australian Pharmacy Council. Retrieved 10 October 2017, from https://www.pharmacycouncil.org.au/our-services/education-providers/accredited-providers/.

CCAPP. (2017a). Accredited International Programs. Retrieved 10 October 2017, from https://ccapp-accredit.ca/international-programs/list-of-international-programs/.
CCAPP. (2017b). International Accreditation Standards for First Professional Degree in Pharmacy Programs. Toronto: Ibid. Canadian Council for the Accreditation of Pharmacy Programs.
Coria, M. M., Deluca, M., & Martinez, M. (2010). Curricular changes in accredited undergraduate programmes in Argentina. *Quality in Higher Education*, *16*(3), 249–255.
Dattey, K., Westerheijden, D. F., & Hofman, W. H. A. (2014). Impact of accreditation on public and private universities: A comparative study. *Tertiary Education and Management*, *20*(4), 307–319.
Dellana, S. A., & Hauser, R. D. (1999). Toward defining the quality culture. *Engineering Management Journal*, *11*(2), 11–15.
Eaton, J. S. (2012). *An overview of U.S. accreditation*. Washington, DC: Council for Higher Education Accreditation CHEA.
El-Jardali, F., Jamal, D., Dimassi, H., Ammar, W., & Tchaghchaghian, V. (2008). The impact of hospital accreditation on quality of care: Perception of Lebanese nurses. *International Journal for Quality in Health Care*, *20*(5), 363–371.
Gaston, P. L. (2014). *Higher education accreditation: How it's changing, why it must* (1st ed.). Sterling, Virginia, USA: Stylus Publishing, L.L.C.
Harvey, L. (2003). The power of accreditation: Views of academics. (The paper is based on a more detailed presentation by the author at the ENQA Seminar on Accreditation in Rome in December 2003).
Harvey, L., & Williams, J. (2010). Fifteen years of quality in higher education. *Quality in Higher Education*, *16*(1), 3–36.
Hou, Y., Morse, R., Ince, M., Chen, H., Chiang, C., & Chan, Y. (2015). Is the Asian quality assurance system for higher education going glonacal? Assessing the impact of three types of program accreditation on Taiwanese universities. *Studies in Higher Education*, *40*(1), 83–105.
International Pharmaceutical Federation—FIP. (2012). *Good pharmacy practice. Joint FIP/WHO guidelines on GPP: Standards for quality of pharmacy services*. The Hague, The Netherlands: International Pharmaceutical Federation.
International Pharmaceutical Federation—FIP. (2014). *Quality Assurance of Pharmacy Education: The FIP global framework* (2nd ed.). The Hague, The Netherlands: International Pharmaceutical Federation.
McDavid, J. C., & Huse, I. (2015). How does accreditation fit into the picture? In J. W. Altschuld & M. Engle (Eds.), *New Directions for Evaluation: vol. 145. Accreditation, certification, and credentialing: Relevant concerns for US evaluators*vol. 145, (pp. 53–69).
Meštrović, A., & Rouse, M. J. (2015). Pillars and foundations of quality for continuing education in pharmacy. *American Journal of Pharmaceutical Education*, *79*(3), 45.
Prisacariu, A., & Shah, M. (2016). Defining the quality of higher education around ethics and moral values. *Quality in Higher Education*, *22*(2), 152–166.
Shaw, C. D., Groene, O., Botje, D., Sunol, R., Kutryba, B., Klazinga, N., et al. (2014). The effect of certification and accreditation on quality management in 4 clinical services in 73 European hospitals. *International Journal of Quality in Health care*, *26*(Suppl. 1), 100–107.
Shaw, C., Groene, O., Mora, N., & Sunol, R. (2010). Accreditation and ISO certification: Do they explain differences in quality management in European hospitals? *International Journal of Quality in Health care*, *22*(6), 445–451.
Sin, C., Tavares, O., & Amaral, A. (2017). The impact of programme accreditation on Portuguese higher education provision. *Assessment & Evaluation in Higher Education*, *42*(6), 860–871.
Van Kemenade, E., Pupius, M., & Hardjono, T. W. (2008). More value to defining quality. *Quality in Higher Education*, *14*(2), 175–185.
Vlasceanu, L., Grunberg, L., & Parlea, D. (2007). *Quality assurance and accreditation: A glossary of basic terms and definitions*. Bucharest: UNESCO.

CHAPTER

REGULATORY AND LEGAL ISSUES IN PHARMACY EDUCATION: CASES IN LATIN AMERICAN COUNTRIES

16

Patricia Acuña-Johnson
University of Valparaiso, Valparaiso, Chile

QUALITY ASSURANCE AS THE DRIVING FORCE IN PHARMACY EDUCATION

Considering that pharmacy practice needs pharmacists with certain competencies, including knowledge, skills, ethical values and principles, and respect for diversity and cultural and social differences, undergraduate curricula must have the necessary institutional structure to train these professionals. Most pharmacy programs (a degree in pharmacy) in Latin American countries have the following characteristics:

- University level;
- Duration between 10 and 12 semesters;
- Curricular structure divided into three cycles or phases: basic, preprofessional, and professional, according to different orientations of the faculty and the country's professional profile. Additionally, there are established experiential practices (usually one or two, depending on the particular pharmacy curriculum and the country as well);
- Minimum mandated content and hours allocated to experiential practices are stipulated by each faculty/country according to the relative significance that each faculty gives to the training cycles. Some may be obligatory and others elective.

The local reality of the country, and especially the history and regulations on higher education, play a very important role when defining the characteristics of pharmacy education. At the same time, the influence of regional and global organizations and their guiding directives as to what the pharmacy curriculum should entail have become increasingly powerful and, in fact, have become the driving forces for curricular innovation (PAHO/WHO, 2016). This framework establishes the minimum quality standards on various quality regulations controlling pharmacy education in Latin American countries.

Pharmacy Education in the Twenty First Century and Beyond. https://doi.org/10.1016/B978-0-12-811909-9.00016-2

In summary, the degree must meet all of the aforementioned requirements and higher education institutions and faculties/schools must count on budgetary and human resources and facilities, including pharmacy practice sites, adapted to each country's needs. The structural features of the pharmacy curriculum are regulated by mandates and regulations at the national level. Quality standards have been established by various agencies, pharmacy school associations, or representatives of the various areas of professional performance in the country. Compliance with standards is verified and promoted by agencies, including those overseeing the quality of education, both public and private; however, the process itself is still voluntary. On the other hand, compliance with national regulations regarding the professional performance of the pharmacist is largely regulated by health codes, technical standards, and provisions that are monitored by national/federal public agencies, depending on the respective ministries of public health in each country.

THE CASE OF BRAZIL

REGULATION OF PHARMACY EDUCATION

Brazil is a Federal Republic of 27 Federal State units, with a population that exceeds 200 million inhabitants. Education at all levels is regulated by the "Law of Guidelines and Bases" of 1996 (MEC, 1996). This law expanded the scope of higher education and as a consequence the courses within pharmacy education (Fig. 1) (Cadastro Nacional da Educação Superior INEP/MEC as cited in CFF, 2008). Undergraduate programs are regulated by the Ministry of Education, and to date there are more than 500 certified pharmacy programs. The vast majority are provided by private institutions that were created in the 2000s (Fig. 2) (Cadastro Nacional da Educação Superior INEP/MEC as cited in CFF, 2008). However, student enrollment has increased with less restrictive and softer entry requirements. Consequently, there is currently a lack of control over the quality of all programs; however, new curricular guidelines were established in 2002 enabling some progress in this regard (CFF, 2002).

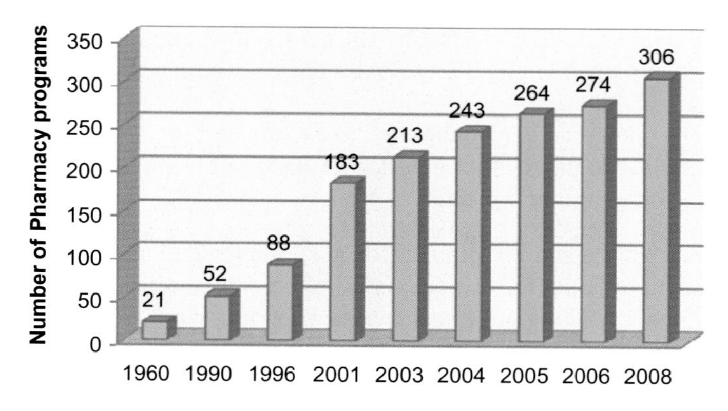

FIG. 1

Evolution of the pharmacy programs offered in Brazil 1960–2008.

Source: Conselho Federal de Farmácia (CFF, 2008).

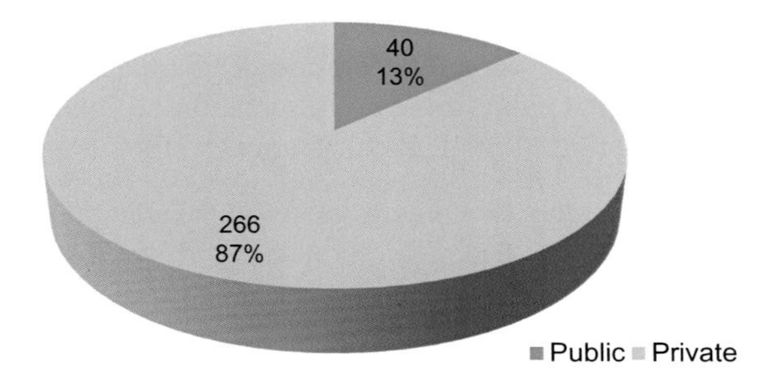

FIG. 2

Administrative liaison of pharmacy programs in Brazil.

Source: Conselho Federal de Farmácia (CFF, 2008).

REGULATIONS AND THEIR INFLUENCE ON STRENGTHENING PHARMACY EDUCATION AND PROGRESS

In 2012, with the aim of reversing the recent retreat in Brazil from the pharmacist's historical role as a health professional, the Federal Council of Pharmacy (CFF), a member of the International Pharmaceutical Federation (FIP), assumed the leadership on this crusade (Frade, 2015). Some of the strategies used for pharmacists' recognition in terms of perception among the community were the building of a modern normative apparatus, aimed at improving the quality of pharmaceutical services provided to the population. The product has the approval of Resolutions 585/2013 and 586/2013 (CFF, 2013a, 2013b). The first one regulates the clinical attributions of the pharmacist regardless of the place where they are adopted. The second one regulates prescription. These two resolutions have greatly contributed to Brazilian pharmacy and its impact on public health. The CFF recognizes that in addition to promoting the value of the pharmacist, these two regulations constitute an important achievement for all citizens, in the so-called Unified Health System (SUS) and for users of private health insurance services (Frade, 2014).

In addition to publishing both of these resolutions, some other strategies and initiatives have been effective:

- Restructuring the Brazilian Medicines Information Center (Cebrim) and regular four-times-a-year publication of the Pharmacotherapeutic Bulletin, to support pharmacists in the development of clinical practice;
- Development of the Pharmaceutical Care Support Program in Health Care (PROFAR) to prepare pharmacists for the implementation of pharmaceutical prescription, management of self-limited health problems, conciliation, review of pharmacotherapy, health education, and pharmacotherapeutic follow-up;
- Financial support for the Clinical Pharmacotherapeutic Webpage[1];
- Agreement with the Evidence-Based Health Portal of the Ministry of Health to offer free access to databases;

[1]The referenced web page is the following: www.farmaceuticoclinico.com.br.

- Creation in February 2014 of the National Forum for the Valorization of Pharmaceutical Profession with representatives of the CFF, the National Federation of Pharmacists (Fenafar), the Interstate Federation of Pharmacists (FEIFAR), the Brazilian Association of Pharmaceutical Education (ABEF), and the National Executive of Students of Pharmacy (Enefar).

This Forum has prioritized political action, seeking to create a legal apparatus that recognizes the pharmacist as an essential professional in the healthcare system. Its first focus was the approval of Law 13.021/14, which changed the concept of the pharmacy in Brazil, transforming the pharmacies into healthcare units that until then were mere commercial drugstores. This new law makes direct reference to the clinical performance of the pharmacist, such as article 13 letter c, establishing an obligation of the pharmacist to carry out pharmacotherapeutic monitoring of patients, including those who are not hospitalized or in hospitals or health centers, both public and private (CFF, 2015).

In summary, the CFF has been the driving force that led to a change in the pharmacy profession, and consequently in pharmacy education. CFF seeks to establish the framework of the professional practice of pharmacists, and seeks to position pharmacists as health professionals, not just distributing medication. Furthermore, the Brazilian Association of Pharmaceutical Education is a very recent creation (almost 3 years ago) and therefore it is essential to articulate the sectors responsible for pharmacy education, health regulatory agencies, professional associations and their scientific societies, and public health policies in order to provide the necessary framework for the development of pharmaceutical services.

Regarding pharmacy education, the pharmacist's rights and duties have increased, and from the pharmacy curriculum point of view, this has involved a great deal of innovation. Considering the new definition and professional scope of the Brazilian pharmacist, the task was to establish minimum and pertinent content, as well as a curricular harmonization between all pharmacy programs. As a result, a so-called integrative curriculum was created, adopting a multidisciplinary, interdisciplinary, and transdisciplinary perspective, without modifying the 4- to 5-year duration of education as is the reality of Brazil, as required in Brazil. The principles that govern the education of the pharmacist in Brazil are stated in the National Curricular Guidelines of the Graduation Courses in Pharmacy (CFF, 2002, CFF, 2016a).

On the other hand, it is important to emphasize that continuing education has acquired a central prominence. Thus all of these changes must be immersed within the framework of a system that guarantees and enables the public to trust the quality of these programs. In 2015, the National Curricular Guidelines that modify the guidelines of the pharmacy programs in Brazil focused mainly on clinical training and, in accordance with the peculiarities of the different regions of the country, was approved and handed over to the Ministry of Education in early 2016. However, the political changes that have taken place in the country in the past 2 years have left these decisions on stand-by. For the time being, the Brazilian Society of Oncology Pharmacists in reference to the Resolution of CFF 623/2016 and the new frame of reference National Curricular Guidelines for the pharmaceutical profession in Brazil (CFF, 2016b) have stated that the complexity of oncological therapies, the inherent risks to professional practice, the need to ensure patient safety, and environmental management, among other aspects, underpin the importance of demanding specific graduation programs for an oncological pharmacist (Sobreira da Silva, 2016).

According to members of the CFF, the 1996 education law needs to be improved, as it leaves open the possibility that some pharmacy programs that do not meet the required quality standards do not have to change, as the Ministry of Education does not have the authority to cease their activities. At the same time, this law allows distance e-learning that is not subject to quality assurance regulation. This type of education has become an alternative to increase resources with greater student enrollment. As an example, according to information from the Brazilian Association of Pharmacy Schools, currently the country has more than 25,000 enrolled in nursing courses in this modality, and pharmacy courses are one of many others that face the same present and future (Dos Santos, 2016, personal communication).

THE CASE OF COSTA RICA

REGULATION OF PHARMACY EDUCATION

According to data provided by the Ministry of Public Education of Costa Rica, to date there are five public institutions of higher education and 54 private entities. In other words, public institutions comprise about 8% and private represent almost 92% of all higher education institutions. As in other Latin American countries, pharmacy education occurs at the university level. Regulation of pharmacy education in particular occurs through two channels, depending on whether the pharmacy program belongs to a public or a private institution. The National Council of Rectors (CONARE) regulates public education through the Office of Planning for Higher Education (OPES) (https://www.conare.ac.cr). Nevertheless, it should be noted that the University of Costa Rica is the only public university with a pharmacy program. Private universities are regulated by the National Council of Private Higher Education (CONESUP) created by Law No. 6693 on November 27, 1981 and published in the Official Gazette, No. 243 on December 21, 1981 (www.mep.go.cr/conesup). CONESUP is not an accrediting body, and as an entity assigned to the Ministry of Public Education it is in charge of regulating and supervising private universities. Also, it authorizes the creation of new universities, opening undergraduate programs, curricular modifications, etc. To date, there are four private faculties/schools of pharmacy.

The current state regulations neither provide a coordination space between the two sectors nor define a common regulatory and supervisory organization. As a result, the quality of education assessed through accreditation processes is carried out by a national accreditation body. The National System of Accreditation of Higher Education (SINAES) is the institution in charge of promoting the permanent improvement of the quality of higher education at an institutional and study programs level. Accreditation is still voluntary, and in Costa Rica today four out of five pharmacy programs are accredited by SINAES (http://www.sinaes.ac.cr/).

REGULATIONS AND THEIR INFLUENCE ON STRENGTHENING PHARMACY EDUCATION AND PROGRESS

As already mentioned, higher education in Costa Rica is regulated by two different bodies depending on whether it is public or private. Specifically, pharmacy education does not have its own regulations, and the accreditation processes ensure compliance with common standards for undergraduate degrees, including the evaluation of their curriculum, faculty, and infrastructure, among many other aspects. Despite this, the Pharmacists Association of Costa Rica in its Organic Law article 1 states that one of its objectives is "to promote the progress of Pharmacy and all related sciences" (COLFAR, 1972). To this end, it has drawn up regulations for the different professional practices that indirectly impact pharmacy education. At the same time, within this organization there is a Professional Development Department that is responsible for continuous pharmacy education or professional certification. This regulation, either for university undergraduate students or for professional development, is considered key to support strengthening pharmacy education in the country. It is important to emphasize that due to an initiative by the Board of Directors of the Association of Pharmacists, the so-called Deans of Pharmacy Commission was created in 2013. This commission is expected to improve the quality of pharmacy education and respond to the health needs of Costa Rica in terms of the competencies of pharmacists (Badilla, 2016). The commission is coordinated by a member of the Board of Directors of the Pharmacists Association and includes the deans from the five pharmacy schools in Costa Rica, i.e., the University of Costa Rica (public) and all four private ones with pharmacy undergraduate programs (the University of Medical Sciences, Universidad Latina, Universidad Iberoamericana and the International University of the Americas). This commission was conceived from the need to create a forum in which every individual academic unit assumes their historical role with respect to their original institutions, along with a commitment to train pharmaceutical professionals to provide the best care for the country. Some additional purposes of this commission are to:

- Ensure the quality of pharmacy education within higher education institutions;
- Define the general competencies of pharmacists in Costa Rica;
- Establish research lines according to pharmacy schools' own interests within the framework of national development;
- Equally disseminate among all pharmacy schools of Costa Rica the commitments of international organizations that are referents in the pharmaceutical field;
- Create a space for reflection among university officials with regard to the future of pharmacy education while preserving their institutional independence.

Another important national public body, the so-called Costa Rican Social Security Fund, is responsible for regulating curricular experiential practices that are conducted in various facilities. These are also known as university students' residences or supervised practices, which are obligatory curricular activities for all the various pharmacy programs and are considered as the final graduation task (http://www.ccss.sa.cr/).

In contrast to these initiatives, pharmacy schools belonging to private institutions have stated that CONESUP regulations somewhat limit curricular modifications. As a result, modifications to the CONESUP regulations have been made to articles 23 and 24, allowing curricular changes for accredited careers to take place with the approval of SINAES but no required consultation with professional associations (MEP, 2016). This decision has already generated important structural problems for pharmacy education. As an example, an accredited pharmacy degree recently eliminated a semester from its curriculum and the Pharmacists Association had no recourse to prevent it or to express its concerns (http://www.ccss.sa.cr/).

THE CASE OF CHILE

REGULATION OF PHARMACY EDUCATION

In 1981, one of the most important modifications to the educational system arose in Chile, with social and economic implications. The reform had implications for the pharmacy degree (chemistry and pharmacy degree) since the law established that all curricula for professional practice and graduate degrees (master's and PhDs) must be conducted at universities only (MINEDUC, 1990). Thus, the chemistry and pharmacy program was a university-level curriculum (as it has been historically), taking at least 5 years to complete (in some schools of chemistry and pharmacy it could take longer, up to 6 years overall). As of 2017, 12 chemistry and pharmacy programs exist, 5 at public universities and 7 at private universities (Table 1). In recent years, important changes in the curricula of chemistry and pharmacy have been carried out due to significant changes in pharmacy practice. However, these curricular modifications have also been influenced by the administrative structures at their respective institutions, explaining the strong curricular foundation in science that prevails in the pharmacy curriculum.

Within the core curriculum, basic science courses are taken to understand drugs starting from their isolation or synthesis until dispensed to patients. Moreover, the final prerequisite for graduation had been for many years an experiential thesis that was carried out in research labs with the faculty/school of chemistry and pharmacy for roughly one year. As a result, involving pharmacy students with patients and the healthcare team occurred too late in their education and was superficial. This situation contrasts with the new responsibilities the health reform has bestowed upon pharmacists. The main changes for the pharmacy practice are contained in the following regulation documents:

- National Medicines Policy (MINSAL, 2004a)
- National Formulary of Medicines Regulation (MINSAL, 2004b)
- National Formulary of Medications (MINSAL, 2006).

Table 1 Faculties or Schools of Chemistry and Pharmacy in Chile to February 2017

University	Category (Public/ Private)	Foundation (Year)	Faculty
U. de Chile	Public	1911[b]	Chemical and Pharmaceutical Sciences
U. de Concepcion	Private	1919	Pharmacy
U. de Valparaiso	Public	1972	Pharmacy
Pontificia U. Catolica	Private	1987	Chemistry
U. Austral de Chile	Private	1994	Sciences
U. Arturo Prat	Public	2000	Health Sciences
U. Catolica del Norte	Private	2000	Sciences
U. Nacional AndresBello[a]	Private	1999	Medicine
U. San Sebastian[a]	Private	2000	Sciences
U. de Santiago	Public	2013	Chemistry and Biology
U. La Frontera	Public	2016	Medicine
U. Bernardo O'Higgins	Private	2017	Engineering, Sciences and Technology

[a]*Programs are given in two different cities.*
[b]*The first Pharmacy course dates from 1833 in the National Institute. It was not until 1911 that it became the School of Pharmacy at the University of Chile.*

The National Medicines Policy has been strategic to the pharmacists' professional development, especially in hospitals and in primary care areas, providing (Sepúlveda, 2008):

- Guaranteed access to and availability of medicines;
- Quality assurance of all medicines;
- Rational drug use;
- A new role for pharmacy and the pharmacist in health reform.

The evolution from a drug-based model to a patient-centered model has added value to the pharmacist's professional practice. Pharmaceutical care and clinical pharmacy now support prescription drug management, and pharmaceutical services are offered in primary healthcare; these among other changes have been part of the modification in health policies in Chile.

Health reform in Chile, including the National Medication Policy, has positioned pharmacists as contributors to achieving therapeutic goals and as promoters of the rational use of medications. Research carried out in 2010 (Núñez & Méndez, 2011) explored sensitivities of pharmacists belonging to different healthcare levels within the metropolitan areas with respect to the implementation of changes due to the new National Medication Policy. The interviewed professionals stated that this policy has given pharmacists and pharmacies an important role in different sectors of the healthcare network. Nevertheless, some difficulties in its application have been cited, such as the absence of different organizational and structural conditions in the various institutional reforms. This has been a challenge for the Ministry of Health officials. Thus, relevant and quality curricula have become a priority for pharmacy schools.

THE IMPORTANCE OF THE QUALITY OF CURRICULA AND THE INSTITUTIONS

In Chile, a wide debate is ongoing among different actors involved in higher education quality assurance at a national level, both at the institutional level and degree programs. A quality assurance model should be able to measure a specific level of knowledge and skills, the students' learning, and the corresponding institutional role. The Chilean Quality Assurance System was established in 2006 (MINEDUC, 2006). On the other hand, the responsible body for verifying and promoting the quality of universities and other higher education institutions, along with undergraduate and graduate degrees, is the National Accreditation Commission (https://www.cnachile.cl). With the exception of medicine and pedagogies, accreditation is still a voluntary process and those who undergo this process do so in order to have a quality certification concerning their internal processes and their results. Law 20,129 establishes a National System for Assuring the Quality of Higher Education. Accreditation of different programs offered by autonomous institutions of higher education includes verifying their quality according to their stated purposes and the corresponding criteria established by both academic and professional communities.

The main bodies of this system are:

- The National Education Council (CNED),
- The National Accreditation Commission (CNA),
- The Ministry of Education, through its Division of Higher Education (MINEDUC).

The activities of the various organizations that make up this system are organized by the Coordination Committee.

THE ACCREDITATION OF THE CHEMISTRY AND PHARMACY CURRICULUM

The curriculum for chemistry and pharmacy shares common characteristics and the emphasis on each of its components is related to the respective mission and vision of the universities and the corresponding academic entities.

Some of the common characteristics of the chemistry and pharmacy curricula in Chile are:

- Generalist, i.e., there is no professional specialization at the undergraduate level;
- Scientific and professional. The emphasis is given by the percentage of courses (credits/hours) taken in three levels during the curriculum: basic sciences, preprofessional, professional, plus experiential at practice sites (community pharmacy is mandatory, and additional practice sites: hospital pharmacy, primary healthcare, industrial pharmacy, cosmetics, clinical analysis laboratories, etc.). In addition, the final requirement for graduating is a one-semester thesis or a longer practice at any of the practice sites (one semester, 5 days a week and 8 hours a day). This is also similar to other countries in Latin America, as seen in the document Basic Plan of Pharmaceutical Education (OPS/OMS, 1999). Table 2 compiles the main aspects to take into account in this regard;
- Once curricular requirements are accomplished, the student is legally allowed to practice in a community pharmacy, hospital pharmacy and primary healthcare system, pharmaceutical and cosmetics industries, regulatory entities, universities, or clinical laboratory, among others;
- Duration of studies lasts from 5 to 6 years, depending on the particular school/faculty.

Furthermore, the changes in health policies observed in the last decade have strongly influenced the professional orientation of the pharmacist, becoming more clinical and patient-centered. At the same time, quality-oriented higher education policies have created an appropriate environment for a new, competency-based approach to curriculum development. In this respect, regional and international organizations have played a leading role. The Pan-American Conference on Pharmaceutical Education at the level of the Americas, and FIP with its global perspective, have guided and supported the schools of chemistry and pharmacy and have proposed a new curriculum. The Joint FIP/WHO Guidelines on Good Pharmacy Practice (FIP/WHO, 2011), the FIPEd Global Competency Framework (FIP, 2012), and the Global Framework for Quality Assurance of Pharmacy Education (FIP, 2014) have been important guidelines and frameworks for pharmacy education at a global level. The two documents

Table 2 Common Characteristics of the Pharmacy Curriculum of Various Programs

Pharmacy Curriculum: Structure	Percentage (%)
Basis Sciences	49–54
Pharmaceutical Sciences	23–32
Biomedical Sciences	13–19
Social, Behavioral, Administrative Sciences	4–7
Integrative Courses	Yes
Preprofessional Experiences	Yes
Thesis or Residences (Longer experiential practice)	6 months[a]

[a] *Eight hours a day from Monday to Friday.*

have been essential for emphasizing specific professional aspects that need to be enhanced in pharmacy students. The recent Nanjing Declaration (FIP, 2016) outlines the main concerns for pharmacy education at present and the near future.

Nonetheless, the current quality standards for the chemistry and pharmacy curriculum go back to 1998 (CNA, 2001). The standards were agreed to by academic faculty officials and leaders representing the different areas of professional practice (Technical Committee), according to the following chemistry and pharmacy profile: "Health Professional, specialist in drugs and other biologically active substances with solid knowledge in biological and chemical sciences with particular emphasis on pharmaceutical sciences, able to participate in actions related to the drug and its application to the individual in order to promote rational drug use and participate in the promotion of public health and improvement of the quality of life."

Quality criteria for all higher education curricula include the following:

- Mission, planning, and continuous quality improvement and evaluation;
- Organization and administration;
- Curriculum;
- Students and academic policies;
- Staff resources;
- Physical and structural facilities and resources;
- External relationships (national and abroad).

According to these criteria, after 19 years discrepancies persist and urgently need to be modified in order to ensure relevant, pertinent, and quality pharmacy programs.

ANALYSIS OF THE SITUATION AT THE PROFESSIONAL LEVEL

As indicated previously, after obtaining the degree, pharmacists can legally practice in any of the professional areas of their interest, although community pharmacy attracts the largest number of professionals (Acuna, 2016). However, with respect to hospital pharmacists, for permanent positions or fixed-term renewable contracts year by year, pharmacists enter through a national or local public application process. Training in hospital pharmacy is certified by the national agency responsible for certification of pharmaceutical specialties, the so-called National Commission for Certification of Pharmaceutical Specialties (CONACEF) created in 2004 (SCHFA, 2012). The certification of a particular specialty is voluntary and not exclusive, i.e., certification of the hospital pharmacy specialty is not necessarily required for hospital pharmacy practice. Currently, the only specialty certified by CONACEF is Pharmacy Management in the Health Care System. Community pharmacy and clinical laboratory specialties are expected to be certified in the near future. CONACEF's Board of Directors is represented by academic bodies, pharmacy practitioner's entities and scientific-professional societies: the Chilean Academy of Pharmaceutical Sciences, the Chilean Pharmacists' Association, scientific societies within the Chilean Pharmacists' Association, and Chilean faculties/schools of pharmacy[2].

[2]Status has considered 5 representatives, although today there are 12 faculty/school/undergraduate programs in Pharmacy (Chemistry and Pharmacy).

On the other hand, as there is not yet a single instance of coordination between the pharmacy schools in the country, it is fundamental and urgent to have a coordinating body bringing together all faculties/schools of pharmacy. Academic leadership is required to establish a common pathway to follow in the short, medium, and long term. In general, academia and the pharmacy profession have mostly followed parallel tracks, and both groups have policies and regulations that support their actions. Academia has developed rather individual initiatives or instrumental networks for curriculum innovation for achieving specific goals. The same is observed in the professional field. However, the National Pharmacists' Association and its scientific-professional association's representatives have played an important role in placing the pharmacist at the center of health and social needs, bringing together health policies and higher education policies.

At the same time, it is necessary to point out the importance of continuing professional development. Voluntary and nonregulating activities are carried out systematically either as postgraduate programs or as courses and diplomas offered every year as a joint effort by both academia and the national pharmacists' association to encourage professional development of graduated pharmacists. First, it is important to highlight two professional master's of science programs in pharmacy. Both the Master's in Pharmacy Management and Hospital Pharmacy (University of Valparaiso), and the Master's in Pharmacy (Andres Bello National University) are linked to undergraduate curricula. These two initiatives are the result of higher education policies that seek to improve the quality of all higher education students (not just pharmacists) and future professionals. However, the necessary communication between the ministries of education and health is lacking, since graduate studies in pharmaceutical sciences/pharmacy are not a requirement when applying for a certain position in the public healthcare system. Therefore, postgraduate studies are voluntary and are seen as a form of professional development that at some point can be recognized in the future. Higher education legislation demands that all postgraduate programs must be accredited or else they cannot exist over time. Thus, graduate and undergraduate programs are conceived under quality assurance standards. On the other hand, two important courses in clinical pharmacy and pharmaceutical care that are well recognized nationally and internationally are the Latin American Course in Clinical Pharmacy (U. Chile) and that in one of the oldest hospitals in Chile (El Salvador). Other continuing pharmacy-developing (CPD) activities are the Diploma in Clinical Pharmacy and Pharmacotherapeutic of the Pontifical Catholic University of Chile, and the Diploma in Management in Pharmacy from the University of Chile. As for professional groups in the clinical field, the Chilean Society of Hospital and Primary Care Pharmacy and the Division of Clinical Pharmacists belonging to the Chilean Society of Intensive Care Medicine stand out (Sepúlveda, 2008).

In addition to many other lifelong learning courses for pharmacy practitioners, for the time being some priority issues to address include the following: increasing the number of and enrollment in pharmacy programs with faculties of different orientations (basic sciences, medicine, engineering, and technology, both public and private), and the influence of this increase on the availability of clinical positions for students' experiential practice (currently a major problem); competencies of the pharmacist; minimum content of pharmacy curricula; and the need to reexamine the standards for the accreditation of curricula as a way of regulating quality.

It should be noted that, regardless of the country and the different institutions with pharmacy education programs, the quality of the training process is strongly linked to the quality of pharmaceutical services delivered as professionals. This not only requires specific knowledge in professional matters, but also attitudes, skills, and values cross-sectionally in a globalized fast-changing world, where the patient is the direct beneficiary of the pharmacist's actions (PAHO/WHO, 2016).

CONCLUSIONS

Latin American variations in the regulations of pharmacy education as seen in some examples were presented in this chapter. All three Latin American countries taken as case studies in this chapter were chosen by the author due to their major social, cultural, political, and economic differences. Regulations have played an important role in the strengthening and guiding of pharmacy education. Despite their differences, all three countries have important issues in common with respect to regulations. As in other cases not illustrated here, none of the regulations have been obstacles nor delayed the advancement of pharmacy education. In general, the Ministry of Education in various countries has played a leading role regarding the new guidelines for pharmacy education. On the other hand, changes in pharmacy practice towards a patient-centered model have been led by the corresponding Ministry of Health. Various norms and regulations (many of them quite similar among each of the different countries) have strongly favored the development of the pharmaceutical profession. Overall, regulations have contributed to the valorization of the profession in all areas of pharmacy practice, especially in hospital pharmacy and primary healthcare pharmacy as well as community pharmacy, although this latter area is not a common issue in many countries. The driving forces have emerged from different pharmacy professional actors, both nationally and internationally. They have contributed to the development of public policies in higher education and in public health. In this regard, the roles of pharmacy professionals representing specific areas of pharmacy practice, national pharmacists' associations and scientific-professional societies, and academia have been crucial.

REFERENCES

Acuna, P. (2016). Pharmacy practice in developing countries. In A. I. Fathelrahman, M. I. M. Ibrahim, & A. I. Wertheimer (Eds.), *Pharmacy practice in Chile* (pp. 403–446): Academic Press, Elsevier.

Badilla, B. (2016). Comisión de Decanos: Un Espacio de Confluencia de la Educación Farmacéutica en Costa Rica [Dean´s Commission: A place of confluence of Pharmacy Education in Costa Rica]. Retrieved January 19, 2017 from Colegio de Farmacéuticos de Costa Rica Website: http://www.colfarma.org.ar/Prensa%20y%20Difusion/Documentos%20BOLETINES/Comisi%C3%B3n%20de%20Decanos%20_19-08-2015_.pdf.

CFF (2002). Diretrizes Curriculares Nacionais do Curso de Graduação em Farmácia. Conselho Nacional da Educação, Câmara Nacional da Educação Superior. Retrieved January 19, 2017 from Ministério da Educação do Brasil Website: http://portal.mec.gov.br/cne/arquivos/pdf/CES022002.pdf.

CFF (2008). Os Desafios da Educação Farmacêutica no Brasil, Conselho Federal de Farmácia, Brasilia, DF. Retrieved January 19, 2017 from Conselho Federal de Farmácia Website: http://cff.org.br, pp. 40–44.

CFF (2013a). Resolução N° 585, 29 agosto 2013, Conselho Federal de Farmácia. Retrieved January 19, 2017 from Conselho Federal de Farmácia Website: http://cff.org.br.

CFF (2013b). Resolução N° 586, 29 agosto 2013, Conselho Federal de Farmácia. Retrieved January 19, 2017 from Conselho Federal de Farmácia Website: http://cff.org.br.

CFF (2015). Pharmaceutical prescription and clinical attributions of the Pharmacist, Compilation of documents, Conselho Federal de Farmácia. Retrieved January 19, 2017 from http://www.cff.org.br/userfiles/file/prescri%C3%A7%C3%A3o%20farmaceutica_AZUL%20(2).pdf, pp. 1–40.

CFF (2016a). Propostas para a elaboração das diretrizes curriculares nacionais para o curso de gradação em farmácia—COMENSINO/CAEF/ABEF. Conselho Federal de Farmácia, Associação Brasileira de Educação Farmacêutica, 10 de Maio, 2016. Retrieved January 19, 2017 from http://www.cff.org.br/userfiles/file/PROPOSTAS%20DE%20DCN%20FARM%C3%81CIA%20-10-05-2016.pdf, pp. 1–15.

CFF (2016b). Entidades de fiscalização do exercício das profissões liberais. Resolução N° 623, de 29 de abril de 2016. Retrieved January 19, 2017 from http://www.cmconsultoria.com.br/imagens/diretorios/diretorio14/arquivo5494.pdf.

CNA (2001). Criterios de Evaluación de Carreras de Química y Farmacia [Assessment Crieria for Chemistry and Pharmacy Graduation]. Retrieved January 19, 2017 from Comisión Nacional de Acreditación Website: http://www.cnachile.cl/Criterios%20de%20carreras/quimicayfarmacia.pdf.

COLFAR (1972). Ley Orgánica N° 5142 de 30 de noviembre de 1972 [Organic Law N°5142 from November 30, 1972]. Retrieved January 19, 2017 from Colegio de Farmacéuticos de Costa Rica Website: http://www.colfar.com/index.php?option=com_phocadownload&view=category&id=9:leyes-y-reglamentos&Itemid=217.

Dos Santos, R. (2016). personal communication, 5 of December of 2016.

FIP (2012). FIPEducation initiatives. Pharmacy education taskforce. A global competency framework, version 1. International Pharmaceutical Federation, FIP Education Initiatives. Retrieved February 27, 2017 from FIP Website: http://www.fip.org/publications.

FIP (2014). Quality assurance of pharmacy education: The FIP global framework. 2nd ed. International Pharmaceutical Federation, FIP Education Initiatives. Retrieved February 27, 2017 from FIP Website: http://www.fip.org/publications.

FIP (2016). Global vision for education and workforce. Global conference on pharmacy and pharmaceutical sciences education. International Pharmaceutical Federation, FIP Education Initiatives. Retrieved February 27, 2017 from FIP Website: http://www.fip.org/publications.

FIP/WHO (2011). Good pharmacy practice. Joint FIP/WHO guidelines on GPP: Standards for quality of pharmacy services. International Pharmaceutical Federation, World Health Organization. Retrieved February 27, 2017 from FIP Website: http://www.fip.org.

Frade, J. (2014). In *El camino hacia la prescripción farmacéutica: el caso de Brasil [The way to pharmacists' prescription]. Presented at the XVI Congreso Farmacéutico Nacional, Septiembre-Octubre, San José, Costa Rica.*

Frade, J. (2015). Estrategias adoptadas por el Consejo Federal de Farmacia para estimular el avance de la Farmacia Clínica en Brasil [Strategies to encourage Clinical Pharmacy development in Brazil. Federal Council of Pharmacy]. *Revista FEFAS: Farmacia Sudamericana*, *19*(1), 10–12. Retrieved January 19, 2017 from https://issuu.com/crfrj/docs/revista_fefas__n__19.

MEC (1996). Ministério da Educação do Brasil.Lei N° 9.394de 20 de dezembro de 1996 Retrieved January 25, 2017 from http://portal.mec.gov.br/seesp/arquivos/pdf/lei9394_ldbn1.pdf.

MEP (2016). Ministerio de Educación Pública de Costa Rica. [Ministry of Public Education of Costa Rica]. Retrieved January 19, 2017 from the Ministry of Public Education Website: http://www.mep.go.cr/circulares_2016.

MINEDUC (1990). República de Chile, Ministerio de Educación. Ley Orgánica Constitucional de Enseñanza N° 18.962. Publicada el 10 de marzo de 1990 [Chilean Republic, Ministry of Education. Constitutional Organic Law of Education N° 18,962]. Retrieved January 19, 2017 from Universidad de Chile Website: http://www.uchile.cl/portal/presentacion/normativa-y-reglamentos/8386/ley-organica-constitucional-de-ensenanza.

MINEDUC (2006). República de Chile, Ministerio de Educación. Ley N° 20.129 de 23 de octubre de 2006. Publicada el 17 de noviembre de 2006. Establece un Sistema nacional de aseguramiento de la calidad de la educación superior [Chilean Republic, Ministry of Education. Law N° 20,129 from October 23, 2006. Published on November 17, 2006. Establishing a national system of quality assurance in higher education]. Retrieved January 30, 2017 from https://leychile.cl/N?i=255323&f=2017-01-28&p=.

MINSAL (2004a). República de Chile, Ministerio de Salud. Política Nacional de Medicamentos para la Reforma de la Salud. Resolución Exenta N°515 de 2 de abril de 2004 [Chilean Republic, Ministry of Health. Drugs' National Policy for Health Reform. Exent Resolution N°515, April 2, 2004]. Retrieved February 27, 2017 from Ministerio de Salud Website: http://web.minsal.cl.

MINSAL (2004b). República de Chile, Ministerio de Salud, Departamento Asesoría Jurídica. Reglamento del Formulario Nacional de Medicamentos. Decreto N°264/03, publicado en Diario Oficial el 16 de marzo de 2004 [Chilean Republic, Ministry of Health, Department of Legal Advice. National Formulary Regulation. Decreet N°264/03, published on the Official Journal on March 16, 2004]. Retrieved February 27, 2017 from http://juridico1.minsal.cl/DTO._264_03.doc.

MINSAL (2006). República de Chile, Ministerio de Salud, Subsecretaría de Salud Pública. Formulario Nacional de Medicamentos. Decreto N°194 de 2005, publicado en Diario Oficial el 10 de Marzo, 2006 [Chilean Republic, Ministry of Health. Undersecretariat of Public Health. Drugs' National Formulary. Decree N°194 2005, published on the Official Journal on March 10, 2006]. Retrieved February 27, 2017 from https://leychile.cl/N?i=247938&f=2013-03-11&p=.

Núñez, P., & Méndez, C. (2011). Implementación de la Política Nacional de Medicamentos de la Reforma de la Salud: Percepción del profesional químico farmacéutico [Implementing the National Drug Policy of the Health Reform: A Pharmacy professional point of view]. *Revista Chilena de Salud Pública*, *15*(1), 21–28.

OPS/OMS (1999). Plan Básico de Educación Farmacéutica. Propuesta de Grupo de Trabajo. Lima, Perú, 6 a 9 de Julio de 1998 [A basic plan for pharmacy education. A proposal from the work group. Lima, Peru, 6–9 of July 1998].

PAHO/WHO (2016). Propuesta de Plan Básico de Educación Farmacéutica y Competencias del Farmacéutico para la práctica profesional. Conferencia Panamericana de Educación Farmacéutica [A basic plan for pharmacy education and competencies for pharmacy practice proposal. Pan-American Conference of Pharmacy Education]. Manuscript for publication.

SCHFA (2012). Requisitos Específicos para la Certificación de Farmacia Asistencial por CONACEF. CONACEF Specific requirements for Pharmacy Health Services. Retrieved January 19, 2107 from the Chilean Society of Pharmacy Health Services. Website: http://schfa.cl/wp-content/uploads/2012/07/CONACEF-REQUISITOS-FCIA.ASISTENCIAL.MC_.M.P.pdf.

Sepúlveda, M. E. (2008). In *Farmacia Asistencial en Chile [Pharmaceutical Health Services in Chile] 53rd National Congress of the Spanish Hospital Pharmacy Society, Valencia, Spain*. Retrieved February 27, 2017 from: http://www.sefh.es/53congreso/documentos/ponencias/ponencia755.pdf.

Sobreira da Silva, M. J. (2016). Atuação do farmacêutico em Oncologia: O que se espera com a exigência de titulação mínima? *Revista Brasileira de Farmácia Hospitalar e Serviços de Saúde*, *7*(2), 4–5.

FURTHER READING

PAHO/WHO (1999). Plan Básico de Educación Farmacéutica. Propuesta del Grupo de Trabajo, Lima, Perú, 1998. [Basic Plan for Pharmacy Education. A proposal from the Task Group, Lima, Peru, 1998. Retrieved December 13, 2016 from PAHO Website: http://www.paho.org/hq/index.php?option=com_content&view=article&id=8374%3A2013-pharmaceutical-education&catid=4831%3Apharmaceutical-education&Itemid=39720&lang=es.

CHAPTER

CURRICULUM DEVELOPMENT: MISMATCH BETWEEN SUPPLY AND DEMAND

17

Bhuvan K.C.

Monash University Malaysia, Subang Jaya, Malaysia

PHARMACY EDUCATION

The fundamental goal of pharmacy education is to provide the necessary knowledge and skills to the students who will serve society as pharmacists and then connect them with the knowledge ecosystem that facilitates them to remain proficient in the profession. A typical pharmacy education degree has three components: science-based, practice/research-based, and practical training components (Guile & Ahamed, 2009). Pharmaceutical sciences form the core of pharmacy education and incorporate pure science and medical science based subjects, such as pharmaceutics, pharmaceutical chemistry, pharmacognosy, pharmacology, anatomy, physiology, and pharmacy practice. Following the science-based and practice/research-based components, a pharmacy student has then to undergo practical training that is either bridged to or leads directly to preregistration training. The pharmacy graduate then becomes registered with the respective pharmacy council or board after following the necessary regulatory requirements (e.g., examination, training). The structure of a pharmacy degree, however, along with regulatory requirements for pharmacists and practice scenarios and roles of pharmacists, differs between countries.

STRUCTURE OF PHARMACY DEGREE

The undergraduate pharmacy degree is offered in various formats, and the curriculum differs for each degree in terms of the balance, preference, and weighting given to science and practice-based subjects.

Generally, the traditional undergraduate course in pharmacy is structured as a full-time, 4-year degree. It is structured around biomedical, pharmaceutical, and health sciences during the first 2 years of the program, and more specific and applied subjects in the third and fourth years (Sosabowski & Gard, 2008). It is taught through lectures, laboratory sessions, tutorials and seminars, supervised practice, and projects; however, these methodologies vary among different universities and countries. A research project–based dissertation, usually in the fourth year, brings together research and analytical skills (Sosabowski & Gard, 2008). Likewise, a practice placement allows students to gain required experience in a clinical setting under experienced supervisor pharmacists (Sosabowski & Gard, 2008). Under

Pharmacy Education in the Twenty First Century and Beyond. https://doi.org/10.1016/B978-0-12-811909-9.00017-4

the traditional undergraduate pharmacy degree format, a preregistration training program of varying length is administered by the pharmacy regulatory body in some countries. Registration as a pharmacist occurs after successful completion of these components.

Doctor of Pharmacy (PharmD) is a professional doctorate degree in pharmacy that comprises at least six years of full-time study to prepare students to be leaders in pharmacy practice (Kreling et al., 2010). Contrary to a traditional BPharm degree, the student must complete a prepharmacy requirement worth certain college or university semester credits before beginning the PharmD program (Kreling et al., 2010; University of Minnesota, 2016). At the University of Minnesota, for example, the core PharmD curriculum covers basic sciences such as physiology, pharmaceutics, and pharmacology and other courses in the first year (University of Minnesota, 2016). Likewise, the second and third year of its PharmD program covers core courses such as pharmacology, medicinal chemistry, pharmacokinetics, pharmaceutics, and pharmacotherapy of particular organ systems, which are combined into intensive courses concentrating on disease management (University of Minnesota, 2016). These second- and third-year courses prepare students for the practice of pharmacy. The final fourth year of PharmD covers advanced pharmacy practice experience through various clinical rotations (University of Minnesota, 2016). These advanced pharmacy practice experiences are carried out in a variety of settings, such as acute, ambulatory, long-term care, and community settings. The modality, electives, and specialization in a PharmD program, however, vary widely among different universities and countries. The differences between a PharmD degree and a regular Bachelor of Science in Pharmacy or Bachelor in Pharmacy degree is that the PharmD degree has a core focus in pharmacy practice, while the BS Pharmacy or the Bachelor in Pharmacy degree covers both pharmaceutical sciences and pharmacy practice in general (University of Minnesota, 2016). Compared to BS Pharmacy or Bachelor in Pharmacy degrees, the PharmD curricula extends by 1 year to cover additional coursework in pharmacotherapy and patient care, with a goal of enhancing clinical skills (Kreling et al., 2010). There are, however, variations among universities offering similar degrees.

Usually, a Master's in Pharmacy (MPharm) degree in different disciplines such as pharmaceutics, clinical pharmacy, hospital pharmacy, industrial pharmacy, pharmacology, and pharmacognosy is a postgraduate degree for pharmacists (Nagavi, 2004). However, there is a different format for the Master of Pharmacy (MPharm). In the UK, it is the entry-level degree for the profession and is considered an undergraduate master. Typically, it is a 4-year, full-time program. For example, the MPharm degree offered by the De Montfort University is a 4-year honors undergraduate degree and has three integrated streams (i.e., pharmaceutical science, body system and clinical studies, and pharmacy practice and healthcare). The degree allows the graduates to sit for the preregistration assessment with the General Pharmaceutical Council (GPhC) following a year of preregistration training (De Montfort University Leicester, 2017). In terms of curriculum, Sosabowski and Gard reported that the UK MPharm program provides the students with theoretical and scientific knowledge along with experimental and clinical expertise. Therefore, unlike pharmacy programs in some other countries, the program does not concentrate purely on scientific aspects before students graduate and enter the pharmacy practice (Sosabowski & Gard, 2008). The main challenge of the UK's MPharm program in the coming years will be to find the right balance between the science and practice aspect within the course, because of the demand of more therapeutics portions to cater to new roles of pharmacists, such as independent prescribing in the UK.

Different countries and universities are running different formats for pharmacy degrees. The BPharm, BPharm (Hons), or Bachelor of Science (BSc) in Pharmacy are still common in many Asian countries, such as India, Bangladesh, Sri Lanka, and Malaysia, as well as in many other countries of the world (Kanke, 2012). The changes in the pharmacy profession, pharmacy practice scenario, and pharmaceutical world have led to a corresponding change in the structure and format of the pharmacy degree in Europe. Hwang et al. in a review reported about the harmonization of many pharmacy programs across Europe after the Bologna Declaration of 1999 and the changes in pharmacy program structure in countries such as the UK (4-year MPharm degree) or France (6-year PharmD degree as professional practice degree), and non-EU states like Switzerland (3-year degree in basic medical or pharmaceutical science followed by a 2-year master's degree in either pharmacy or industrial pharmaceutical sciences) (Hwang, Hale, & Kim, 2014). The PharmD program is considered to be a professional Doctor of Pharmacy degree, and is recognized as a standard pharmacy degree in the United States. In some Asian countries, the PharmD program has been launched to meet the needs for advanced practitioners and patient care skills in the area of pharmacy (Kheir et al., 2008). The PharmD program is also offered in countries such as Saudi Arabia, Canada, Qatar, United Arab Emirates, Lebanon, and India. However, in some countries, such as India, there are both a PharmD as a first degree and postbaccalaureate PharmD degree (Kheir et al., 2008). Moreover, not having a regional or international accreditation of the PharmD degree seems to be one of the problems of the PharmD degree program outside the United States (Kheir et al., 2008).

Change in the focus of the pharmacy profession from pharmaceutical products to pharmaceutical services, greater interaction with other healthcare professions, and involvement of pharmacists in disease-state management have mainly underpinned the changes in the format of the pharmacy degree (Wiedenmayer et al., 2006). These changes in pharmacy education have been facilitated and regulated by the pharmacy councils or boards, pharmaceutical societies, pharmacy guilds, and other professional bodies and universities. At the crux of these different pharmacy-degree formats are the balance, weighting, and emphasis of pharmacy education on pharmaceutical sciences and pharmacy practice.

DEMAND AND SUPPLY OF PHARMACY WORKFORCE

FACTORS AFFECTING THE DEMAND AND SUPPLY OF PHARMACY WORKFORCE

The ability to provide required pharmaceuticals and pharmacy services in each country and global market depends on a competent workforce, appropriate environment and infrastructure, and well-integrated institutions. The global demand for pharmaceutical products, pharmacists, and pharmaceutical services, however, is the key force that shapes the supply of qualified pharmacists.

1. The global supply of qualified pharmacists, however, is skewed towards different factors and varies across countries and regions. As per the Global Pharmacy Workforce report from the International Pharmaceutical Federation (FIP), the number of pharmacists per 10,000 population ranges from as low as 0.02 in Somalia to 25.07 in Malta, while the mean number equates to 6.02 pharmacists per 10,000 population (International Pharmaceutical Federation (FIP), 2012). Thus, the first factor that affects the global demand and supply of the pharmacy support workforce is the high regional (geographical) variation in demand and supply of qualified pharmacists.
2. Furthermore, if one looks at the number of pharmacists against the global disease burden, the African region has the least number of pharmacists to serve for a standard of 10,000 population,

despite having 30% of the global disease burden (International Pharmaceutical Federation (FIP), 2015). In contrast, countries with the lowest disease burden (as measured by disability-adjusted life years (DALYs) per 1000 population) such as Singapore have a good supply of pharmacists, at 144 pharmacists per 10,000 population (International Pharmaceutical Federation (FIP), 2015). Thus, the second factor that needs to be taken into account is the mismatch between the need and supply of pharmacists.

3. The third factor to be considered is the demand and supply of a pharmacy support workforce. Medicines have to be procured, transported, supplied, and stored in an appropriate facility before being dispensed to the end users. Pharmacies need adequately trained staff who can perform these duties so that the pharmacists can devote more time to patient care activities. These types of staff are called the pharmacy support workforce and are commonly known as pharmacy technicians. In practice, however, there is a mismatch between demand and supply of these technicians. In countries such as Japan, these pharmacy support workforces are nonexistent, while in Pakistan these pharmacy technicians comprise almost two-thirds of the workforce (Connelly, 2014; International Pharmaceutical Federation (FIP), 2012). Similarly, in Nepal's case, the pharmacy technicians or assistants that were schooled to replace the untrained people running retail drug shops went on to do higher studies in pharmacy. Thus, in practice there is a shortage of trained pharmacy assistants in Nepal and most of the retail pharmacies (i.e., community pharmacies) are still run by people who are not formally trained in pharmacy.
4. The fourth factor is gender distribution in the pharmacy workforce. There are differences and variation across countries when it comes to pharmacy workforce and gender distribution (Connelly, 2014). There is a higher percentage of female pharmacists in European and African/Eastern Mediterranean regions, while a higher percentage of male pharmacists are in the pharmacy workforce of the Southeast Asian and Western Pacific region (International Pharmaceutical Federation (FIP), 2012). Furthermore, more females are graduating as pharmacists and joining the global workforce, and as per the FIP report (2012), women constituted 54.9% of the pharmacist workforce globally (International Pharmaceutical Federation (FIP), 2012). Thus, a review of traditional models of pharmacy profession and practice and innovative policies are required so that the profession can gain a positive boost from this gender shift in the pharmacy workforce (Gardner & Stowe, 2007).
5. The fifth factor that impacts the global demand and supply of pharmacists is the lack of balanced growth in various areas of pharmacy, such as the pharmaceutical industry, community pharmacy, hospital pharmacy, research, administration, NGOs, and academic sectors. In South Asian countries such as India, Pakistan, Nepal, Bangladesh, and Sri Lanka, different branches of pharmacy such as industrial pharmacy and pharmaceutical product development and marketing are well established and absorb most of the pharmacy graduates. Areas such as community pharmacy, hospital pharmacy, and clinical pharmacy, however, are not well established in these countries. Most of the hospitals in these countries do not run their own hospital pharmacy, so there are not many pharmacists working in the hospital and clinical pharmacy sector. Likewise, community pharmacies in countries such as Pakistan and India are run as sales-oriented retail pharmacies, without providing much in the way of pharmacy services (Aslam, Bushra, & Khan, 2012; Basak & Sathyanarayana, 2009). This environment has impacted the overall quality use of medicines in these countries.

All of these factors have contributed towards the imbalance in pharmacy workforce production, distribution, and the overall growth of the pharmacy sector. They have led to a skewed distribution of pharmacists across the different regions, and lack of growth in some vital areas of pharmacy (such as hospital and clinical pharmacy, and community pharmacy). They have also led to:

a) Oversupply of pharmacists in some areas and regions, while causing undersupply in other areas and regions;
b) A "brain drain" of pharmacists; and
c) Hampering of the qualitative growth of the pharmacy profession.

LABOR MARKET FOR PHARMACY SERVICES

The FIP's global pharmacy workforce report (2015) states that the aspiration of many countries towards Universal Health Coverage (UHC) means a demand for more health workforce, including pharmacists (International Pharmaceutical Federation (FIP), 2015). It also reports on the increase in the density of pharmacists in all the WHO regions, with the highest mean percentage change in pharmacist density in the Western Pacific and Eastern Mediterranean regions (International Pharmaceutical Federation (FIP), 2012). It suggests, however, the need to do much more in terms of delivery of pharmacists and pharmacy services in low-income countries, as there exists a linear association between the total number of pharmacists and the income level of the countries (International Pharmaceutical Federation (FIP), 2012). Thus, pharmacy colleges and health institutions of low-income countries have dual challenges: producing enough pharmacists to meet the country's heath needs, and ensuring qualitative growth in the pharmacy profession.

The demand and supply of the pharmacy workforce in individual countries must be seen in the context of the country's population, local disease burden, and the economic situation of the country. Moreover, the pharmacy workforce production and management and delivery of pharmacy services must align with the country's health policies and strategies. The US Bureau of Labor Statistics projects that employment of pharmacists and pharmacy assistants will grow by 3% and 8% respectively in 2014–2024 (Bureau of Labor Statistics, 2015). There appears to be an increasing demand for advanced pharmacy services in the United States, especially within community pharmacies and hospital/clinical pharmacies (Hulisz & Brown, 2014). Likewise, a Pharmaceutical Group of European Union (EU) report (2016) shows an increasing number of community pharmacies in EU countries and the increasing need for specialized community pharmacy services in these countries (Pharmaceutical Group of the European Union, 2016). Thus there seems to be an increasing demand for advanced pharmacy and pharmaceutical care services in the Organisation for Economic Co-operation and Development (OECD) countries.

This increasing demand in the OECD countries is for both regular pharmacy services and advanced pharmacy services (Pharmaceutical Group of the European Union, 2016). Regular pharmacy services include dispensing of medicines, patient counseling and education, and medication management, but there is an ever-increasing demand for advanced pharmacy services such as chronic disease management, medicine use review, homecare services, aged care services, and specialized pharmaceutical care services (OECD, 2015; Pharmaceutical Group of the European Union, 2016).

Similarly, there is an increasing demand for pharmacists and pharmacy services in low-income countries. There are pharmacists available to work but there are not enough jobs for these pharmacists.

For example, there is a need for more pharmacists to enhance the pharmaceutical manufacturing capacity, as well as to ensure quality use of medicines in many African countries, but the institutions to deliver these services are lacking due to economic problems. In South Asian countries, there is a need for pharmacists to work in community pharmacies, hospital pharmacies, and the public health sector, but again there are not enough jobs in these areas as they are occupied by those with minimal training in pharmacy (e.g., pharmacy technician).

PHARMACY CURRICULUM, PHARMACEUTICAL EXPERTISE AND PHARMACY SERVICES

In general, a pharmacy curriculum needs to reflect the pharmaceutical expertise and pharmacy services needed by the healthcare system. The health workforce, which is an important component of a healthcare system, is affected by several factors, such as healthcare financing, health policy, and the general sociopolitical and socioeconomic environment of each individual country. Thus there seems to be significant differences across countries or regions when it comes to the harmonization between pharmacy curriculum and the demand for pharmaceutical expertise and pharmacy services of the healthcare system.

Ideally, a pharmacy curriculum should reflect the latest trends and practice in the areas of pharmaceutical manufacturing, pharmacy practice (hospital, clinical, community and regulatory pharmacy), pharmaceutical research (new drug delivery, newer formulations and pharmacognosy), and public health. But, in reality, some of these sectors are well developed while others are lagging behind within a single country. This unevenness is reflected in the pharmacy curriculum as well. For example, pharmaceutical manufacturing and the drug development sector are relatively better in India due to the involvement of big private pharmaceutical manufacturers. This is not, however, the same case with the hospital pharmacy, clinical pharmacy, and community pharmacy in India. So, the undergraduate pharmacy curriculum in India is sound and well-designed when it comes to subject areas such as pharmaceutics, dosage form and design, industrial pharmacy, medicinal and pharmaceutical chemistry, and quality assurance.

To increase the coverage of healthcare systems, the systems in South Asian countries such as India, Nepal, and Pakistan are in need of a larger healthcare workforce, including pharmacists. There is a huge demand for pharmacists who can work in hospital pharmacy, community pharmacy, and advanced clinical settings. Producing such pharmacists requires an extensive theoretical and practical training of pharmacy students in the areas of pharmacy practice, clinical pharmacy, and pharmaceutical care. The undergraduate pharmacy curricula in some countries as depicted in Table 1, however, mostly lack adequate practical training in hospital/clinical pharmacy and community pharmacy. Undergraduate pharmacy students are posted for just a few weeks (i.e., 1 to 4 weeks training) in a hospital during the BPharm course, while many schools do not send students for community pharmacy training. Therefore, many pharmacy schools' curricula in the South Asian countries lack proper hospital, community, and clinical pharmacy training. Similarly, many hospitals in these countries do not run a hospital pharmacy of their own; instead they rent the hospital premises to the private sector to run a retail pharmacy in the hospital. These hospital-linked retail pharmacies focus more on sales and supply of medicines and do not provide patient counseling, drug information services, medication review, and other hospital pharmacy services. Moreover, some of the hospitals in India and Nepal still do not have a drug information and pharmacovigilance unit, patient counseling and education unit, therapeutic drug monitoring

Table 1 Pharmacy Curriculum Coverage in Different Countries

Pharmacy Programs	Country	Pharmacy Practice Based Subjects	Remarks
University Institute of Pharmaceutical Sciences, Punjab University	India	• Health Education (blended with Anatomy and Physiology course) • Pharmaceutical Jurisprudence • Clinical Pharmacy • General and Dispensing Pharmacy	Strong lab-based training in the area of pharmaceutics, pharmacognosy, and pharmacology Limited community pharmacy based education and training
Web page: http://pharma.puchd.ac.in/			
JSS College of Pharmacy, JSS University	India	• Pharmaceutical Jurisprudence and Management • Pharmacy Practice • Social Pharmacy and Behavioral Science	At least 150h (over 4 weeks) of industry or hospital or community pharmacy training
Web page: http://jssuni.edu.in/JSSWeb/WebHome.aspx			
School of Health and Allied Sciences, Pokhara University	Nepal	• Hospital Pharmacy • Clinical Pharmacy • Pharmacoeconomics and Management • Social Pharmacy and Pharmaceutical Jurisprudence • Pharmacy Practice	Only two weeks of hospital and retail pharmacy training
Web page: http://pu.edu.np/university/school-of-health-allied-sciences/			
Faculty of Medicine Galle, University of Ruhuna	Sri Lanka	• Pharmacy Law and Ethics • Hospital and Clinical Pharmacy • Community Pharmacy • Management and Economics • Marketing and Accounting	Provisions of clinical orientation program where pharmacy students need to undergo clinical attachments in different wards of hospital Some modules on community pharmacy practice

Continued

Table 1 Pharmacy Curriculum Coverage in Different Countries—cont'd

Pharmacy Programs	Country	Pharmacy Practice Based Subjects	Remarks
Web page: http://www.medi.ruh.ac.lk/			
School of Pharmaceutical Sciences, Universiti Sains Malaysia	Malaysia	• Pharmaceutical Management and Marketing • Social and Public Health Pharmacy • Clinical Pharmacy Practice • Forensic Pharmacy and Ethics • Medication Counseling Practice • Hospital Pharmacy • Community Pharmacy	Provisions of pharmacy practice training in different organizations from year two of BPharm program Compulsory provisions of 1 year of housemanship at hospital or industry or retail pharmacy
Web page: http://www.pha.usm.my/index.php/ms/			
School of Pharmacy, University of Otago	New Zealand	• Principles of Pharmacy Practice Courses • Quality Use of Medicines • Professional Pharmacy Practice Courses	One year of internship at a pharmaceutical establishment
Web page: https://www.pharmacy.umn.edu/			
Faculty of Pharmacy, University of Sydney	Australia	• Social Pharmacy • Pharmacy Practice • Pharmacy Skills and Dispensing • Integrated Dispensing Practice • Pharmacy Services and Public Health • Pharmacy Management • Professional Practice	Provisions of specialized clinical pharmacy subjects Clinical placement in hospital and clinical pharmacies and a preregistration training

Web page: http://sydney.edu.au/pharmacy/			
College of Pharmacy, University of Minnesota	US	• Pharmaceutical Care (Foundation/Skills Lab) • Foundation of Social and Administrative Pharmacy • Community-Practice Pharmacy Experience • Institutional-Practice Pharmacy Experience • Community Practice and Ambulatory Care	Adequate clinical pharmacy and practice-based components
Web page: https://www.pharmacy.umn.edu/			
Faculty of Pharmacy, Uppsala University	Sweden	• Pharmacoepidemiology and Health Economics • Pharmaceutical Care and Pharmaceutical Legislation • Applied Pharmacy Practice	Integrated pharmacy practice internship provision in a community pharmacy where students are paid during the internship
Web page: http://katalog.uu.se/organisation/?orgId=FF			
Faculty of Health Science, Nelson Mandela Metropolitan University	South Africa	• Pharmacy Profession and Environment • Clinical Placement	Adequate pharmacy practice exposure with clinical placement during undergraduate studies and compulsory 1 year of community services (pharmacy) after completion of the 4-year BPharm degree
Web page: http://health.nmmu.ac.za/			

unit, total parenteral nutrition, and in-patient compounding unit. The pharmacy schools cover these applied pharmacy skills in theory, but there are no practice settings for students to become trained in these areas.

The pharmacy education in countries such as Malaysia, Singapore, New Zealand, Australia, and many OECD countries covers both theoretical and practical components in the area of pharmacy practice. The pharmacy curriculum in these countries covers a long period of training in hospital pharmacy and community pharmacy, so the student has both theoretical and practical exposure in these areas (either integrated in the curriculum or separated in a full year of preregistration training). The healthcare system in many of the OECD or high-income countries, however, is still in need of pharmacists who can run disease management programs, carry out home medication reviews, run pharmacist-managed clinics, perform medication management in rest homes for the elderly population, and carry out prescribing/deprescribing (Pharmaceutical Group of the European Union, 2016). Moreover, pharmacists need additional or specialized training so that they can provide such advanced services. Except for the Doctor of Pharmacy (PharmD) program, the undergraduate pharmacy curriculum in many countries does not envision producing pharmacists who can manage to provide direct patient care services. Instead, they aim to produce pharmacists who can work in hospital pharmacy or community pharmacy settings to provide traditional services (i.e., product-oriented services). So, can a community pharmacist or a hospital/clinical pharmacist run independent or collaborative services such as disease management, medication review, travel health, or an immunization program? Whether we need to train future undergraduate pharmacy students in these areas, or whether we can leave these areas for a postgraduate pharmacy program is an open question. Both the pharmacy school and pharmacy council have to work out a plan to cater to societies' needs for these types of specialized pharmacy services.

The healthcare systems in both developed and developing countries are exposed to ups and downs in the economic environment. There seems to be an ever-increasing pressure on the healthcare system due to "resource crunch." This resource crunch has put extra pressure on the governmental pharmaceutical benefits schemes, as they have to manage medicines and other pharmaceutical expenditure on a very tight budget. Pharmaceutical agencies must make choices about government spending on vaccines, cancer medicines, and other medications that are publicly funded. Moreover, community pharmacists have to deal with healthcare insurance systems and publicly funded or subsidized healthcare systems. Thus, pharmacists need to know about the intricacies and functioning of healthcare systems, healthcare financing provisions and health insurance systems, and pharmacoeconomic evaluation methods. The curriculum of undergraduate and postgraduate pharmacy needs to cover some of these components in detail. Moreover, the subjects of social and administrative pharmacy, which cover some of these components, are still not part of the undergraduate pharmacy curriculum in many countries. A gap exists in the pharmacy curriculum in the areas of public health pharmacy, management, and financing, which covers topics such as health systems, healthcare financing, health service organizations, pharmaceutical benefits schemes, and pharmacoeconomics.

BRIDGING THE GAP

There is an increasing demand for a larger health workforce, including pharmacists, especially in low-income countries. Likewise, there is a demand for more specialized and innovative pharmacy services in OECD countries (OECD, 2015; Pharmaceutical Group of the European Union, 2016). There are challenges ahead for the pharmacy education sector: increasing the number of pharmacists; ensuring qualitative growth in the pharmacy profession; and catering to society's needs for specialized pharmacy services. To meet these challenges, pharmacy schools have to:

1. Incorporate into the undergraduate pharmacy curriculum adequate and structured training in hospital pharmacy, community pharmacy, and clinical settings courses.
2. Liaise with the Pharmacy Council, Ministry of Health, and other healthcare institutions such as government hospitals, private hospitals and clinics, retail pharmacies, and nongovernmental organizations' healthcare facilities to create pharmacy practice practical sites.
3. Have an adequate number of preceptors who train pharmacy students in these facilities so that pharmacy students have proper exposure and can work in these areas.
4. Review curriculum and offer elective pathways so that the students or pharmacists can train themselves further in a specialized area of pharmacy practice and gain honors points/status in a particular area that one specializes in.
1. The respective pharmaceutical societies or councils and professional bodies have to work together with the pharmacy education sector to harmonize pharmacy education standards. These stakeholders of health also have to create an environment for the pharmacy sector where a pharmacist can provide different pharmaceutical care services and be reimbursed for these services.

CONCLUSION

Society's or the health sector's need for pharmaceutical products and pharmacy services changes with time. There is a demand for pharmacists who can deliver pharmaceutical products and quality pharmacy services in low-income countries. Likewise, there is a growing demand for individualized and specialized pharmacy services in the developed world. In many countries, however, pharmacy education is still evolving to meet these growing demands. The pharmacy curriculum, especially in low-income countries, lacks the coverage, resources, and vision to meet these demands. Similarly, in developed countries, the resilience of the pharmacy curriculum has been tested by society's need for specialized and individualized patient care services. The pharmacy education sector has to play a more proactive role and collaborate with the health sector to develop a curriculum that is more resilient and addresses the current practice needs.

REFERENCES

Aslam, N., Bushra, R., & Khan, M. U. (2012). Community pharmacy practice in Pakistan. *Archives of Pharmacy Practice*, *3*(4), 297.

Basak, S. C., & Sathyanarayana, D. (2009). Community pharmacy practice in India: Past, present and future. *Southern Medical Review*, *2*(1), 11–14.

Bureau of Labor Statistics. (2015). Occupational outlook handbook: Pharmacists. Retrieved from https://www.bls.gov/ooh/healthcare/pharmacists.htm.

Connelly, D. (2014). Taking stock of pharmacy: A breakdown of global workforce data. *The Pharmaceutical Journal*, *293*.

De Montfort University Leicester. (2017). Pharmacy MPharm (Hons). Retrieved from http://www.dmu.ac.uk/study/courses/undergraduate-courses/pharmacy-mpharm-hons-degree/pharmacy-mpharm-hons.aspx.

Gardner, S. F., & Stowe, C. D. (2007). The impact of a gender shift on a profession: Women in pharmacy. Paper presented at the Forum on Public Policy Online.

Guile, D., & Ahamed, F. (2009). Modernising the pharmacy curriculum: A report for the modernising pharmacy careers pharmacist undergraduate education and pre-registration training review team. Retrieved from London, http://discovery.ucl.ac.uk/1545760/.

Hulisz, D., & Brown, D. (2014). The future of pharmacy jobs—Will it be feast or famine? Retrieved from http://www.medscape.com/viewarticle/823365.

Hwang, C., Hale, K., & Kim, H. (2014). Pharmacy practice in Europe. Pharmacy practice.

International Pharmaceutical Federation (FIP) (2012). FIP Global pharmacy workforce report. Retrieved from Portugal, http://apps.who.int/medicinedocs/documents/s20206en/s20206en.pdf.

International Pharmaceutical Federation (FIP) (2015). FIP Global pharmacy workforce intelligence: Trends report. Retrieved from The Hague, https://www.fip.org/files/fip/PharmacyEducation/Trends/FIPEd_Trends_report_2015_web_v3.pdf.

Kanke, M. (2012). Pharmacy Education in Asia and the Asian Assoc of Schools of Pharmacy. Retrieved from Boston: http://www.aacp.org/governance/SIGS/global/Documents/Pharmacy%20Education%20in%20Asia.pdf.

Kheir, N., Zaidan, M., Younes, H., El Hajj, M., Wilbur, K., & Jewesson, P. J. (2008). Pharmacy education and practice in 13 Middle Eastern countries. *American Journal of Pharmaceutical Education*, *72*(6), 133.

Kreling, D. H., Doucette, W. R., Chang, E. H., Gaither, C. A., Mott, D. A., & Schommer, J. C. (2010). Practice characteristics of bachelor of science and doctor of pharmacy degreed pharmacists based on the 2009 National Workforce Survey. *American Journal of Pharmaceutical Education*, *74*(9), 159.

Nagavi, B. (2004). Clinical pharmacy in India. In G. Parthasarathi, K. Nyfort-Hansen, & M. C. Nahata (Eds.), *A textbook of clinical pharmacy practice—Essential concepts and skills* (1st ed., pp. 1–8). Chennai, India: Orient Longmen.

OECD. (2015). Health at a glance 2015: OECD indicators. Retrieved from Paris, http://apps.who.int/medicinedocs/documents/s22177en/s22177en.pdf.

Pharmaceutical Group of the European Union. (2016). The roles of the pharmacist in the context of an ageing and mobile population. Retrieved from Saint-Gille, http://healthworkforce.eu/wp-content/uploads/2016/02/Getov_Ilko.pdf.

Sosabowski, M. H., & Gard, P. R. (2008). Pharmacy education in the United Kingdom. *American Journal of Pharmaceutical Education*, *72*(6), 130.

University of Minnesota, College of Pharmacy. (2016). Curriculum. Retrieved from https://www.pharmacy.umn.edu/degrees-programs/doctor-pharmacy/curriculum.

Wiedenmayer, K., Summers, R. S., Mackie, C. A., Gous, A. G., Everard, M., & Tromp, D. (2006). *Developing pharmacy practice: A focus on patient care.* World Health Organization and International Pharmaceutical Federation. pp. x, 87–x, 87.

FURTHER READING

JSS University. (2015). Syllabus: Bachelor of Pharmacy Course. Retrieved from Mysore, https://jssuni.edu.in/JSSWeb/UDData/Docs/Pharmacy-B-PHARM.pdf.

Pokhara University. (2005). Syllabus: Bachelor of Pharmaceutical Sciences. Retrieved from Pokhara, http://www.cct.edu.np/userfiles/file/B_Pharmacy%20Syllabus-(I-VIII).pdf.

University of Ruhuna. (2014). Student handbook: Bachelor of Pharmacy. Retrieved from Faculty of Medicine, University of Ruhuna.

CHAPTER

LEADERSHIP IN PHARMACY EDUCATION

18

Lisa M. Nissen, Judith A. Singleton
Queensland University of Technology, Brisbane, QLD, Australia

The requirements of the pharmacy profession are changing globally, moving from a supply function to a more integrated health service delivery model. To optimize its contribution to the health sector, the pharmacy profession needs to demonstrate leadership, not only in health service delivery, but also in the ongoing preparation of new practitioners taking up these new extended or expanded roles. This chapter discusses the strategic direction that leaders in pharmacy education need to take in light of the challenges of a complex health system, and the subsequent implications for curriculum design and delivery. Finally, it provides the reader with the strategic steps required to bring about these changes in their own degree programs. To execute these strategies, the authors argue that pharmacy educators require a thorough understanding of systems thinking. They recommend that leaders of pharmacy educational institutions adopt a relational leadership approach to best guide the process and manage the negative consequences of organizational change that come with any shift in an organization's strategic direction.

LEADERSHIP IN PHARMACY EDUCATION

Health systems are complex, continually experiencing change. The pharmacy profession needs to be able to respond to this continually changing environment and adapt appropriately. This requires pharmacy graduates to have both the skills and the resilience to adapt to changing roles and a changing professional landscape. Hence, educators must envision a way of educating future pharmacists that delivers these capabilities. To achieve leadership in pharmacy education, a soft-systems thinking approach is required. This approach requires one to think about a problem or task holistically, recognizing that what you may take to be the "whole" may itself be part of an even larger whole (Checkland, 2000). As described by Checkland (2012, p. 466), "any entity called 'a system' may also contain within itself, functional sub-systems, and may itself, as a whole, be a functional part of a wider system." This methodology has as its underpinning core construct the notion of a system as an entity able to adapt to environmental "shocks" through performance monitoring of system components and effective communication via complex feedback loops (Checkland, 2012). Environmental "shocks" in health systems include skills mix reviews in response to budgetary contractions with resultant extended or expanded roles. Key factors that have a negative impact on the quality of healthcare delivery are budgetary constraints, limited resources, system inefficiencies, and increasing complexity in the overall healthcare system (Weberg, 2012). Bearing in mind the key tenet of soft-systems thinking, which is that any

Pharmacy Education in the Twenty First Century and Beyond. https://doi.org/10.1016/B978-0-12-811909-9.00018-6

"whole" system has emergent properties (i.e., any "whole" system is more than the sum of its parts), it is important to appreciate the importance of multidisciplinary healthcare delivery since each health system comprises so much more than the individual contributions of each health discipline. This holistic view of health systems should therefore guide our approach to the education of pharmacy students.

Leaders in pharmacy education need to be "connected" to the healthcare system in some way—and without an understanding of the major drivers of the healthcare system at both a local and global level, pharmacy education leaders risk creating visions and plans that push their individual system away from the bigger healthcare system and create organizational "anxiety." Leadership in pharmacy education therefore requires engagement with not only the profession and its respective national and international professional organizations, but also the wider healthcare sector and its stakeholders.

The first international pharmacy education report was delivered by FIP in 2013 (International Pharmaceutical Federation (FIP), 2013). It provided a baseline of global pharmacy education at the time and reported on pharmacy education initiatives around the world. A key message from this report was the need for alignment between pharmacy education and society as a whole to deliver desired patient health outcomes globally. In 2016 FIP held the first global conference on Pharmacy and Pharmaceutical Sciences Education, delivering "a coherent global vision for professional pharmacy education and workforce development" (International Pharmaceutical Federation (FIP), 2016, p. 4) aimed to align with the UN Sustainable Development Goals and in particular Goal 3—Good Health and Well-Being (United Nations (UN), 2015). To deliver leadership in pharmacy education, pharmacy academics need to be aware of the international drivers of the pharmacy workforce and pharmacy education.

It is also important that pharmacy academics understand the academic institutional systems in which they operate, and the context in which pharmacy schools deliver their programs in the higher education space (Dean, 2002). Connections with other health disciplines' schools and faculties are important for engendering a multidisciplinary approach to healthcare delivery and fostering the notion of multidisciplinary healthcare teams.

Pharmacy educators face the constant challenge of balancing the pressures of the academic world and evolving teaching and learning strategies with the constantly changing, hypercompetitive health sector (both public and private). With the automation of dispensing functions in both the public and private sectors, pharmacists have been able to reallocate time previously spent on technical functions to clinical roles. Changes in the skills mix in the public health sector have seen pharmacists' time freed up to undertake new and expanded scope roles. Examples of these new roles in public hospitals include an admissions role in hospital emergency departments and prescribing pharmacists in hospital preadmission clinics. In these new roles, the pharmacist conducts a full patient medication history and writes up the patient's medication chart (prescribes). In the community setting pharmacists are now prescribing, vaccinating, conducting health checks (e.g., blood pressure, blood cholesterol, blood glucose, and INR (International Normalised Ratio) monitoring) and working as team members in general practice clinics conducting medication reviews. These are only a few examples of the innovative roles community pharmacists around the world are now undertaking. All of these roles have evolved over the last two decades, and new roles will continue to evolve. Providing the pharmacy profession with graduates who have the requisite skills and confidence to undertake new roles in their future careers (roles that perhaps have not even been imagined at this point) will require strong and effective leadership from the pharmacy academic sector.

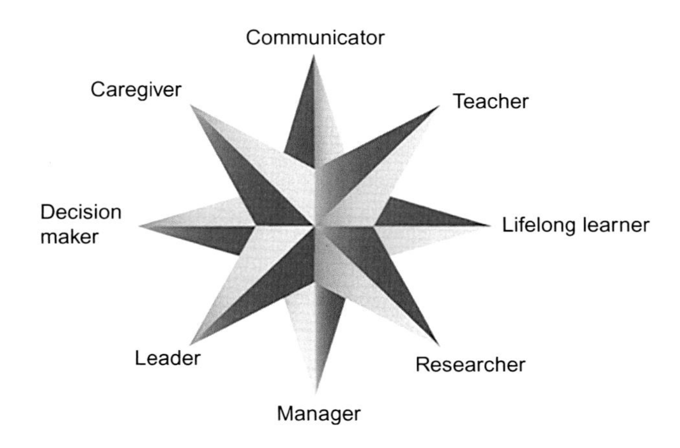

FIG. 1

The eight-star pharmacist model.

The seven-star pharmacist concept, introduced by the World Health Organization (WHO), articulates the skills and attributes necessary for pharmacists to undertake extended and expanded roles as effective members of the healthcare team. In 2000 FIP endorsed this concept in its policy statement on Good Pharmacy Education Practice (International Pharmaceutical Federation (FIP), 2000). The seven attributes listed are caregiver, decision maker, communicator, manager, lifelong learner, teacher, and leader. An eighth attribute, researcher, was added in 2006 (Wiedenmayer et al., 2006) (Refer to Fig. 1).

In the current hypercompetitive pharmacy environment, pharmacy educators need to produce workforce-ready graduates meeting employers' expectations. Skills that employers have identified as being the most desirable in graduates are leadership, the ability to work in a team, the ability to make decisions and solve problems, interpersonal skills, and communication skills (both written and verbal) (NACE (National Association of Colleges and Employers), 2017). Leadership is one of the roles depicted in the eight-star pharmacist model. It is an important attribute for pharmacists in their practice and, equally, an important attribute in heads/deans of pharmacy schools. Traditional views of leadership that emerged postindustrialization were "based on the assumption that the world is knowable, and planning and control brings about desired outcomes" (Plowman & Duchon, 2008, p. 129). The top-down, hierarchical, command-and-control leadership approach was perceived to be desirable to control uncertainty and keep the organization operating like a well-oiled machine. However, this traditional view of what leadership should look like does not fit with today's reality of healthcare organizations. The complexity of the healthcare system requires healthcare organizations operating within it to be in themselves complex, adaptive organizations. Authoritarian, top-down controlling leadership is no longer considered appropriate in knowledge-intensive workplaces such as healthcare organizations (Senge, 1994). Leadership literature describes these types of leaders as "heroic" leaders—heroic, "superman" types who save the organization and save the day. The old, heroic type of leader has been described by Eicher (1997) as a lone omnipotent leader with superior knowledge and a fear of failure (who will therefore expend much energy in keeping up appearances at all costs, including blaming others), and as one who views subordinates as inferiors. This top-down leadership style therefore presents the risk of the leader being hailed as a hero in the light of organizational success or hailed as a villain in the light of organizational failure. Consequently, heroic leadership produces stressed, unhappy leaders who lack legitimacy in the eyes of their employees and other stakeholders (Crevani, Lindgren, & Packendorff, 2007). In reaction to top-down, heroic leadership, new forms of leadership have emerged in which the key is relationships rather than dominance and control (Drath, 2001). Uhl-Bien (2006) lists several of these new approaches appearing in the leadership literature, including distributed (Gronn, 2002), distributive (Brown & Gioia, 2002), shared (Pearce & Conger, 2003), postheroic (Fletcher, 2004), and complexity (Marion & Uhl-Bien, 2001). These leadership constructs, while having a common premise that leadership is shared rather than enacted by one formal, "heroic" leader, vary widely. In healthcare, alternative approaches to heroic leadership have mostly been transformational, postheroic leadership or distributed leadership (Fulop, 2012). The postheroic transformational leader empowers followers to participate in the leadership process by taking responsibility and gaining knowledge, encourages innovation, and seeks input and consensus in decision-making (Eicher, 1997; Fletcher, 2004). It is a leadership perspective based on dynamic, "collective construction processes" within a group of people (Crevani et al., 2007). Another relatively new leadership approach discussed in healthcare leadership literature is relational leadership (Fulop, 2012; Fulop & Mark, 2013; Uhl-Bien, 2006). Relational leadership theory is defined as a "social influence process through which emergent coordination (e.g., evolving social order) and change (e.g., new approaches, values, attitudes, behaviors, ideologies) are constructed and produced" (Uhl-Bien, 2006, p. 655). Relational leadership explores the *relational* dynamics of leadership and organizing. Rather than viewing people working in organizations as separate individuals, this theory depicts leadership as a social construct that emerges from the human connections and networks within organizations (Uhl-Bien, 2006). A multidisciplinary systematic review of leadership outcomes in nursing literature concluded that relational leadership produced more frequent and more positive outcomes (including improved staff satisfaction) compared with task-focused leadership (Cummings et al., 2010). Today's leaders of healthcare organizations must eschew the traditional, command-and-control leadership style and adapt a more relational, collaborative leadership style. If they do not, their organizations risk being unable to adapt or evolve quickly enough to remain relevant in the current and emergent healthcare environment (Weberg, 2012). Understanding this changed requirement of healthcare leaders is of paramount importance in developing pharmacy curricula that will produce graduates with the requisite skill sets to take up these leadership roles in the future. As with healthcare organizations, pharmacy schools must also be able to adapt quickly to produce these workforce-ready graduates for this changing pharmacy professional landscape. This therefore would suggest that leaders in pharmacy education also adopt a relational leadership approach. But what does this relational leadership look like and how do pharmacy academic leaders enact it?

Relational leadership may be understood as a reciprocal relationship whereby leaders and followers interrelate in order to understand an issue, then determine what needs to be done and how to proceed (Douglass & Gittell, 2012). In an environment of mutual respect and shared goals, this synthesis of knowledge from the whole team ensures a holistic approach to understanding an issue. The importance of mutual respect in this interrelationship cannot be understated—it facilitates the emotional connection that increases the likelihood that each party will respect the needs and insights of the other. This in turn ensures optimal knowledge sharing, achievement of shared goals, and holistic, situational sense-making. The relational leader creates a workplace culture that provides a "safe" environment for these reciprocal interrelationships to take place. Fletcher's conceptualization of "fluid expertise" sheds light on what a relational leadership interaction might look like.

> "[P]ower and/or expertise shifts from one party to the other, not only over time but in the course of one interaction. This requires two skills. One is a skill in empowering others; an ability to share—in some instances even customizing—one's own reality, skill, knowledge, etc. in ways that made it accessible to others. The other is skill in being empowered: an ability and willingness to step away from the expert role in order to learn from or be influenced by the other."
>
> **Fletcher (1999, p. 64).**

Relational leaders establish this culture of reciprocal knowledge sharing and sense-making through the way they give, seek, and receive help (Schein, 2009). This leadership style values being ethical and inclusive. Relational leaders acknowledge the diverse talents of their followers and trust the relational process to bring effective thinking to the socially responsible changes staff agree they want to work towards (shared goals). A relational leadership approach by heads/deans of pharmacy schools is more likely to deliver positive outcomes in terms of graduate outcomes and staff satisfaction as pharmacy schools reevaluate how they will produce graduates with the requisite skills described previously, including effective leadership skills.

The ability to change practice is essential in a complex healthcare system undergoing constant environmental shocks. The emergence of new, extended, or expanded roles for pharmacists brings with it a large degree of ambiguity, the potential for increased responsibility on the part of the pharmacist, and a degree of risk. Real-life healthcare problems are not neat and well-structured. Students must therefore develop the skills to handle "messy," ambiguous, poorly defined problems, and make sense of them (Stinson & Milter, 1996). Rosenthal, Austin, and Tsuyuki (2010) argued that the ultimate barrier to pharmacy practice change may actually be pharmacists. They identified five key traits of practicing pharmacists related to patient care that would impede practice change. These traits were:

- Lack of confidence
- Fear of new responsibility
- Paralysis in the face of ambiguity
- Need for approval
- Risk aversion (Rosenthal et al., 2010, p. 39)

These five traits will hinder the profession moving forward, and therefore it is an urgent priority for pharmacy educators to address ways to change or remove these traits in pharmacy graduates. These traits will hinder pharmacists coping with the continually changing complex adaptive system that is the health system.

As discussed earlier, any complex system by its very nature has emergent properties. Dealing with these emergent properties requires healthcare professionals to be flexible, demonstrate effective problem-solving skills, and exhibit a high level of emotional intelligence. Leading these complex healthcare organizations will require critical thinking and problem-solving skills (Frankel, Louizos, & Austin, 2014; International Pharmaceutical Federation (FIP), 2000), and also the ability to work independently. These types of skills cannot be taught in a traditional didactic style of content delivery. Frankel et al. (2014) suggested standardizing the admissions processes for pharmacy schools to attract students "who possess innate critical-thinking skills and leadership qualities." Teaching students "skills" and teaching students "knowledge" are diametrically opposed, and require a different mode of content delivery and a reimagining of pharmacy curriculum design. This leads us therefore to argue that leadership in pharmacy education requires acceptance that pharmacy schools must move away from the traditional pharmacy curriculum with its didactic mode of content delivery and emphasis on teaching knowledge, towards an active learning environment with an emphasis on teaching skills and developing personal attributes such as tolerance to ambiguity, resilience, and self-confidence. Leadership in pharmacy education therefore requires leadership in curriculum design and mode of delivery.

LEADERSHIP IN CURRICULUM DESIGN AND DELIVERY

Current pharmacy curricula deliver learning outcomes for pharmacists' roles *today*. Leaders in pharmacy curriculum development are identifying learning outcomes for pharmacists' roles of the *future* and designing curricula to achieve these outcomes. Leadership in curriculum design and delivery therefore requires pharmacy educators to be innovative. The leadership skills described previously that are necessary for leaders of complex healthcare systems are the same leadership skills required in leaders of pharmacy academic institutions. As with any change process, leading change in pharmacy curriculum design will be challenging. Decisions on aspects of curriculum redesign including mode of delivery should be evidence-based, and therefore pharmacy educators should continue to conduct rigorous research to monitor if learning outcomes address workforce skills desirable to employers. The key to leading curriculum design and delivery is engaging with *all* stakeholders, not just industry stakeholders, to ensure our graduates meet not only pharmacy workforce needs but, most importantly of all, meet the needs of patients.

Curriculum redesign requires the "new" curriculum to be clearly articulated in a framework that demonstrates both horizontal and vertical integration of subjects in the year levels of the degree program. The new curriculum should map to agreed standards for that country or province (e.g., in Australia pharmacy curricula are mapped to the Australian Pharmacy Council's accreditation standards) (Australian Pharmacy Council Ltd, 2012), and should align to appropriate, "authentic" assessments. All subjects or courses in a program should follow the key criteria set out in the curriculum design map—there should be a uniform approach across a degree program as to the curriculum (the "what") and the mode of content delivery (the "how"). Developing a new curriculum design without considering the instructional practices (mode of delivery) needed to deliver it effectively risks sabotaging the entire curriculum redesign implementation (Mooney & Mausbach, 2008). Redesigning a new pharmacy curriculum is more than simply producing a curriculum map or framework. It also includes determining what knowledge and skills pharmacy students require to be workforce-ready, and then providing pharmacy lecturers with proven practices or strategies that will work in their subject area to deliver these previously identified knowledge and skills. As discussed earlier, pharmacy academics need to find strategies to remove or reduce the five traits identified in pharmacists by Rosenthal et al. (2010) that inhibit practice change: lack of confidence, fear of new responsibility, paralysis in the face of ambiguity, need for approval, and risk aversion. When developing a new curriculum, rigorous professional development for teaching staff must be embedded in the process, along with the provision of assistance from learning designers to help staff implement innovative and engaging activities for students that are embedded in pedagogy. To ensure a continuity of approach across the entire degree program, all members of the pharmacy teaching team need to operate as a professional, learning community of practice (Mooney & Mausbach, 2008). Effective communities of practice demonstrate optimal knowledge management by encouraging knowledge sharing and facilitating the creation of new knowledge (Hildreth & Kimble, 2004; Wenger, McDermott, & Snyder, 2002). Establishing a community of practice will ensure that ideas are shared, teaching strategies are evaluated, and suggestions for improvement shared and acknowledged. Ultimately, successful achievement of course learning outcomes by students is a result of the interplay between the curriculum, the teaching methods used (mode of content delivery) and the engagement of the students themselves and their subsequent learning efforts (Meyers & Nulty, 2009). Determining if desired learning outcomes have been achieved requires evaluation of assessment items and student's academic results. Assessment items need to indicate to academics if there is any improvement in the way students acquire, process, and synthesize knowledge.

The WHO Vancouver Consultancy (International Pharmaceutical Federation (FIP), 2000) highlighted the need for a move away from the traditional, didactic mode of content delivery (with its passive transfer of knowledge) in pharmacy curricula, and for students to actively participate in the learning process. Active participation has been encouraged in university curricula through the introduction of teaching and learning strategies such as active learning (or activity-based learning), gamification, student-centered learning, problem-based learning, enquiry-based learning, and case-based learning, to name a few. A UK study of curriculum design attributes that increased student performance and engagement in a first-year undergraduate cohort identified four key attributes: active learning, timely feedback, relevance of course content to future job, and challenge (Bovill, Bulley, & Morss, 2011). These identified attributes are applicable to all levels of the pharmacy curriculum.

Of the many curriculum redesign initiatives being undertaken globally, this chapter presents a curriculum redesign strategy introduced into the Bachelor of Pharmacy (Hons) degree program at Queensland University of Technology (QUT) in 2015. In this reenvisioned, integrated curriculum, clinical cases are introduced in the early years of the degree program, and subject areas such as pharmacology, physiology, pharmacokinetics and pharmacodynamics, and pharmaceutics are integrated under a topic area (usually a clinical area). For example, a patient-focused integrated Respiratory unit would include an outline of various types of respiratory conditions, their pathophysiology, the pharmacology and pharmacokinetics of the drugs used to treat these conditions, and any pharmacodynamic and pharmaceutic considerations. This integration of subjects previously taught as standalone subject areas, using case-based, problem-based, or enquiry-based learning strategies, and delivered in an active learning environment provides students with a real-world context. Each week in a workshop setting (active learning environment) students work through formative patient cases of increasing complexity receiving feedback from tutors. A scaffolded approach is used with these patient cases to support student engagement and learning. The tutor works through a patient case with the students watching and listening. Next, the class works through a patient case with the tutor guiding but the students doing the work. Finally, the students work in small groups on their own to solve a patient case with the tutor bringing the class back together afterwards to discuss the case and provide feedback on the students' performances. This type of curricula meets all four of the key attributes for increasing student enhancement and engagement identified in the UK study described earlier. The workshops are conducted in an active learning environment, feedback is on-the-spot so therefore timely, the patient cases are relevant to future real-world practice, and the content is challenging. By their authenticity, these types of curricula increase student engagement. Evidence also suggests that students in integrated curricula utilizing problem-based teaching strategies become better self-directed learners (Jones, Higgs, de Angelis, & Prideaux, 2001). Having identified key attributes and skills needed to produce workforce-ready pharmacy graduates, and having identified that the acquisition of these skills and attributes requires a redesign of the traditional pharmacy curriculum, the authors now consider how this paradigmatic shift might be achieved.

STRATEGIC STEPS

Scholarship of Teaching and Learning (SoTaL) research is very important for guiding policy and practice and also for guiding strategies for curriculum redesign in pharmacy programs. Unfortunately, there is little evidence-based, Scholarship of Teaching and Learning (SoTaL) research in the literature to guide strategies to achieve this paradigmatic shift in the way we teach pharmacy students (Frankel et al., 2014). Consequently, the authors have drawn upon leadership literature to determine the most effective leadership style for the health system and for pharmacy educators, and then looked to curriculum redesign literature from Education to inform the most effective process for pharmacy education leaders to affect change in their programs. A three-phase process is recommended. Phase I involves an internal environment scan, Phase II involves planning and development—an in-depth curriculum review and then redesign, and Phase III is the implementation and evaluation phase of the new curriculum.

PHASE I: THE INTERNAL ENVIRONMENT SCAN

This phase is one of reflection and evaluation. It is a period of reflection for all the teaching team on how the curriculum is currently delivered, the culture of the department, team weaknesses and strengths, and team resources and capabilities. It is also a period of self-reflection on the part of the head/dean of the pharmacy school on their leadership style. Importantly, this phase should also include an extensive, in-depth stakeholder consultation to gain an understanding of the drivers of the profession, and the profession's requirements for workforce-ready graduates. Findings from the reflective phase should then be evaluated to inform the curriculum redesign process.

There are many scholarly articles in health literature on the importance of self-reflection in health professionals' practice (Hanya, Yonei, Kurono, & Kamei, 2014; Lonie, 2010; Lonie & Desai, 2015; Yusuff, 2015). Self-reflective practice enables practitioners to identify what they do and the habits they have formed in carrying out their daily work routines and examine these habits objectively to understand what purpose they serve and why they persist in order to identify if, and where, a change in practice is required (Taylor, 2010). Taylor (2010, p. 39) describes reflection as "the throwing back of thoughts and memories, in cognitive acts such as thinking, meditation, and any other form of attentive consideration, in order to make sense of them, and to make contextually appropriate changes if they are required." This process requires time—time away from the busyness of one's work day—and quiet. To achieve this, the reflector needs to make a commitment to the process, and make time in their schedule to step away for a period of quiet time for reflection. This reflective process should be ongoing, not only because it will contribute to the curriculum redesign strategy, but also because it will be necessary to evaluate the process (measured by team's feedback), and the outcomes (measured by student satisfaction and learning outcomes, and employers' feedback on the quality of the graduates). It is not within the scope of this chapter to describe in detail how a pharmacy academic team should implement self-reflective practice, if they do not already do so. There is much literature already on self-reflective practice for healthcare practitioners; however, the REFLECT model proposed by Taylor (2010) is a good starting point. The steps in this model (outlined here) should be considered a reflective "flow" rather than a series of consecutive steps.

*R*eadiness—be prepared to make the commitment to take time out of your busy schedule to reflect
*E*xercising thought—turning on and tuning into your thoughts
*F*ollowing systematic processes—to reduce the complexity of reflective thoughts break them into manageable components
*L*eaving oneself open to answers—reflection may not necessarily provide "truth" or correct answers so the reflector needs to remain open to suggestions and alternative solutions to problems/issues being reflected upon
*E*nfolding insights—taking insights from multiple sources and synthesizing these with present understandings
*C*hanging awareness—gathering and assessing insights raises the possibility that change may be required
*T*enacity in maintaining reflection—making and sticking to a commitment to reflect on an ongoing basis requires tenacity when faced with competing workplace goals

This phase lays the important foundation for the curriculum review and redesign process. Without effective leadership and a corporate culture that nourishes and supports knowledge management (knowledge sharing and the creation of new knowledge), the whole process is doomed to failure. The second important component of this phase is the departmental resource audit—are there sufficient academic staff with the requisite teaching skills to deliver this newly envisioned curriculum? If not, does the department have the financial resources to recruit new staff or provide training for incumbent staff to develop their skills? Does the university have adequate teaching spaces and technologies (e.g., good WiFi for internet access) to support the pedagogy? Thirdly, there must be a thorough consultation with all pharmacy stakeholders to gauge their opinions and requirements of pharmacy graduates. This very process also alerts the profession and industry that your university is progressive and inclusive—the consultation process itself may help drive student recruitment for your new program in the future. These three components need to be undertaken *before* you embark upon Phases II and III.

PHASE II: PLANNING AND DEVELOPMENT

Once the foundations are in place, a thorough review of the old curriculum can then take place leading into the curriculum redesign process. The planning and development phase should be consultative, drawing on insights from the entire team. The leader then has the final say on what will actually be delivered—this is an enactment of relational leadership. School "retreats" where staff all come together off-campus are ideal opportunities for brainstorming what the new curriculum will look like and what will be the department's strategy for going forward with its development and implementation. When redesigning the new curriculum, it is important to continually refer to the list of topic areas required by the accreditation body for the relevant Bachelor of Pharmacy program—this list must be reviewed regularly to ensure no topic area is overlooked. It is also very important to ensure there is a smooth horizontal and vertical integration across the semesters/terms of the program and the topics/concepts covered. Students will struggle if assumed knowledge areas have never actually been taught in previous subjects and they are launched straight into a more advanced level.

The development component of Phase II should be thorough, and sufficient time must therefore be allowed for it to take place. When developing the new curriculum, engaging if possible the help of a teaching and learning expert with experience in curriculum design is helpful. This will also speed up the process and keep the development phase on track. In summary, aim for:

1) Delivery of didactic knowledge-based content in the form of videos, podcasts or lecture notes delivered online that the students can view before class
2) An active-learning, workshop environment for face-to-face contact time with lots of activities based on patient cases that consolidates the preworkshop content
3) Ensure the workshop activities are authentic (realistic and likely to be encountered in the workplace), timely feedback is provided to students, and the activities are challenging but scaffolded

Also, there needs to be a consistency in teaching strategies and mode of delivery across the program—audits need to be conducted in Phase III to ensure all teaching staff understand what is required in the delivery of this new curriculum.

PHASE III: IMPLEMENTATION AND EVALUATION

This phase is perhaps the most difficult—this is where "the rubber hits the road." Things may not always go as planned but constructive, blame-free self-reflection can help the team and the implementation process identify things that went well, those things that perhaps didn't go as well as planned, and things that need to be improved in moving forward. Evaluation should involve looking carefully at each assessment item for each subject and identify questions and concepts where a large number, or a specific group (e.g., culturally and linguistically diverse students) have scored poorly. Re-examine how these concepts or topics are being taught—is a new strategy required here? Evaluation should be a constructive process. The quality of the leadership is immensely important for this phase. Teams will be stressed and perhaps feeling overloaded; support, encouragement, and thanks from the team leader can make all the difference to the team during this phase, and give them the motivation needed to continue to put energy into the continued roll-out of the new curriculum.

Teaching in workshops utilizing active learning can be very rewarding for teaching staff and we need to keep this in mind—students tend to be more engaged in these types of teaching settings, and this energy is invigorating for the teaching staff delivering the content. Developing activities that are fun makes the session more enjoyable for everyone—students and teachers.

CONCLUSION

Embarking on any new journey is never easy—it requires thought and planning. Making the paradigmatic shift in a pharmacy degree curriculum from a traditional didactic mode of delivery with lecture-tutorial format to an active learning environment with a workshop format may at first seem daunting. However, as FIP and the WHO have indicated, the time for change is now—otherwise we risk our pharmacy graduates being unable to take up the new roles awaiting them. In this chapter, the authors have described some of the advanced-scope roles pharmacists are undertaking, the skills required of our graduates to meet employers' requirements and patients' needs, and the type of leadership approach required to drive the change in the profession and in academic institutions. Leading change in pharmacy education requires leading change in curriculum design and delivery, and the authors have described one example of what this new pharmacy curriculum might look like. Finally, the authors outlined the strategic steps required to achieve this change. We wish you luck on your curriculum redesign journey!

REFERENCES

Australian Pharmacy Council Ltd. (2012). *Accreditation standards for pharmacy programs in Australia and New Zealand (effective from 1 January 2014).* Canberra, Australia: Australian Pharmacy Council Ltd.

Bovill, C., Bulley, C. J., & Morss, K. (2011). Engaging and empowering first-year students through curriculum design: Perspectives from the literature. *Teaching in Higher Education*, *16*(2), 197–209. https://doi.org/10.1080/13562517.2010.515024.

Brown, M. E., & Gioia, D. A. (2002). Making things click: Distributive leadership in an online division of an offline organization. *The Leadership Quarterly*, *13*(4), 397–419. https://doi.org/10.1016/S1048-9843(02)00123-6.

Checkland, P. (2000). Soft systems methodology: A thirty year retrospective. *Systems Research and Behavioral Science*, *17*(S1), S11–S58. https://doi.org/10.1002/1099-1743(200011)17:1+<::AID-SRES374>3.0.CO;2-O.

Checkland, P. (2012). Four conditions for serious systems thinking and action. *Systems Research and Behavioral Science*, *29*(5), 465–469. https://doi.org/10.1002/sres.2158.

Crevani, L., Lindgren, M., & Packendorff, J. (2007). Shared leadership: A postheroic perspective on leadership as a collective construction. *International Journal of Leadership Studies*, *3*(1), 40–67.

Cummings, G. G., MacGregor, T., Davey, M., Lee, H., Wong, C. A., Lo, E., et al. (2010). Leadership styles and outcome patterns for the nursing workforce and work environment: A systematic review. *International Journal of Nursing Studies*, *47*(3), 363–385. https://doi.org/10.1016/j.ijnurstu.2009.08.006.

Dean, J. O. (2002). Leadership requires perspective. *American Journal of Pharmaceutical Education*, *66*(1), 86–87.

Douglass, A., & Gittell, J. H. (2012). Transforming professionalism: Relational bureaucracy and parent–teacher partnerships in child care settings. *Journal of Early Childhood Research*, *10*(3), 267–281. https://doi.org/10.1177/1476718X12442067.

Drath, W. H. (2001). *The deep blue sea: Rethinking the source of leadership. vol. 1.* San Francisco: Jossey-Bass.

Eicher, J. P. (1997). Post-heroic leadership: Managing the virtual organization. *Performance Improvement*, *36*(2), 5–10. https://doi.org/10.1002/pfi.4140360203.

Fletcher, J. K. (1999). *Disappearing acts: Gender, power and relational practice at work.* Cambridge: MIT Press.

Fletcher, J. K. (2004). The paradox of postheroic leadership: An essay on gender, power, and transformational change. *The Leadership Quarterly*, *15*(5), 647–661. https://doi.org/10.1016/j.leaqua.2004.07.004.

Frankel, G., Louizos, C., & Austin, Z. (2014). Canadian educational approaches for the advancement of pharmacy practice. *American Journal of Pharmaceutical Education*, *78*(7), 143. https://doi.org/10.5688/ajpe787143.

Fulop, L. (2012). Leadership, clinician managers and a thing called "hybridity" *Journal of Health Organization and Management*, *26*(5), 578–604. https://doi.org/10.1108/14777261211256927.

Fulop, L., & Mark, A. (2013). Relational leadership, decision-making and the messiness of context in healthcare. *Leadership*, *9*(2), 254–277. https://doi.org/10.1177/1742715012468785.

Gronn, P. (2002). Distributed leadership as a unit of analysis. *The Leadership Quarterly*, *13*(4), 423–451. https://doi.org/10.1016/S1048-9843(02)00120-0.

Hanya, M., Yonei, H., Kurono, S., & Kamei, H. (2014). Development of reflective thinking in pharmacy students to improve their communication with patients through a process of role-playing, video reviews, and transcript creation. *Currents in Pharmacy Teaching & Learning*, *6*(1), 122–129.

Hildreth, P. M., & Kimble, C. (2004). *Knowledge networks: Innovation through communities of practice*. Hershey: Idea Group Publishing.

International Pharmaceutical Federation (FIP) (2000). FIP statement of policy on good pharmacy education practice. Retrieved from https://fip.org/www/uploads/database_file.php?id=188&table_id=.

International Pharmaceutical Federation (FIP) (2013). FIPEd global education report. Retrieved 6/9/17, from http://www.fip.org/files/fip/FIPEd_Global_Education_Report_2013.pdf (Archived by WebCite® at http://www.webcitation.org/6tGpM1kSO).

International Pharmaceutical Federation (FIP) (2016). Transforming our workforce. Retrieved 6/9/2017 from http://www.fip.org/files/fip/PharmacyEducation/2016_report/FIPEd_Transform_2016_online_version.pdf (Archived by WebCite® at http://www.webcitation.org/6tGiwxCf4).

Jones, R., Higgs, R., de Angelis, C., & Prideaux, D. (2001). Changing face of medical curricula. *The Lancet*, *357*(9257), 699–703. https://doi.org/10.1016/S0140-6736(00)04134-9.

Lonie, J. M. (2010). Learning through self-reflection: Understanding communication barriers faced by a cross-cultural cohort of pharmacy students. *Currents in Pharmacy Teaching & Learning*, *2*(1), 12–19. https://doi.org/10.1016/j.cptl.2009.12.002.

Lonie, J. M., & Desai, K. R. (2015). Using transformative learning theory to develop metacognitive and self-reflective skills in pharmacy students: A primer for pharmacy educators. *Currents in Pharmacy Teaching & Learning*, *7*(5), 669–675.

Marion, R., & Uhl-Bien, M. (2001). Leadership in complex organizations. *The Leadership Quarterly*, *12*(4), 389–418. https://doi.org/10.1016/S1048-9843(01)00092-3.

Meyers, N. M., & Nulty, D. D. (2009). How to use (five) curriculum design principles to align authentic learning environments, assessment, students' approaches to thinking and learning outcomes. *Assessment & Evaluation in Higher Education*, *34*(5), 565–577. https://doi.org/10.1080/02602930802226502.

Mooney, N. J., & Mausbach, A. T. (2008). *Align the design: A blueprint for school reform*. Massachusetts, USA: Association for Supervision and Curriculum Development.

NACE (National Association of Colleges and Employers) (2017). Job Outlook 2016: Attributes employers want to see on new College Graduates' resumes Retrieved 27/1/2017, 2017, from NACE, http://www.naceweb.org/s11182015/employers-look-for-in-new-hires.aspx (Archived by WebCite® at http://www.webcitation.org/6o12Okb1C).

Pearce, C. L., & Conger, J. A. (2003). *Shared leadership: Reframing the hows and whys of leadership. vol. 1*. Thousand Oaks, Calif: Sage Publications.

Plowman, M. A., & Duchon, D. (2008). Dispelling the myths about leadership: From cybernetics to emergence. In M. Uhl-Bien & R. Marion (Eds.), *Complexity leadership part 1: Conceptual foundations* (pp. 129–153). Charlotte, North Carolina, USA: Information Age Publishing.

Rosenthal, M., Austin, Z., & Tsuyuki, R. T. (2010). Are pharmacists the ultimate barrier to pharmacy practice change? *Canadian Pharmacists Journal/Revue des Pharmaciens du Canada*, *143*(1), 37–42. https://doi.org/10.3821/1913-701X-143.1.37.

Schein, E. H. (2009). *Helping: How to offer, give, and receive help. vol. 1*. San Francisco: Berrett-Koehler Publishers.

Senge, P. M. (1994). *The fifth discipline fieldbook: Strategies and tools for building a learning organization*. New York: Currency, Doubleday.

Stinson, J. E., & Milter, R. G. (1996). Problem-based learning in business education: Curriculum design and implementation issues. *New Directions for Teaching and Learning*, *1996*(68), 33–42. https://doi.org/10.1002/tl.37219966807.

Taylor, B. J. (2010). *Reflective practice for healthcare professionals: A practical guide. vol. 3* (3rd ed.). New York; Maidenhead: Open University Press.

Uhl-Bien, M. (2006). Relational leadership theory: Exploring the social processes of leadership and organizing. *The Leadership Quarterly*, *17*(6), 654–676. https://doi.org/10.1016/j.leaqua.2006.10.007.

United Nations (UN) (2015). Sustainable development goals. Retrieved 6 September 2017, from United Nations (UN), http://www.un.org/sustainabledevelopment/sustainable-development-goals/ (Archived by WebCite® at http://www.webcitation.org/6tGIV3Qlu).

Weberg, D. (2012). Complexity leadership: A healthcare imperative. *Nursing Forum*, *47*(4), 268–277. https://doi.org/10.1111/j.1744-6198.2012.00276.x.

Wenger, E., McDermott, R. A., & Snyder, W. (2002). *Cultivating communities of practice: A guide to managing knowledge*. Boston: Harvard Business School Press.

Wiedenmayer, K., Summers, R. S., Mackie, C. A., Gous, A. G. S., Everard, M., Tromp, D., … Federation, I. P. (2006). Developing pharmacy practice: A focus on patient care: Handbook/Karin Wiedenmayer. [et al.]. Retrieved from https://www.fip.org/files/fip/publications/DevelopingPharmacyPractice/DevelopingPharmacyPracticeEN.pdf.

Yusuff, K. B. (2015). Does self-reflection and peer-assessment improve Saudi pharmacy students' academic performance and metacognitive skills? *Saudi Pharmaceutical Journal*, *23*(3), 266–275. https://doi.org/10.1016/j.jsps.2014.11.018.

CHAPTER 19

INTERPROFESSIONAL EDUCATION IN PHARMACY: REVIEW OF CASE STUDIES

Tahir M. Khan*,†, Allah Bukhsh*,†

**Monash University Malaysia, Subang Jaya, Malaysia, †University of Veterinary & Animal Sciences, Lahore, Pakistan*

BACKGROUND AND HISTORICAL PERSPECTIVE OF INTERPROFESSIONAL EDUCATION

Transition of health professional education in the 21st century has become imperative. Rapidly advancing health technology and increased disease burden have made it very difficult for clinicians practicing alone to provide optimum patient-centered care, without the involvement of other healthcare providers (Buring et al., 2009; Page et al., 2009; Reeves, Boet, Zierler, & Kitto, 2015). The complex healthcare system and the massive prevalence of chronic diseases have led to an appreciation of the need for change in multiple health practice areas, including pedagogy, e.g., Interprofessional education (IPE), competency-based training, and health workforce education (Page et al., 2009). Thus improvement in community health-related outcomes requires the identification and implementation of all the possible changes from the perspective of education and training (Buring et al., 2009).

IPE is not a new phenomenon; however, the initiation and history of IPE practice has not been properly documented. IPE initiatives have been undertaken over the past seven decades, starting in the late 1940s. Since the late 1960s, there has been an increasing interest in interprofessional collaborative practice in the fields of primary care, community-based care, palliative care, and others, with the goal of ensuring a safe, accessible, high-quality, and patient-focused approach (FIP, 2015). The United States provided substantial funding during the 1970s to develop and promote interdisciplinary programs, resulting in the incorporation of interdisciplinary education in academic programs. The Institute of Medicine (IOM) in its first conference, held in 1972, urged that all academic health centers had an "obligation" to nurture collaborative practice among different professionals in the healthcare team, a team which is to be built around the "personal needs of patients" (National League for Nursing, 2015). During the 1980s, the Veterans Administration (VA) promoted an interdisciplinary professional training program for geriatric care (Baldwin, 1996). In the UK, the need for IPE was recognized in the mid-1980s, with the establishment of the Center for the Advancement of Interprofessional Professional Education (CAIPE) in 1987 (Buring et al., 2009). After the 1990s, to increase collaboration among different healthcare professionals, importance was placed upon students from healthcare disciplines other than medicine. During this era the need for interdisciplinary education among healthcare professionals was highlighted by many organizations, including the Robert Wood Johnson Foundation

Pharmacy Education in the Twenty First Century and Beyond. https://doi.org/10.1016/B978-0-12-811909-9.00019-8

and Hartford Foundation (Baldwin, 1996; Clark, 1997; Page et al., 2009). In 2003, Health Canada undertook its first IPE initiative with Collaborative Patient-Centered Practice (Buring et al., 2009). From the start of the 21st century, substantial efforts have been made in the implementation and promotion of IPE by various organizations worldwide (e.g., Canadian Interprofessional Health Collaborative, 2009; European Interprofessional Practice and Education Network, 2013; Institute of Medicine, 1972, 2003, and 2008; Interprofessional Education Collaborative (IPEC), 2011; and World Health Organization (WHO), 2010) (Dominguez, Fike, MacLaughlin, & Zorek, 2015).

HISTORICAL PERSPECTIVE OF INTERPROFESSIONAL EDUCATION IN PHARMACY

Implementation of a sustainable IPE approach in the healthcare system is not possible without understanding the historical perspective of IPE (Page et al., 2009). To maximize the beneficial outcomes of IPE from the patient's perspective, it was noted that the concept must also be included and implemented by practicing pharmacists. The American Association of Colleges of Pharmacy (AACP) developed a strategic plan in 2004 for the implementation of IPE in institutions that taught pharmacy. A year later, the barriers for implementing IPE in the PharmD curriculum among pharmacy institutes were analyzed by the AACP's Council of Faculties task force, based on which core competencies were devised. In 2007, the Professional Affairs Committee of AACP emphasized the importance of implementing IPE within different healthcare practice areas, in addition to the classroom environment. The AACP strongly endorsed interprofessional competencies required for healthcare professionals, as mentioned in the IOM report, and directed all institutions teaching pharmacy to include IPE in their curriculum (Kroboth et al., 2007; Page et al., 2009).

In the late 2000s, 18 institutions in the United States initiated advanced IPE courses in healthcare education. After 2007, any school seeking accreditation for their PharmD program in the United States was required to devise the objectives of its curriculum parallel with the IOM report, which states that "all health professionals should be educated to deliver patient-centered care as members of an interdisciplinary team, emphasizing evidence based practice, quality improvement approaches, and informatics." (Accreditation Council for Pharmacy Education, 2006; CoQoHCi America, 2001; Page et al., 2009). A brief timeline summary of historical IPE initiatives in Europe and the United States is presented in Fig. 1.

DEFINITIONS

- *(Uni) Disciplinary*: "One provider working independently to care for a patient. There is little awareness or acknowledgment of practice outside one's own discipline. Practitioners may consult with other providers but retain independence" (Page et al., 2009).
- *Multidisciplinary*: "Different aspects of a patient's care are handled independently by appropriate experts from different professions. The patient's problems are subdivided and treated separately, with each provider responsible for his/her own area" (Page et al., 2009).
- *Transdisciplinary*: "Requires each team member to become familiar enough with the concepts and approaches of his/her colleagues to 'blur the lines' and enable the team to focus on the problem with collaborative analysis and decision-making" (Page et al., 2009).

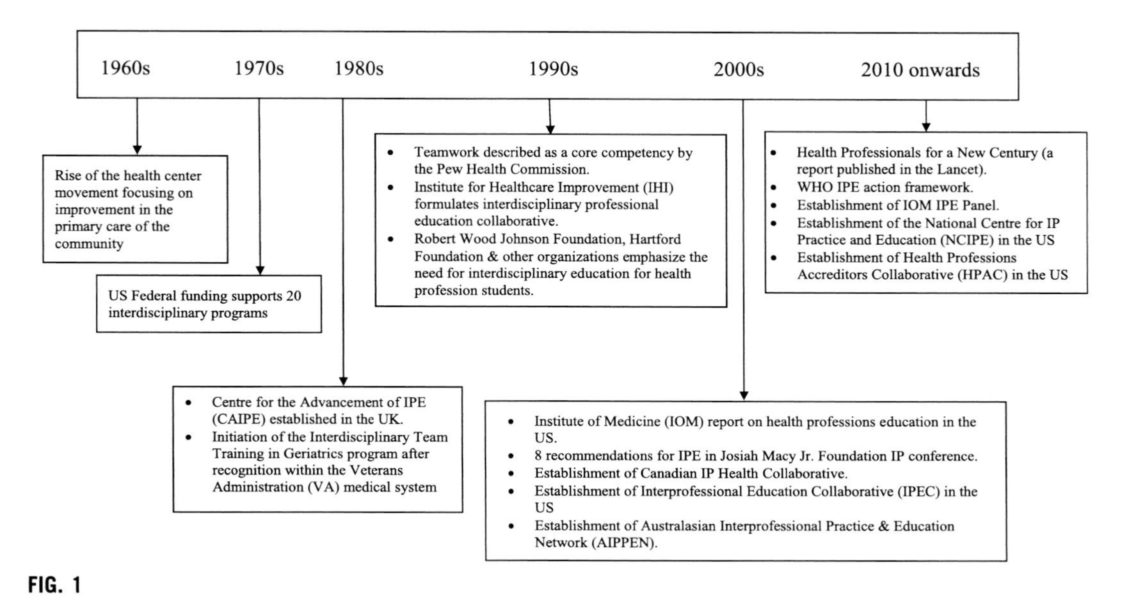

FIG. 1

Timeline of IPE initiatives in the United States and Europe.

Adapted from FIP. (2015). Interprofessional education in a pharmacy context: Global report 2015 and Page, R.L., Hume, A.L., Trujillo, J.M., Leader, W.G., Vardeny, O., Neuhauser, M.M., ... Cohen, L.J. (2009). Interprofessional education: Principles and application a framework for clinical pharmacy. Pharmacotherapy: The Journal of Human Pharmacology and Drug Therapy 29(7), 879.

- *Interdisciplinary/interprofessional*: "The provision of health care by providers from different professions in a coordinated manner that addresses the needs of patients. Providers share mutual goals, resources, and responsibility for patient care. The term interprofessional is used to describe clinical practice, whereas the term interdisciplinary is often used to describe the educational process. Either term may be used when referring to health professions education and practice" (Page et al., 2009).
- *Interprofessional teamwork*: "When different health and/or social professionals who share a team identity work closely together in an integrated and interdependent manner to solve problems and deliver services" (FIP, 2015).
- *Interprofessional collaborative practice*: "When healthcare workers from different professional backgrounds work together with patients, families, carers, and communities to deliver the highest quality of care" (FIP, 2015).
- *Collaborative pharmacy practice*: "The advanced clinical practice where pharmacists collaborate with other healthcare professionals in order to care for patients, carers, and the public" (FIP, 2015).
- *Interprofessional education*: "When members of two or more health and/or social care professions (e.g., dentistry, medicine, nursing, pharmacy) engage in learning with, from, and about each other to improve collaboration and the delivery of care. The term 'Interprofessional' is used to describe clinical practice" (FIP, 2015).

- *Interdisciplinary education*: "When members of different disciplines engage in collaborative interactive learning for a range of purposes (e.g., to understand complex interdisciplinary issues, to explore different disciplinary roles and contributions). The term 'Interdisciplinary' is often used to describe the educational process" (FIP, 2015).
- *Multiprofessional education or multidisciplinary education*: "When members of two or more professions learn alongside one another; in other words, parallel rather than interactive learning" (FIP, 2015).

THE NEED FOR INTERPROFESSIONAL EDUCATION

The services of more than one healthcare professional are required today due to the increasing complexity of diseases as well as challenging healthcare needs (Bridges, Davidson, Odegard, Maki, & Tomkowiak, 2011). Indeed, the shortage of professional manpower strongly underlines the need for interprofessional collaborative practice. According to the WHO, the healthcare work force is extremely low all over the world (FIP, 2015). Additionally, the growing sophistication of health technology and medication therapies supports the need for interprofessional approaches (Abu-Rish et al., 2012; Darragh, Huddleston, & King, 2009; Grace, McLeod, Streckfuss, Ingram, & Morgan, 2016; Simons, Ziviani, & Copley, 2011). The provision of optimum patient care is a shared goal of all healthcare providers, which can be achieved with higher rates of patient satisfaction and in a cost-effective manner if individual healthcare professionals work together as a collective unit, utilizing each other's skills (Barceló et al., 2010; Helitzer et al., 2011; Janson et al., 2009; Morey et al., 2002; Taylor, Hepworth, Buerhaus, Dittus, & Speroff, 2007; Weaver et al., 2010; Young et al., 2005). Currently healthcare professionals are constantly being assigned to cater to the healthcare needs of rapidly growing complex health issues. As such, the incorporation of IPE in health professional education will be a major contribution towards the challenging task of reshaping the health workforce for the benefit of the ailing community (Hood et al., 2014; Kyrkjebø, Brattebø, & Smith-Strøm, 2006).

Expanding health professional institutions may increase the number of healthcare professionals working in the community individually, but this will not fulfill the need for quality and healthcare relevancy. The incorporation of IPE is thus an attempt to reform the training and education of health professionals to improve the relevance, quality, and number of healthcare professionals. To achieve this, collaborative efforts are required from health ministries and educational institutions for the incorporation and implementation of IPE, so that healthcare providers can work efficiently and transform the fragmented healthcare system into a uniform, strengthened, and collaborative system (Dominguez et al., 2015). The concept of IPE is also to be incorporated into undergraduate healthcare programs in order to shift the focus from a single discipline to multidisciplinary and integrated patient care (Hood et al., 2014).

IPE has been considered a foundation that will lead towards a collaborative and integrated practice, resulting in improved health-related patient outcomes. In light of this, IPE should ideally involve present and future healthcare professionals at the undergraduate level as well as after licensing, in continuing professional development (CPD) sessions/programs, which will translate to a strengthening of the healthcare system (FIP, 2015).

BASIC AND ESSENTIAL REQUIREMENTS FOR ESTABLISHING INTERPROFESSIONAL EDUCATION

In order to provide patient-focused and transdisciplinary interprofessional care, students and healthcare practitioners will have to learn interprofessional skills to become more productive in the system. Strong communication skills are key to enhance collaborative working and to manage barriers. Leadership is another important skill required for IPE, in order to efficiently manage the healthcare team to achieve the common objective of optimum patient care. Working together as a team for a defined common patient care objective could be considered a vital competency for IPE (Buring et al., 2009). Additionally, clinical competency in the relevant field, problem-solving skills, and respecting the contributions and knowledge of other healthcare professionals are integral to its success (Barker & Oandasan, 2005; Karim & Ross, 2008; Toner, 2006).

ESSENTIAL REQUIREMENTS FOR IPE

- Communication skills
- Leadership
- Teamwork
- Clinical competency
- Problem solving skills

Although many factors must be taken into account when designing the core characteristics of an ideal IPE model, the most important is to identify which health disciplines are crucial for IPE and its intended outcomes. One should also be cognizant of the fact that pharmacists have not been considered as essential team members, especially when potential contributions of other healthcare professionals are also being evaluated when designing the respective IPE model (Reeves et al., 2008). Indeed, an ideal IPE team should consist of students from medicine, pharmacy, nursing, nutrition, and clinical social work (Reeves et al., 2008).

THE CURRENT GLOBAL IMPLEMENTATION OF INTERPROFESSIONAL EDUCATION (CASE STUDIES FROM ESTABLISHED PHARMACY PROGRAMS IN THE UNITED STATES, UK, AUSTRALIA, AND MALAYSIA)

Pharmacists play a vital role not only in the provision of patient care in multidimensional healthcare teams, but also as facilitators in the provision of IPE (D'amour & Oandasan, 2005; Davies, Horne, Bennett, & Stott, 1993; Greene, Cavell, & Jackson, 1996). Many national pharmacy organizations have taken initiatives for the ratification and articulation of policies and procedures backing IPE. However, IPE has not been implemented and delivered effectively in academic institutions and clinics (Barnsteiner, Disch, Hall, Mayer, & Moore, 2007), which can be correlated with a decline in the quality of patient care. Additionally, the shortage of healthcare professionals within their respective healthcare fields has compromised interprofessional patient care in day-to-day practice (Barnsteiner et al., 2007; Jacobs, 1987).

An established IPE infrastructure is in place at universities across the United States. Most of the IPE activities require coursework, student organization activities, and service learning activities (e.g., seminars and workshops), where it was noted that average student hours for IPE activities were 15 ± 16 for exposure activities, 12 ± 9 for immersion activities, and 21 ± 45 for competence activities (Congdon, 2016).

In 2011, a survey of 116 US pharmacy education institutes revealed that 78% of colleges listed IPE as a curricular goal (Jones et al., 2012). A systematic review of IPE studies published from 2005 to 2010 reported a wide array of IPE educational activities being adopted in English-speaking countries (Fig. 2), with the most commonly adopted strategies being small group discussions (57.8%), followed by case- or problem-based learning (48.2%) and large group lectures (36.1%) (Abu-Rish et al., 2012).

The concept of IPE practice has been gaining popularity among pharmacy and other healthcare institutions in Malaysia over the past few years. The National University of Malaysia organized a teaching and learning conference based on the theme of IPE in 2012, leading to the development of interprofessional cocurriculum design (FIP, 2015). Additionally, a successful cocurricular module was introduced to provide more emphasis on the concept of IPE for first-year students in healthcare disciplines. A series of prescribing skills workshops using the "jigsaw learning" technique, a cooperative learning technique in which students teach part of the regular curriculum to a small group of interdependent peers (Moskowitz, Malvin, Schaeffer, & Schaps, 1983), have also been included as a part of the pharmacy curriculum. (FIP, 2015).

BARRIERS TO THE IMPLEMENTATION OF INTERPROFESSIONAL EDUCATION: A GLOBAL PERSPECTIVE

Although the concept of IPE is not novel and has been around for decades, barriers to its implementation have been identified at both individual and organizational levels (Erickson, McHarney-Brown, Seeger, & Kaufman, 1998; Harvan et al., 2009; Meleis, 2016; Pecukonis, Doyle, & Bliss, 2008). Loss of professional identity is one of the traditional concerns with IPE models. There is also the issue of attitudinal barrier observed among practitioners who have been educated and trained in traditional educational programs with distinctive boundaries around other healthcare professionals. This isolation can negatively affect the practitioners' beliefs and values regarding other healthcare professionals and their contributions to patient care. Limitations related to fiscal resources, insufficient interdisciplinary faculty, inadequate logistics, and lack of leadership and administrative support are some of the major organizational and operational barriers (Finch, 2000; FIP, 2015; Gilbert, 2005). Profession-centrism and the continuous chronicle of medical privilege are the most dogmatic barriers to IPE, which need to be replaced with equity and transdisciplinary narratives (Meleis, 2016). Indeed, academic scheduling, logistics, and inadequate financial support were observed as main challenges to the implementation of IPE among 16 US medical schools in 2016 (West et al., 2016). These barriers can be overcome by educating and training students and healthcare professionals to implement transformative IPE using a collaborative approach, and empowering all players equally.

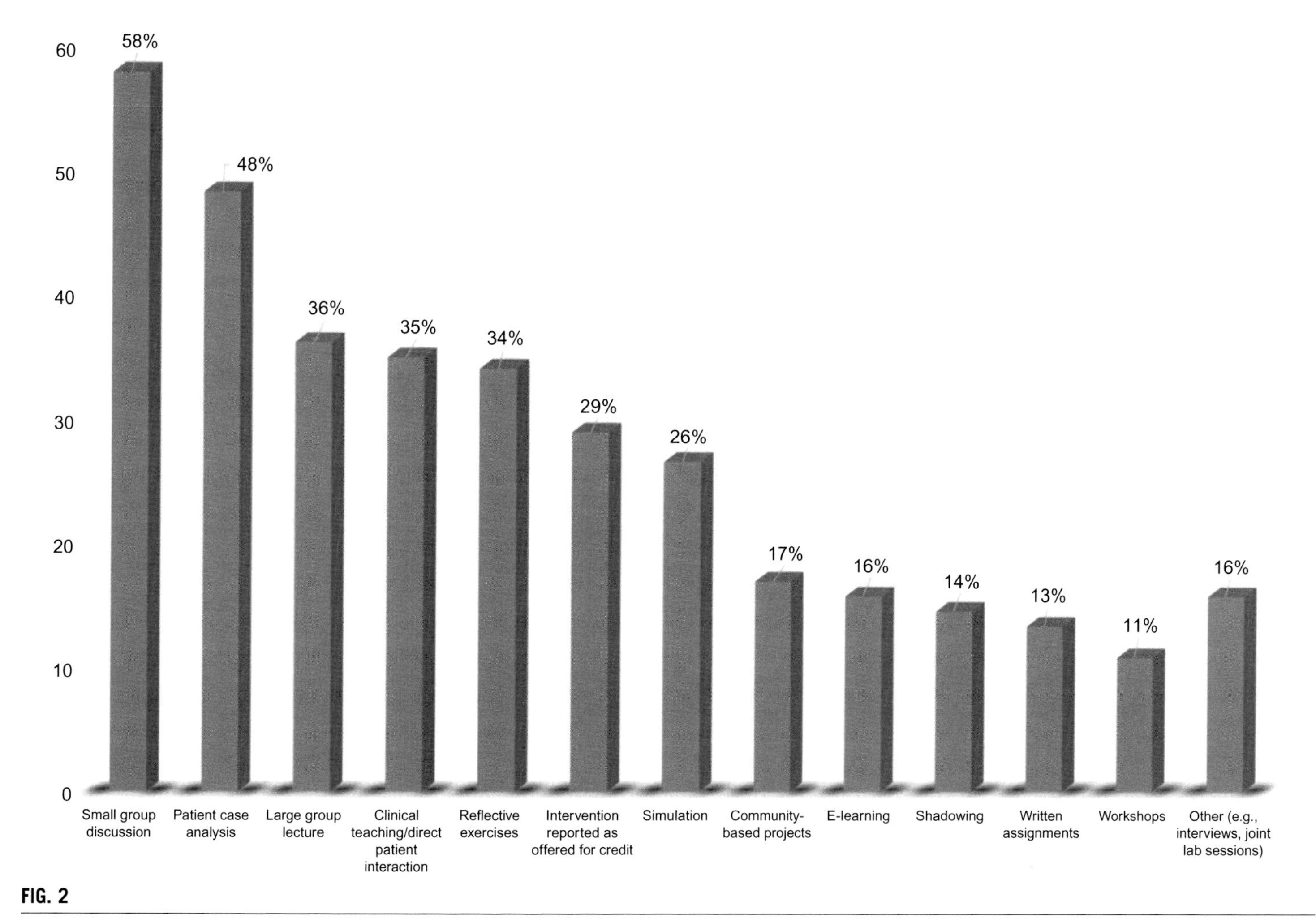

FIG. 2

IPE educational strategies adopted in US, Canada, UK, Australia, and Sweden.

BARRIERS TO IPE

- Loss of professional identity
- Attitudinal barrier
- Limited Fiscal resources
- Insufficient interdisciplinary faculty
- Inadequate logistics
- Lack of leadership and administrative support
- Profession centrism

THE CURRENT GLOBAL IMPLEMENTATION OF INTERPROFESSIONAL EDUCATION (CASE STUDY FROM 12 INSTITUTIONS IN 4 SOUTH ASIAN ASSOCIATION FOR REGIONAL COOPERATION COUNTRIES)

A survey was conducted between August 2016 to November 2016 in pharmacy academic institutions in SAARC countries to explore current IPE perspectives, different IPE strategies in practice, and barriers towards IPE implementation. The questionnaire used was adopted from previous studies (Dominguez et al., 2015; FIP, 2015), which was filled by either the head or a senior faculty member of the institution. The questionnaire was mailed to three randomly selected pharmacy institutions from each SAARC country, which were approved by their respective pharmacy councils. Twelve pharmacy institutions from four SAARC countries (Pakistan, India, Nepal and Bangladesh) responded to the survey (response rate 50%).

SAARC is a geopolitical union of Southeast Asian and Eastern Mediterranean countries, which includes Afghanistan, Bangladesh, Bhutan, India, Nepal, Maldives, Pakistan, and Sri Lanka. As of 2015, SAARC countries cover 3% of the world's area, 21% of the world's population, and 9.12% of the global economy. The survey revealed that the most frequent IPE methodology in practice was interdisciplinary social work/community services (83%), followed by theoretic or didactic IPE teaching as a part of the curriculum, small group work sessions, and collaborative workshops with other students/staff from health science disciplines (Fig. 3). Less frequently adopted strategies included hospital rotations in ambulatory care, emergency care, and all other institutional settings (17%), nursing homes/assisted living visits (17%), and multidisciplinary tutor teams in hospital trainings (33%) (Fig. 3).

PROPOSED MODEL FOR IPE IN PHARMACY PROGRAMS IN DEVELOPING COUNTRIES

An effective interprofessional education program for healthcare students of IP teams could be an ideal solution to tackle complex and challenging medical issues (Bridges et al., 2011). The main objective of the IPE program is to develop the attitude, skills, knowledge, and behaviors which are essential for collaborative practice (Reeves, 2009). In developed countries, different IPE models have been successfully incorporated into the curricula of their professional degree programs (Dominguez et al., 2015; FIP, 2015; Humphris, 2011; Lakhani & Anderson, 2008; Lee et al., 2016), and are customized and

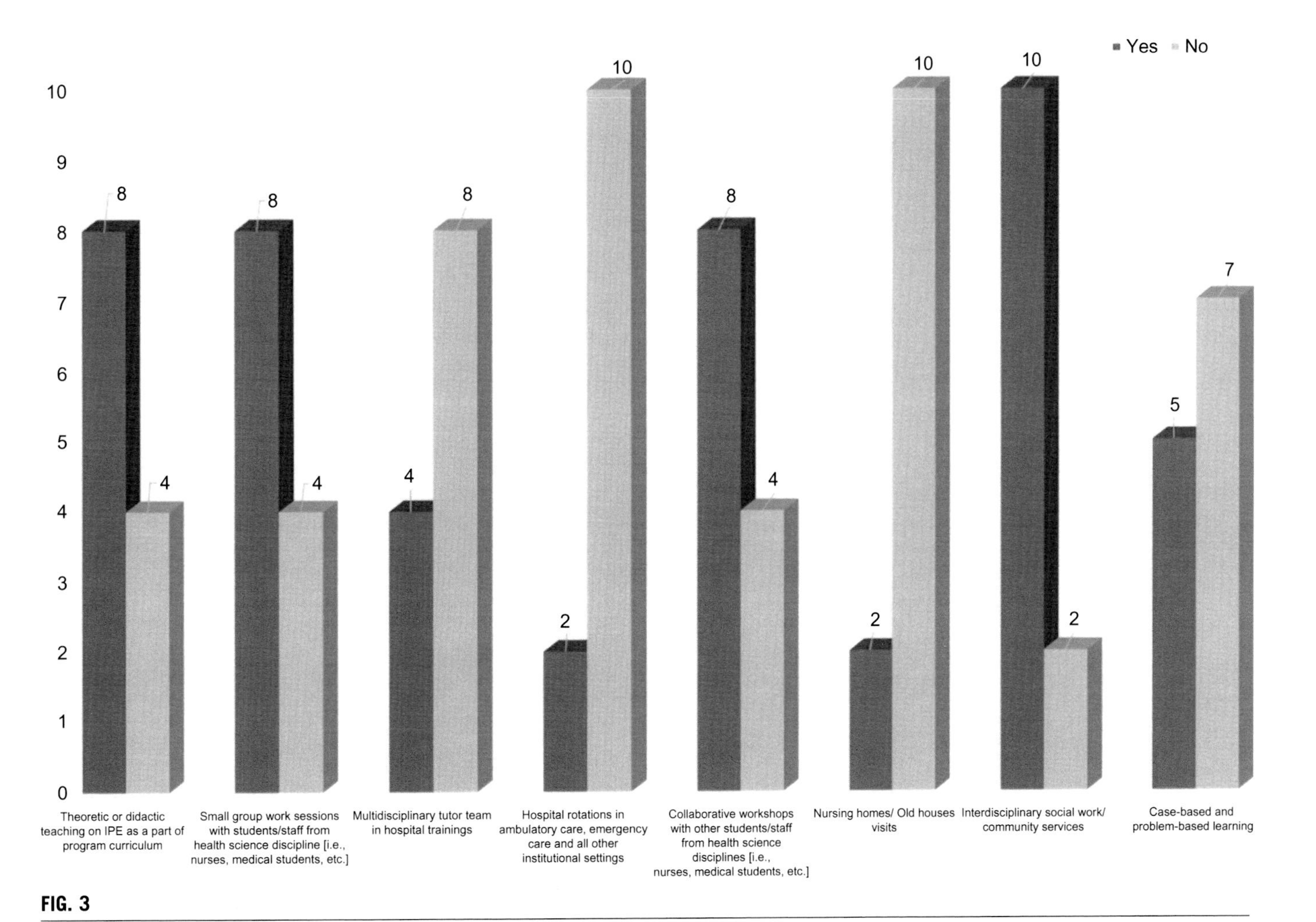

FIG. 3

IPE methods in practice in 12 pharmacy institutions of 4 SAARC countries.

*(**Note:** Nursing homes/old house in SAARC countries are recognized as assisted living/retirement homes in developed countries.)*

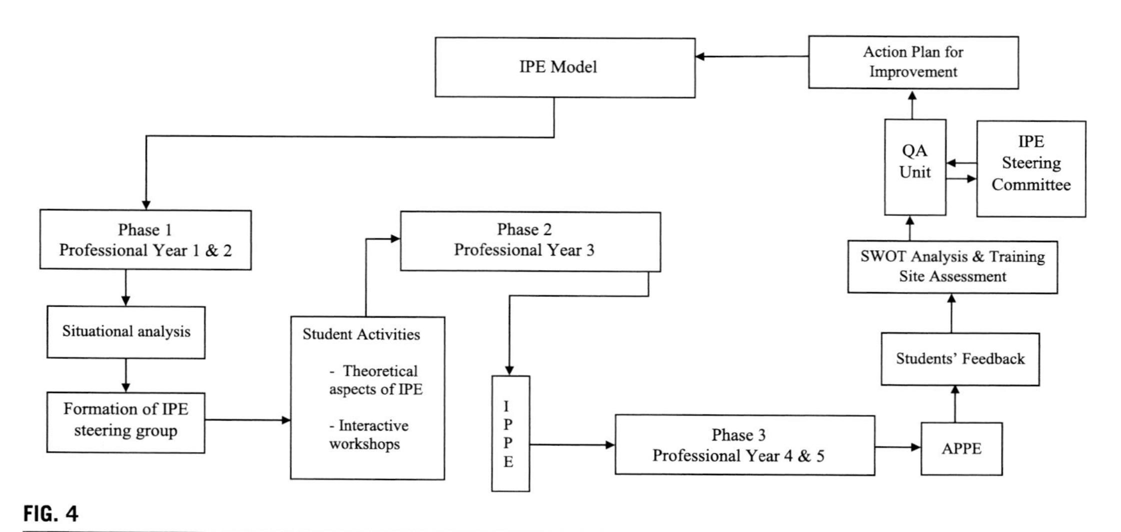

FIG. 4

Proposed model for IPE in pharmacy programs in developing countries

designed, keeping in view the available infrastructure, facilities, and barriers. This has, however, proved challenging in developing countries (e.g., SAARC countries). We thus propose an IPE model (Fig. 4) for institutions offering pharmacy programs in developing countries (especially SAARC countries). This model was designed based on the current scenario of IPE methodologies, while being cognizant of the barriers to its implementation in pharmacy education institutions in SAARC countries. However, other developing countries with similar characteristics can make use of the model. The proposed IPE model will follow an interactive three-phase model (see Fig. 4), which can be adopted by undergraduate pharmacy students. Each phase is designed to build IP collaborative skills and teamworking abilities and attitudes among students (Grace et al., 2016).

In Phase I, the university will form an IPE steering group made up of multidisciplinary tutors and health workers (including medical doctors, dentists, pharmacists, nurses, dietitians, and clinical psychologists), which will design the possible IPE approaches while keeping in view the current situation of the university (Bridges et al., 2011; Lee et al., 2016). In this phase year 1 and 2 pharmacy students will be introduced to the basic concepts of IPE, and theoretical aspects of effective team cooperation and collaboration during classroom-based activities (Lakhani & Anderson, 2008). Additionally, 2- to 3-day interactive workshops presenting information about IPE core competencies and the role of IPE at the global and regional levels, as well as an overview of different IPE models, will help to build teamwork experience among the students.

Phase II is oriented from theory to practice, as initial learning from phase I will be applied to practice-based settings (hospitals and community pharmacies/community-based programs). This phase will include introductory pharmacy practice exposure (IPPE) in the form of case presentations and joint club sessions (problem-solving, case study approaches, joint planning, and team-building exercises). Year 3 students will visit patients at their homes or point of care, and will have interactive sessions with practitioners involved in the patient's healthcare (Lakhani & Anderson, 2008).

Phase III will foster the skills and experience of year 4 and 5 pharmacy undergraduate students, gained during phase II, in the form of advance pharmacy practice experience (APPE). It will involve practice at ambulatory care, emergency care, and all other institutional settings. This phase will include special tasks like listening to patients with communication difficulties (e.g., patients with laryngectomy, stroke, and Parkinson's disease). Real patient case scenarios, situational awareness, leadership, empowerment, and communication skills will also be included to develop students' IP skills in communication and teamwork (Grace et al., 2016). This will ensure that students encounter a range of health and social care providers and become empowered to engage in the system and suggest appropriate changes to enhance multidisciplinary working (Reeves, 2009). Finally, all pharmacy students will be required to write about each phase of their IPE learning and how it will impact and reflect in their future practice. An evaluation will be undertaken to analyze the students' attitudinal changes towards the IP healthcare team before and after participation in the program.

CONCLUSION

IPE will help reform and revolutionize healthcare education and practice, which seems impossible to achieve without substantial understanding of the theoretical and practical aspects, as well as pedagogical approaches. This chapter attempts to give a brief overview and historical perspective of IPE in developed countries and the SAARC region. The challenges faced in pharmacy institutions in SAARC countries include financial and regulatory constraints, lack of appreciation for the role of other healthcare professionals, traditional culture, and lack of enforcement of IPE for health and educational departments; these issues are also being faced in developed countries. Administrative and financial support, IP program infrastructure, experienced faculty, and the promotion of a collaborative culture among the different healthcare professions are the key elements to ensure the success of IPE programs. A three-phase interactive IPE model has been suggested for pharmacy institutions in developing countries. There are plenty of opportunities for pharmacy professionals to play a collaborative and emerging role within the healthcare team and improve its effectiveness between health and social care professionals to ensure better patient care in both institutional and community settings.

REFERENCES

Abu-Rish, E., Kim, S., Choe, L., Varpio, L., Malik, E., White, A. A., et al. (2012). Current trends in interprofessional education of health sciences students: A literature review. *Journal of Interprofessional Care*, *26*(6), 444–451.

Accreditation Council for Pharmacy Education. (2006). Accreditation standards and guidelines for the professional program in pharmacy leading to the Doctor of Pharmacy Degree [electronic Resource]: Adopted January 15, 2006: Released February 17, 2006: Effective July 1, 2007: Accreditation Council for Pharmacy Education.

Baldwin, D. W. C. (1996). Some historical notes on interdisciplinary and interprofessional education and practice in health care in the USA. *Journal of Interprofessional Care*, *10*(2), 173–187.

Barceló, A., Cafiero, E., de Boer, M., Mesa, A. E., Lopez, M. G., Jiménez, R. A., et al. (2010). Using collaborative learning to improve diabetes care and outcomes: The VIDA project. *Primary Care Diabetes*, *4*(3), 145–153.

Barker, K. K., & Oandasan, I. (2005). Interprofessional care review with medical residents: Lessons learned, tensions aired—A pilot study. *Journal of Interprofessional Care*, *19*(3), 207–214.

Barnsteiner, J. H., Disch, J. M., Hall, L., Mayer, D., & Moore, S. M. (2007). Promoting interprofessional education. *Nursing Outlook*, *55*(3), 144–150.

Bridges, D. R., Davidson, R. A., Odegard, P. S., Maki, I. V., & Tomkowiak, J. (2011). Interprofessional collaboration: Three best practice models of interprofessional education. *Medical Education Online, 16.*

Buring, S. M., Bhushan, A., Broeseker, A., Conway, S., Duncan-Hewitt, W., Hansen, L., et al. (2009). Interprofessional education: Definitions, student competencies, and guidelines for implementation. *American Journal of Pharmaceutical Education, 73*(4), 1.

Clark, P. G. (1997). Values in health care professional socialization: Implications for geriatric education in interdisciplinary teamwork. *The Gerontologist, 37*(4), 441–451.

Congdon, H. B. (2016). Interprofessional education (IPE) practices at universities across the United States with an established IPE infrastructure in place. *Journal of Interprofessional Education & Practice, 5*, 53–58.

CoQoHCi America. (2001). *Crossing the quality chasm: A new health system for the 21st century.* Washington, DC: Institute of Medicine.

D'amour, D., & Oandasan, I. (2005). Interprofessionality as the field of interprofessional practice and interprofessional education: An emerging concept. *Journal of Interprofessional Care, 19*(sup1), 8–20.

Darragh, A. R., Huddleston, W., & King, P. (2009). Work-related musculoskeletal injuries and disorders among occupational and physical therapists. *American Journal of Occupational Therapy, 63*(3), 351–362.

Davies, J. G., Horne, R., Bennett, J., & Stott, R. (1993). Doctors, pharmacists and the prescribing process. *British Journal of Hospital Medicine, 52*(4), 167–170.

Dominguez, D. G., Fike, D. S., MacLaughlin, E. J., & Zorek, J. A. (2015). A comparison of the validity of two instruments assessing health professional student perceptions of interprofessional education and practice. *Journal of Interprofessional Care, 29*(2), 144–149.

Erickson, B., McHarney-Brown, C., Seeger, K., & Kaufman, A. (1998). Overcoming barriers to interprofessional health sciences education. *Education and Health, 11*(2), 143.

Finch, J. (2000). Interprofessional education and teamworking: A view from the education providers. *British Medical Journal, 321*(7269), 1138.

FIP. (2015). Interprofessional education in a pharmacy context: Global report 2015.

Gilbert, J. H. V. (2005). Interprofessional learning and higher education structural barriers. *Journal of Interprofessional Care, 19*(sup1), 87–106.

Grace, S., McLeod, G., Streckfuss, J., Ingram, L., & Morgan, A. (2016). Preparing health students for interprofessional placements. *Nurse Education in Practice, 17*, 15–21.

Greene, R. J., Cavell, G. F., & Jackson, S. H. D. (1996). Interprofessional clinical education of medical and pharmacy students. *Medical Education, 30*(2), 129–133.

Harvan, R. A., Royeen, C. B., Jensen, G. M., Royeen, C., Jensen, G., & Harvan, R. (2009). Grounding interprofessional education in practice and theory. In *Leadership in rural health interprofessional education & practice.* Boston: Jones and Bartlett Publishers.

Helitzer, D. L., LaNoue, M., Wilson, B., de Hernandez, B. U., Warner, T., & Roter, D. (2011). A randomized controlled trial of communication training with primary care providers to improve patient-centeredness and health risk communication. *Patient Education and Counseling, 82*(1), 21–29.

Hood, K., Cant, R., Baulch, J., Gilbee, A., Leech, M., Anderson, A., et al. (2014). Prior experience of interprofessional learning enhances undergraduate nursing and healthcare students' professional identity and attitudes to teamwork. *Nurse Education in Practice, 14*(2), 117–122.

Humphris, D (2011). Interprofessional education: A UK perspective.

Jacobs, L. A. (1987). Interprofessional clinical education and practice. *Theory Into Practice, 26*(2), 116–123.

Janson, S. L., Cooke, M., McGrath, K. W., Kroon, L. A., Robinson, S., & Baron, R. B. (2009). Improving chronic care of type 2 diabetes using teams of interprofessional learners. *Academic Medicine, 84*(11), 1540–1548.

Jones, K. M., Blumenthal, D. K., Burke, J. M., Condren, M., Hansen, R., Holiday-Goodman, M., et al. (2012). Interprofessional education in introductory pharmacy practice experiences at US colleges and schools of pharmacy. *American Journal of Pharmaceutical Education, 76*(5), 80.

Karim, R., & Ross, C. (2008). Interprofessional education and chiropractic. *Journal of the Canadian Chiropractic Association*, *52*, 766–778.

Kroboth, P., Crismon, L. M., Daniels, C., Hogue, M., Reed, L., Johnson, L., et al. (2007). *Getting to solutions in interprofessional education: Report of the 2006–2007 Professional Affairs Committee*. AJPE.

Kyrkjebø, J. M., Brattebø, G., & Smith-Strøm, H. (2006). Improving patient safety by using interprofessional simulation training in health professional education. *Journal of Interprofessional Care*, *20*(5), 507–516.

Lakhani, N., & Anderson, E. (2008). Interprofessional education: Preparing future pharmacists for 2020. *The Pharmaceutical Journal*, *280*(7501), 571–572.

Lee, B., Shinozaki, H., Bouphavanh, K., Tokita, Y., Makino, T., Matsui, H., et al. (2016). A plan for embedding an interprofessional education initiative into an existing programme in a Southeast Asian university. *Journal of Interprofessional Care*, *30*(3), 401–403.

Meleis, A. I. (2016). Interprofessional education: A summary of reports and barriers to recommendations. *Journal of Nursing Scholarship*, *48*(1), 106–112.

Morey, J. C., Simon, R., Jay, G. D., Wears, R. L., Salisbury, M., Dukes, K. A., et al. (2002). Error reduction and performance improvement in the emergency department through formal teamwork training: Evaluation results of the MedTeams project. *Health Services Research*, *37*(6), 1553–1581.

Moskowitz, J. M., Malvin, J. H., Schaeffer, G. A., & Schaps, E. (1983). Evaluation of a cooperative learning strategy. *American Educational Research Journal*, *20*(4), 687–696.

National League for Nursing. (2015). Guide to effective interprofessional education experiences in Nursing Education.

Page, R. L., Hume, A. L., Trujillo, J. M., Leader, W. G., Vardeny, O., Neuhauser, M. M., et al. (2009). Interprofessional education: Principles and application a framework for clinical pharmacy. *Pharmacotherapy: The Journal of Human Pharmacology and Drug Therapy*, *29*(7), 879.

Pecukonis, E., Doyle, O., & Bliss, D. L. (2008). Reducing barriers to interprofessional training: Promoting interprofessional cultural competence. *Journal of Interprofessional Care*, *22*(4), 417–428.

Reeves, S. (2009). An overview of continuing interprofessional education. *Journal of Continuing Education in the Health Professions*, *29*(3), 142–146.

Reeves, S., Boet, S., Zierler, B., & Kitto, S. (2015). Interprofessional education and practice guide No. 3: Evaluating interprofessional education. *Journal of Interprofessional Care*, *29*(4), 305–312.

Reeves, S., Zwarenstein, M., Goldman, J., Barr, H., Freeth, D., Hammick, M., et al. (2008). Interprofessional education: Effects on professional practice and health care outcomes. *Cochrane Database of Systematic Reviews*, *1*(1).

Simons, M., Ziviani, J., & Copley, J. (2011). Explanatory case study design: Application in paediatric burns health services research. *International Journal of Therapy & Rehabilitation*, *18*(5).

Taylor, C. R., Hepworth, J. T., Buerhaus, P. I., Dittus, R., & Speroff, T. (2007). Effect of crew resource management on diabetes care and patient outcomes in an inner-city primary care clinic. *Quality & Safety in Health Care*, *16*(4), 244–247.

Toner, J. A. (2006). Effective interprofessional education—Argument, assumption & evidence. *Journal of Interprofessional Care*, *20*(2), 217–218.

Weaver, S. J., Rosen, M. A., DiazGranados, D., Lazzara, E. H., Lyons, R., Salas, E., et al. (2010). Does teamwork improve performance in the operating room? A multilevel evaluation. *The Joint Commission Journal on Quality and Patient Safety*, *36*(3), 133–142.

West, C., Graham, L., Palmer, R. T., Miller, M. F., Thayer, E. K., Stuber, M. L., et al. (2016). Implementation of interprofessional education (IPE) in 16 US medical schools: Common practices, barriers and facilitators. *Journal of Interprofessional Education & Practice*, *4*, 41–49.

Young, A. S., Chinman, M., Forquer, S. L., Knight, E. L., Vogel, H., Miller, A., et al. (2005). Use of a consumer-led intervention to improve provider competencies. *Psychiatric Services*, *56*, 967–975.

CHAPTER

20 DEBATABLE ISSUES AND FUTURE DISCUSSIONS IN PHARMACY EDUCATION

Albert I. Wertheimer

College of Pharmacy, Nova Southeastern University, Ft. Lauderdale, FL, United States

INTRODUCTION

There are numerous debatable issues and opportunities for future discussions regarding pharmacy as a profession, as well as pharmacy education in particular. It seems as though some topics are too controversial to bring to the fore, or perhaps some others are not mentioned because solutions are seen as impossible or too costly. And there is even the possibility that stakeholders fear that changes may have a negative impact on their situation, and therefore they prefer the far-from-perfect status quo.

TEACHING FOR PRACTICE EXPECTATIONS TODAY OR FOR THE FUTURE

Perhaps the most pressing question is whether we should teach pharmacy students for practice expectations today or teach for what our projections of practice will be in 20 years. There are pluses and minuses for each approach. Teaching with a focus on current needs is easy to accomplish, as we understand the environment in which pharmacy is practiced today, both in the community and in the hospital (Sonnedecker, 1963). Our graduates will feel confident and will have subject mastery over contemporary matters, but they may be obsolete in 20 years when new practice modalities arise, and when newer financial and organizational characteristics will be felt. The alternative is to take a large risk and teach for the future, just as the hunter aims for the expected trajectory of the target. This has major potential pitfalls. Our predictions could be far from the mark, doing a disservice to our graduates and/or we have the possibility of causing dissatisfaction and frustration among our graduates in the coming years, when the practice environment has not yet reached the level of professionalism they were expecting. It is not clear what a curriculum would resemble to hedge our bets, as they say, and teach for the nearer-term future.

Pharmacy Education in the Twenty First Century and Beyond. https://doi.org/10.1016/B978-0-12-811909-9.00020-4

CONTROLLING THE NUMBER OF INCOMING STUDENTS TO MATCH THE EXPECTED WORKFORCE NEEDS

If that were the only problem we face, our task would be easy. However, there are additional questions of equal or greater importance, such as controlling the number of incoming students. This is a delicate issue and there is no simple universal answer. We want students enrolling in pharmacy study to demonstrate high levels of achievement in their previous studies and yet certainly do not want to produce more students than the job market can absorb. If a large surplus of graduates were to be produced, salaries would decline and there might be some unemployment or underemployment, which is most undesirable, since the most qualified students would pursue different areas of study at the university once this information were to be made public. There is probably general agreement that it is wise to match expected workforce needs with enrollment figures. But who should do this and is this best for society?

Individual schools of pharmacy are not eager to reduce their enrollments, since tuition fees help to provide funds for their diverse activities. This is of special importance to nonpublic or nonstate institutions, where nearly all of their revenue comes from tuition payments. State owned and operated facilities receive most of their income from State funds transferred from the Ministry of Health or Ministry of Education in most countries. Of course, they receive the usually reduced student tuition funds and the other large sources of income are from gifts and donations, as well as revenue from research grants and contracts earned by their faculty members. Size often dictates power and prestige and a large alumni group generates influence. The association of schools of pharmacy does not have the authority to work on this. If they attempted to establish student enrollment quotas at various schools, they would, most likely, be prosecuted by the antitrust authorities, since this is in restraint of trade, little different from a situation in which soda manufacturers agreed how to share the market. And, in any case, the nongovernment-owned schools would not support this intervention (Crighton, Toscano, Barone, & Colaizzi, 2016).

The accreditation body does not have the authorization to undertake efforts in this area. They must inspect and review schools regarding their students' success, their resources, etc., and award accreditation approval to schools that demonstrate effective operation. The various national pharmacists' associations have no mandate for any activities in such an area, and governmental agencies also have no remit to undertake activity in this realm. State governments could limit the budget allocations to State-owned facilities within their respective State, but there is little likelihood that all or even a majority of States would cooperate. And just consider the harm if, through some mechanism, pharmacy student enrollments were able to be reduced and that these reductions overshot the target goals, creating a pharmacist shortage. That would result in bidding wars to employ pharmacists, raising salaries, but with the unfortunate effect of raising medication prices for everyone to cover the increased cost of pharmacist salaries.

EFFECTIVE STRATEGIC PLANNING AND MARKETING OF THE EMERGING CONCEPTS

Next, we will address the future of pharmacy and pharmacy education. We need to utilize strategic planning. Corporations do it, governments do it, some families do it, the military does it, and probably some professions do it. Strategic planning is much more complicated than it sounds. We must consider the impact on all of the constituencies we come into contact with. We will begin thinking of strategic planning as realistically as possible. For example, just as the tail cannot wag the dog, we have limits on what we might change in the overall healthcare delivery system. There is a lesson to be learned from the "pharmaceutical care" concept failure. The designers of the concept neglected to perform any market research, an important and vital process for possibly introducing any new goods or services. For example, we would expect insurers and other healthcare payers to be willing to pay for pharmaceutical care services, but everyone reading this chapter knows that health insurers will only pay for something that is cost-effective. In other words, they would gladly pay $5.00 if that cost saved them $10 or even $8.00, but no pharmacoeconomic studies were conducted. Similarly, physicians would accept it if it had no negative impact on their incomes, but at the moment, physicians are paid for managing the overall outcomes of patients, so it would be most unlikely that physicians would cede managing patient outcomes to others. And then, an insufficient selling job was done to educate the average community pharmacist and point out the possible advantages of using the pharmaceutical care practice model. So, if a community pharmacist were to have been asked by a physician or nurse or patient: "What is this pharmaceutical care stuff?" it would be unpredictable as to what answer they might receive, if any (Zellmer, 2015).

Effective strategic planning looks to see where we want to be in, let us say, 10 years, but one could plan for 3 years or 5 years as well. Once we know this goal, we must determine a strategy to arrive there. It might be one or a combination of educational reforms, hiring of advertising agencies or public relations firms, or it could be to increase educational standards or duration, change the degree, or even require a bachelor's degree for entry to the pharmacy school. It could mean submitting to continuing competency examinations on a periodic basis to maintain one's licensure, etc. When we have figured out what mix of inputs are desired, it is logical to estimate a budget for what all of the chosen inputs will cost and the next step is to figure out where that money will come from. That may require a special one-time assessment to all members of the pharmacists' associations or requested contributions from biopharmaceutical companies or some combination of funding sources. Then the endeavor must be organized with responsibilities shared among the involved parties (Aileron, 2011). There should be an evaluation plan to monitor the campaign so that midcourse corrections may be made, if necessary. Then the active portion of the activity is begun, which includes receiving feedback (market research) from other parties and professions. If we plan efficiently, we have a better chance of succeeding in our goal quest.

Not every goal is possible, but there is no harm in considering every possible option. Some goals are not affordable or practical due to traditions, customs, the political or economic systems present, failures from previous related attempts, or for a host of other reasons. Actually, pharmacy education is too important to be left solely in the hands of pharmacy educators. Consider the fact that up to 25 years ago, pharmacy education in most countries could be accurately described as applied chemistry, with the bulk of coursework in the chemistry-related areas. Schools had many chemists on their faculties and many of those people became deans of colleges. Well, if asked what courses are most important, it is very probable that chemists will indicate that chemistry courses are the most important. Fortunately, we have come to recognize that the goal of pharmacy education is not to prepare street-corner chemists, but rather to prepare someone with the patient as their principal interest and focus (Zuckerman, 2012).

Then we have the matter of strategic planning for the profession. It is neither logical nor reasonable for the profession to undertake its own strategic planning without input from other related stakeholders, such as physicians, nurses, public health agencies, health planners, insurance leaders, etc. While we might know what we would like to offer the public, our offerings must be compatible with the healthcare scene in 20 to 30 years. Each of our brother or sister professions in the health sciences is also changing, evolving, and planning, and these efforts must be coordinated before we can have positive expectations. In addition, we must be flexible in providing sufficient latitude and space to enable pharmacy leaders and educators to conduct planning that takes into consideration the economic environment, the political situation, and traditions and cultural characteristics of each region and the country (Khandoobhai & Weber, 2014).

WHO SHOULD STUDY PHARMACY AND WHAT TOPICS ARE TO BE TAUGHT?

This leads to another unsolved matter. Who should study pharmacy? Historically, students with excellent grades in math and chemistry and other sciences were encouraged to enroll in pharmacy. But, just as the roles and obligations of a pharmacist have evolved from mastery of chemistry and the making of flawless ointments toward a focus on the patient in our new clinical pharmacy orientation, so too have the desired characteristics of pharmacy students. Yes, we have moved from the product to the patient. Chemistry is important, of course, but far less important than skills in communicating with patients. Therefore, a desirable student to enter pharmacy study should like people and talking to people, be empathetic and patient, and enjoy counseling and educating. He or she should feel gratified and professionally fulfilled if he or she solves a therapeutic question or problem. Naturally, this new pharmacy student cannot be selected from currently available predictive tests. The new admissions test will have to be created and tested for its accuracy in identifying ideal candidates for study.

Who should be encouraged to study pharmacy? Traditionally, students with high math and chemistry grades were suggested to enter pharmacy school. That is probably a fine match if our goal is to prepare research scientists for the biopharmaceutical industry. But as we all know, about 90 percent of pharmacy graduates obtain employment in community pharmacy venues. In such an ambulatory care environment, knowledge about double bonds and bonding angles is as important as poetry classes for pharmacists. In the opinion of this chapter author, the best correlates or predictors of community pharmacist success or professional fulfillment would be empathy, excellent communication skills and liking people. Each individual pharmacy practitioner is an ambassador for the entire profession to that individual patient. The ability to answer questions, make suggestions and comfort patients when needed is a valuable, precious skill. People leave the physician's office not sure whether it was 4 pills 3 times a day or 3 pills 4 times a day and whether the MRI should be done before the bloodwork at the laboratory or vice versa. And if the patient was told that surgery might be needed for themselves or for a spouse or child, they need to hear that this is a common procedure that is routinely performed in hospitals all over the world every day with very, very few negative outcomes. Double bond information would not be particularly helpful here.

Let's move on and talk about a topic of importance to all of us: economics/finance. For the most part, pharmacists are paid for their distributive function with no attention paid to their cognitive efforts. We would likely be trusted more by the population if they understood the pharmacist would not gain financially from selling of a product: that payments were made by capitation or salary. If we find a way to separate the pharmacist's income from medicine sales, we have a more wholesome situation.

The inverse to that last question is what can be sold in nonpharmacy outlets and what cannot be sold in the nonpharmacies. There are many vested interests seen here, so resolution of this matter needs many years and it is likely to be a costly battle. Perhaps there needs to be two or three types of shops, such as the licensed community pharmacy that we all are familiar with, and perhaps health and beauty aides.

The range of answers is immense; depending on location, the answers vary greatly. In some countries, pharmacies sell only prescribed and over-the-counter (OTC) medications. Others have school supplies, first-aid items, and some cosmetics. And then there are the ultralarge shops that sell foods, gifts, appliances, tobacco products, toys, detergents, hardware, party items, greeting cards, etc. There is no simple answer as to which model is correct. What is correct in one place may be inappropriate in another place. So, probably no total harmonization or standardization can take place in this area, at least in the immediate future.

Today, there is no real agreement internationally on what is the role of pharmacists, and this impasse makes things even more difficult. For many years the pharmaceutical chemists rose into dean positions and their influence on the pharmacy curriculum was to have as much pharmaceutical chemistry as possible (WHO, 1990). In some countries pharmacists are prepared for industrial positions, while in other countries they may be educated for roles in community or hospital pharmacy. Clearly, students aiming for these different areas of responsibility would be wise to study different subject matter at University.

We are faced with many issues, questions, and often problems. Many of these are similar to solving a quadratic equation, where we need to learn some information and trends before we can proceed. For example, should pharmacy educators teach for skills required today to create an effective practitioner, or should we teach for what we expect to be the practice environment in 15 to 20 years? It is easy to teach the skills that are currently required, and it is more difficult to predict future practice characteristics and teach for competency then. This latter choice involves a great deal of frustration for new graduates until such time as the practice has evolved to more closely resemble the predicted future practice environment.

Thirty years ago, the conventional wisdom was that the science, theories, rules, and formulae were to be taught by faculties and the applied material was to be taught in actual practice experiences, such as in an internship or residency. This barrier or divide has evaporated, as actual practice examples, cases, and scenarios are probably the best way to teach principles that will be remembered by the student, as they are anchored to something the student can grasp and picture.

So, who will be the brave person to formally suggest that we reconsider the admission tests and prepharmacy study subject requirements? And who should be responsible for revising the curriculum to replace some of the physical sciences with social and behavioral subjects, to learn the techniques from social psychology and medical sociology? Change is always difficult, and this would be no exception (Gable, 1974; Harding, Nettleton, & Taylor, 1990).

WHO SHOULD OWN A PHARMACY AND WHAT PRODUCTS SHOULD BE SOLD THERE?

Let us turn our attention in some other directions. One question that has not been completely solved is "Who should own a pharmacy?" In the United States, for many years, it has been any licensed pharmacist or groups of pharmacists, or companies or corporations, or partnerships that employ a properly licensed pharmacist as the pharmacist in charge, responsible for all professional and legal obligations. Should the State or government agencies own pharmacies? In some countries, one must be a pharmacist, who is limited to ownership of one or two or some small number of shops (Institute for Local Self-Reliance, 2014). There are pros and cons to be said for each model. The actual studies to determine which policy is optimal have not been done, and actually one would not expect a significant difference in professional or ethical conduct among any of these formats, as it is reasonable to assume that the owner pharmacist would act with equal integrity as the nonowner responsible pharmacist, since both risk loss of licensure for any misbehavior.

To untie product sales from income will be difficult, for several reasons. Change is always difficult since we have no idea how it will impact us personally, or what it might do to the image of the pharmacist. It should be possible, however, and let us assume that it can be successfully accomplished. That leads to the next question: What should be sold in a community pharmacy?

That raises a controversial and awkward question, but let's consider it. Some of the most developed countries practice a rigid system of pharmacy and drug control with rigorously enforced regulations about dispensing practices, refill limits, various schedules for controlled substances, staff qualifications, with in-person pharmacy inspections from the regulatory authorities, record-keeping requirements, and only a limited number of products that may be sold OTC. One must wonder whether there are any fewer overdoses, adverse events from drug interactions, incidences of abuse, or other problems in the numerous countries where one may walk into a community pharmacy and purchase nearly any pharmaceutical product without the need for a doctor's prescription, and usually from a clerk with some elementary or high-school education, with no pharmacist present. An intriguing question, at least.

THE USE OF AUTOMATION AND PARAPROFESSIONALS ON THE FUTURE JOB MARKET PLANNING FOR PHARMACISTS

The use of automation, and robotics in particular, is expanding as automation prices fall and as salaries for persons along with fringe benefits increase. In essence, this is a related question to asking about the impact of the ever-wider use of pharmacy technicians (The American Society for Automation in Pharmacy, 2018). The simple matter is that technicians cost less than fully qualified pharmacists and this logic is guiding the expanded use of paraprofessionals in hospitals, in medical and dental practices, and elsewhere across the board. Consider this example. If a pharmacist can dispense a prescription in 5 min for a labor cost of $8.00, and a technician can do it in 4 min for a labor cost of $2.50, it makes perfect sense for a pharmacy to hire additional technicians before hiring a more expensive additional pharmacist. It still makes economic sense if the pharmacist must spend under 1 min to check the technician's work. So, someone needs to think about the use of automation and paraprofessionals in the future job-market planning for pharmacists, and perhaps there are necessary curricular modifications, such as interpersonal relations and management, since there are employees to be managed, trained, and led. The future pharmacist must learn this somewhere.

OPPORTUNITIES SEEM TO BE SLIPPING AWAY FROM OUR GRASP

It is often said that one cannot see the forest because the trees impede the view. This may be happening right now in pharmacy. If one looks up from the dispensing counter for a moment, they will see trends that are becoming established at this very moment. In recent years, optometrists have been given the right to prescribe prescription-requiring drugs, as have nurse practitioners and physician's assistants. While pharmacists have been campaigning for pharmaceutical care, this has happened under their noses. Well, we cannot turn back the clock of societal progress, but another opportunity seems to be slipping away from our grasp. Most of the newest drugs are biotechnology products, which are often made of peptides or proteins, both of which are destroyed by the oral route of administration, therefore requiring that they be injected. Today, someone in the physician's office is administering those injected drugs. An ideal and less costly alternative is to have such parenteral drugs administered at the pharmacy, where no appointment would be required; less time away from work would be needed; the cost would be less; and physician's offices would be less crowded with people who do not really need to see a fully qualified physician. The community pharmacy would require some minor remodeling work to build a few small private booths in the back similar to the fitting rooms found at a clothing store. This identical solution can be proposed for administration of other specialty drugs, the fastest-growing segment of the medication marketplace. Many of these injections for cancers and other medical problems are not proteins or peptides but nevertheless could be most efficiently administered at a pharmacy. This includes drugs for hemophilia, osteoporosis, rheumatoid arthritis, long-acting contraceptives, and others requiring injected or infused medications.

MILLIS COMMISSION REPORT: PHARMACISTS FOR THE FUTURE

A little over 40 years ago, a seminal report on pharmacy education was published in the United States. It was the report of the Millis Commission, titled *Pharmacists for the Future*, and its 14 findings and recommendations merit repeating here: (Study Commission on Pharmacy, 1975)

1. Among other deficiencies is the unavailability of adequate information for those who consume, prescribe, dispense, and administer drugs.... Pharmacists are seen as health professionals who can make an important contribution to the healthcare system of the future by providing information about drugs to consumers and health professionals. Education and training of pharmacists now and in the future must be developed to meet these important responsibilities.
2. The concept is to be advanced that pharmacy should be conceived basically as a knowledge system that renders a health service by concerning itself with understanding drugs and their effects.
3. They believe that a pharmacist must be defined as an individual who is engaged in one of the steps of a system called pharmacy.... A pharmacist is characterized by the common denominator of drug knowledge and the differentiated additional knowledge and skill required by his/her particular role.
4. The system of pharmacy cannot be described as either effective or efficient in developing, organizing, and distributing knowledge and information about drugs.
5. Major attention should be given to the problems of drug information to find who needs to know, what he needs to know, and how these needs can best be met with speed and economy.

6. There is a common body of knowledge, skill, attitudes, and behavior which all pharmacists must possess... The objectives of pharmacy education must be stated in terms of both the common knowledge and skill and of the differentiated and/or additional knowledge and skill required for specific practice roles. This can be done only by stating a series of limited educational objectives which, if met in sequential order, will accomplish both common and differentiated objectives.
7. The following three educational objectives recommended: (a) mastery of knowledge and the acquisition of skills which are common to all of the roles of pharmacy practice; (b) mastery of additional knowledge and the acquisition of the additional skill needed for those differentiated roles requiring additional pharmacy knowledge and experience; (c) Acquisition and mastery of additional knowledge other than pharmacy.
8. Every school of pharmacy must promptly find and provide appropriate practice opportunities for its faculty members having clinical teaching responsibilities so that they may serve as effective role models for their students.
9. It is the opinion of the Study Commission that schools of pharmacy curricula should be based upon the competencies desired for their graduates rather than upon the basis of knowledge available in the several relevant sciences.
10. The greatest weakness of the schools of pharmacy is a lack of an adequate number of clinical scientists who can relate their specialized scientific knowledge to the development of the practice skills required to provide effective, efficient, and needed patient services. It is recommended that support be sought for a program to train a modest number of clinical scientists for pharmacy education.
11. We suggest that one of the first steps in reviewing the educational program of a college of pharmacy should be weighing the relative emphasis given to the physical and biological sciences against the behavioral and social sciences in the curriculum for the first professional degree.
12. Those schools with adequate resources should develop, in addition to the first professional degree, programs of instruction at the graduate and advanced professional level for more differentiated roles of pharmacy practice.
13. It is the opinion of the Study Commission that the optimal environment for pharmacy education is the university health sciences center, for the full range of knowledge, skill, and practice can be found there. But it is to be noted that not all schools require this environment.
14. It is the opinion of the Study Commission that all aspects of credentialing of pharmacists and pharmacy education, and the quality of pharmacy education, would be enhanced by the services of a National Board of Pharmacy Examiners... that the major organizations involved in pharmacist and pharmacy accountability and specialty credentialing join in the formation of a committee to study the necessity and the feasibility of creating a National Board of Pharmacy Examiners.

PROFESSIONAL ISSUES, CONTINUING PROFESSIONAL DEVELOPMENT, AND PHARMACY SPECIALTIES

The clinical scientist was envisioned to be as comfortable by the patient's bedside as in the laboratory. That is a tall order, which may or may not be achievable. A demonstration project in creating such a clinical pharmacy scientist was conducted with about 15 pharmacy graduates with at least 2 years of experience who entered a PhD program in the social and administrative sciences at the University of Minnesota in the early 1980s. There is further information about that later in the chapter (Wertheimer, 2006).

There are numerous definitions describing a profession, as opposed to an occupation. Most of those definitions have several concepts in common. A profession should be self-policing, practitioners should hold the patient's interests ahead of their own, it must be the principal master of a specific body of knowledge, and membership in that group should have entry limitations and, in exchange, the practitioners must demonstrate their competency. That is usually accomplished through State licensing examinations and required continuing education annual requirements. A well-regarded medical educator once said that continuing education as it existed in the 1980s was neither continuing, nor education.

One suggestion to demonstrate confidence in the mind of the public and to prove continuing competency for pharmacists throughout their careers is to require passage of periodic examinations. For example, one might have to sit for a practice-oriented examination every 10 years. The examination would not ask about the Kreb's cycle, or inorganic chemistry, or pharmacognosy, but rather about evidence-based clinical questions likely faced by pharmacists in everyday practice. One might have up to 2–3 years to repeat the examination until successful passage. If the exam cannot be passed within some reasonable period of time, that pharmacist would no longer be a licensed pharmacist. This author does not know when this will happen, but he is totally certain that it will take place within the next 20 years.

We have briefly mentioned pharmacy specialization and credentialing earlier in this chapter, and now we can explore it in greater detail. Many professions attempt to emulate the practice of medicine. Physicians in many countries are well compensated, regarded with ample respect, and are trusted by the society. Many years ago, in the 20th century, various groups of physicians gathered together to form specialist societies. Today, the societies number in the midtwenties, with many additional subspecialties. Once we had, for example, only cardiologists, but now we have interventional cardiologists, pediatric cardiologists, geriatric cardiologists, and further specialists in nuclear medicine, valve treatment, cardiac catheterization, and many more. Pharmacy now has about 10 specialty areas in which clinicians can take an examination and present a review of their practice experience (Board of Pharmacy Specialties, 2016). Successful candidates are considered (specialty) board certified. They exist in ambulatory practice, nuclear pharmacy, psychiatric pharmacy, etc. This specialization generally begins after the first professional degree (PharmD) when a recent graduate enters a residency or fellowship training program, usually for 2 years. This is usually followed by a staff position in this area of specialization at a clinic or hospital. Some of these clinicians move up the career ladder at hospitals to become directors of specific services and many others join the faculty ranks at schools of pharmacy. At the moment, the numbers are low but it is likely that this proportion will increase. Medicine now has a problem that there are too many specialists and not enough numbers of primary-care physicians. Knowing that this can easily happen, we must be vigilant in how many specialty training opportunities we operate. Specialty board certification generally translates to a higher salary and better working conditions. But like the pharmaceutical care matter discussed earlier, we can only provide what the market is willing to pay for, and not what we'd like to offer.

THE ISSUE OF PHARMACEUTICAL CARE AND THE IMPLEMENTATION OF COST-EFFECTIVE PHARMACY-BASED SERVICES

That leads to the topic of medication therapy management (MTM) and something in the United States called "provider status." The only piece of "pharmaceutical care" to survive is called MTM. It is a service provided by pharmacists in which the patient makes an appointment with a pharmacist to review the patient's medications. The patient is asked to bring all of their medications in a bag with them to the consultation session. Such a session often takes 45 min, but can be as brief as 30 min and some sessions have been known to exceed an hour. In essence, the pharmacist asks the patient what the intended use is for each item, independent of whether it is a prescribed drug, an OTC, or a supplement or nutraceutical product.

Items that are no longer needed or beneficial can be discarded with no future use. This streamlining of a patient's medication use often saves money and prevents serious adverse drug effects. Many seniors use 15–18 products, including vitamins and other supplements, all of which have the possibility of interfering with each other. The patient often saves money, buying fewer medications in the future, and the payer or health insurer sometimes saves money when drug-drug interactions can be prevented. Some insurers pay for this service since they see it as cost-effective, especially for very elderly patients with complex illnesses and many, many medications. The fee is routinely in the range of US$50.00 (Burns, 2014).

If the pharmacist can obtain an approval as an accepted service provider, then he/she can offer this service to the millions of Medicare and Medicaid beneficiaries and be paid by the agency. Without that approval and a provider number, the pharmacist losses a potentially large income stream.

Another avenue pursued by some pharmacists is the use of a joint practice agreement. Certainly, the majority of community pharmacists do not participate in this, but a small, energetic minority is pioneering this effort in which a local, usually primary-care, physician authorizes in advance the right to a nearby known pharmacist to issue refills or prescribe drugs in specified situations. For hypertensive patients, the pharmacist may dispense the next bottle of medications if the blood pressure is about the same as last time. If it has risen, the pharmacist is authorized to dispense the next higher dose of the same medication. This is usually done for refills of chronic disease medications, such as for hypertension or diabetes, among others, where the pharmacist can test blood pressure or blood glucose levels, for example. In its most basic form, the physician delegates authority to one specific pharmacist to handle certain specified medical conditions with a narrow range of treatment options. This adds to the positive image and reputation of a pharmacist in community practice, more as a healthcare professional and less as a merchant.

In the UK for the last several years, community pharmacists have been paid by the local health authorities from the NHS budget to handle trivial diseases. This is cost-effective for the health authority since the GP's office is less crowded, patients wait shorter times, and most of these minor ailments are self-limiting in the first place, so little harm can be expected. Patients seem to like it and health money is usually saved. This is an example of a worldwide trend to use persons who might be a bit lesser trained but cheaper, if the delegation is seen as safe for the population.

A related trend is the use of high-tech. We see it every day in using an ATM at the bank instead of chatting with a bank teller, ordering airplane or train tickets online, or shopping online rather than in person at the shop. Next, we will see patients picking up their prescribed medicines in a type of vending machine, negating the need to speak with the pharmacist. The noted futurist Alvin Tofler when considering these trends said that the increased use of high-tech will leave a void where persons want to discuss their health or purchase with a real, live person. He said that this growth of high-tech will create a demand for "high touch," or contact with a fellow human. Perhaps this is a void where some pharmacists can fulfill such a role. The pharmaceutical care concept proved to be a failed concept and is no longer mentioned by pharmacy leaders or planners. It was a popular cause in the early 2000s, but it has not been accepted by physicians, insurers, most pharmacists, and other stakeholders. Fortunately, the clinical pharmacy movement of the 1970s, of patient-centered care, continues to advance throughout the world. It is worth thinking about, even though many persons will be unwilling to pay extra for personal service.

PRODUCING SECOND CLASS OF PHARMACISTS

Periodically, we hear or read about a proposed second class of pharmacists: not a technician, but a junior pharmacist, akin to the nurse practitioner in a physician's office or in a clinic. This junior pharmacist could be prepared to independently, that is, without immediate supervision, dispense refills, answer questions about OTC products, teach patients how to do self-injections, use blood pressure testing devices, etc. This scenario would free up the pharmacist to do more cognitive services such as therapeutic problem solving, MTM and patient counseling, especially for newly diagnosed patients with chronic conditions. The Swedish have trained "prescriptionists" for many years and they have staffed pharmacies in tiny villages, areas minimally populated north of the Arctic Circle and elsewhere. Perhaps there is something here to be modified and adapted (Pharmacy Technician Certification Board, 2015).

GLOBAL STANDARDS FOR THE FIRST PROFESSIONAL DEGREE IN PHARMACY AND OTHER ISSUES

An issue that has never been adequately studied and policy made about is the goal of the first professional degree in pharmacy. In many countries, the first professional degree, i.e., B.S. or PharmD, prepares a graduate for community pharmacy or hospital pharmacy practice. In other locations, all possible pharmacy-related jobs are expected to be handled by such a first-degree pharmacist. Yet, some places have a 1- or 2-year additional master's degree for positions in the pharmaceutical industry, in hospital administration, or in management in chain pharmacy corporations and in regulatory matters, among others. There are no uniform international standards, and there does not appear to be any significant attention devoted to this question. As a rule, formal education is not wasted, but requiring pharmacy graduates to spend one or two additional years at the university may not be cost-effective. Consider a prospective student thinking about pharmacy study for 7 years and comparing it with medicine or dentistry of the same length of time. This could damage future enrollment numbers. Whatever decision is reached, it would be wise to have global agreement to enable professionals to move among countries as the market dictates.

On the topic of pharmacy education, the deans of faculties of pharmacy have traditionally been pharmacists, but there are a growing number of persons credentialed in other, related professions such as medicine or chemistry who have been selected as deans of pharmacy schools. A most ambitious project would be to determine whether it is necessary for a dean to be a member of the same profession. More than likely, there are positive and negative examples of both sides. Perhaps an individual personality characteristic determines success as a dean. We simply do not know the answer, meaning that policy must wait until the policy can be informed with facts.

Now and then, new job descriptions are generated in order to solve or correct some void and/or need. For example, during the current decade it has become apparent that more persons with skills in the pharmacovigilance area will be needed within the pharmaceutical industry. This is a need that was recognized by the biopharmaceutical companies, and since there were no experienced graduates from pharmacy schools, the industry had to train its own personnel. Another area where the private sector created a function and demand for capable professionals is in the realm of managed care pharmacy, with work on comparative effectiveness, technology assessment, and pharmaco-economics. This has the purpose of aiding insurers and payers to select the optimal drug products for their formularies. Most of the time, new innovations emanate from university research laboratories and the graduates are then able to bring those new skills to the industry. In these two examples, pharmacy schools will have to learn from the industrial side and teach students who might have career aspirations in such specialty areas. While we see examples of industry employees teaching at universities, it is not a bad idea for academics to spend time on occasion in the industry and vice versa. When both sides understand the needs and abilities of the other side, it is more probable that useful progress may be made, often jointly.

Study Commissions in the UK, United States, Europe, Canada, and via the World Health Organization have convened task forces and committees to study and report on what the responsibilities of the pharmacist might resemble.

Most report similar findings that it is a waste of time and money to have the pharmacist count pills and label bottles and sell medications to the patient. That could be taken care of by robots or technicians, freeing up pharmacist time and attention to be focused on serious medication problems, drug history taking, or designing multiple drug regimens to minimize possible adverse events. Some have stated that pharmacists could detail physicians objectively about newly marketed products, teach nurse practitioners about prescribing and interactions, and volunteer at faculties of pharmacy to increase the amount of real-world experience, as opposed to material gleaned only from textbooks.

THE SELECTION OF FACULTY DEANS

The last matter to be discussed is a very controversial one, akin to religion or politics, where most involved parties hold strong opinions and where it is most unlikely that discussions or conversations can sway one's thinking. That topic is the selection of faculty deans (Salary.com, 2017). In Europe, the position of dean is filled via an election of faculty members eligible to vote. The term of office is usually from 2 to 4 years and most universities have policies preventing any one person from serving more than two consecutive terms in that office. In North America, the typical policy is for the provost or chancellor to appoint a dean, usually for a 4–5 year term, and there is little mention of any number of permitted consecutive terms in office. Someone could serve for 15 or 20 or more years if their supervisor is satisfied with their performance. After having the opportunity to observe both systems, this writer prefers the European system, for a number of reasons. It forces faculty members to learn firsthand some of the issues, battles, and work a dean must accomplish, and what latitude he/she has regarding budgets, etc. Moreover, it keeps things honest. By that I mean that if the dean treats a colleague unfairly, it is only a matter of time before that colleague or a friend will be in the dean position, to obtain their revenge. This system nearly guarantees that there will be greater collegial and mutually respectful relationships. The only material shortcoming of the system is the existence of a learning curve. One probably does not have sufficient skills and expertise on their first day in office. That means that there will be some inefficiencies during the first several months of each new dean's tenure in office. However, the staff in the dean's office who continue from administration to administration can probably assist in such circumstances.

The North American system gives great power to a dean who has been in office for 15 or more years. More than likely, most newer faculty hires were overseen by him or her, and they might have encouraged rivals or persons with opposing views to leave the institution. By 15 years, there are the inescapable differences that occur in various little (or larger) questions. It takes a very secure, accomplished, and mature individual to ignore these differences in perspective and not take them personally. In fact, as a general rule of thumb, it is wisest to hire or select a dean who already has achieved great feats in research and teaching as a professor. Such a person can be fulfilled by the vicarious accomplishments of his academic team. Otherwise, there is the unfortunate possibility that the dean will be a competitor with his colleagues instead of a source of support and encouragement.

There are probably many more debatable issues and future discussions that might be considered, but those reviewed in the preceding pages could keep one occupied for a lengthy period of time. It is hoped that reading this chapter has provided you with some ideas and perspectives not considered previously, that might assist you in making superior decisions and choices.

REFERENCES

Aileron. (2011). Five Steps to a Strategic Plan, Forbes, 10/24. https://www.forbes.com/sites/aileron/2011/10/25/five-steps-to-a-strategic-plan/#3f12a3005464 (accessed 6 September 2017).

American Society for Automation in Pharmacy, 2018 website, (assessed April 2017).

Board of Pharmacy Specialties, (2016) www.bps.org. Washington, DC.

Burns, A. (2014). Medication therapy management in pharmacy practice: Core Elements of an MTM Model, version 2.0. *Journal of the American Pharmacists Association*, *49*(3), 341–353.

Crighton, M, Toscano, M, Barone, J and Colaizzi, J. (2016). Are Pharmacy Schools Growing Too Fast? Pharmacy Times, 15.

Gable, F. B. (1974). *Psychosocial pharmacy: The synthetic society*. Philadelphia: Lea and Febiger.

Harding, G., Nettleton, S., & Taylor, K. (1990). *Sociology for pharmacists: An introduction*. London: Macmillan.

Institute for Local Self-Reliance. (2014), Pharmacy ownership laws, Washington https://ilsr.org/rule/pharmacy-ownership-laws/ (accessed 6 September 2017).

Khandoobhai, A., & Weber, R. (2014). Issues facing pharmacy leaders in 2014: Suggestions for pharmacy strategic planning. *Hospital Pharmacist*, *49*(3), 295–302.

Pharmacy Technician Certification Board. (2015) Pharmacy Technician's Letter, Pharmacy Technician Certification Board (PTCB), Frequently asked questions, Stockton, Calif.

Salary.com. 2017 Dean's job description. www.salary.com?Dean-of-Pharmacy-Salary.html, (assessed March 2017).

Sonnedecker, G. (Ed.), (1963). *Kremers and Urdang's History of Pharmacy* (3rd ed., pp. 203–206). Philadelphia: Lippincott.

Study Commission on Pharmacy. (1975). *Pharmacists for the future: The report of the Study Commission on Pharmacy*. Ann Arbor: Health Administration Press.

Wertheimer, A. (2006). In D. Worthen (Ed.), *The Millis Study Commission on Pharmacy: A roadmap to a Profession's Future*. New York: Haworth Press. Chapter 5.

World Health Organization (WHO). (1990), The role of the Pharmacist in the Healthcare System, Report of a WHO Consultative Group, New Delhi, 13–16 December 1988, Geneva: World Health Organization.

Zellmer, W. (Ed.), (2015). *Pharmacy Forecast 2016-2020*. American Society of Health-System Pharmacists: Bethesda.

Zuckerman, A. (2012). *Healthcare strategic planning* (3rd ed.). Ann Arbor: Health Administration Press.

CHAPTER

CONCERNS AND CHALLENGES IN PHARMACY EDUCATION: MIND THE GAPS

21

Mohamed Izham Mohamed Ibrahim*, Ahmed Ibrahim Fathelrahman†

**College of Pharmacy, Qatar University, Doha, Qatar, †College of Pharmacy, Taif University, Taif, Saudi Arabia*

"Education is the most powerful weapon which you can use to change the world."
Nelson Mandela (Former President of South Africa and Political Activist)

INTRODUCTION

At the time of writing this chapter, most of the pharmacy colleges are in the new academic session (i.e., the fall semester). Every academic year, pharmacy colleges continue to prepare to produce new graduates and some will become pharmacy leaders. The colleges are preparing tomorrow's pharmacists today, producing the "8-Star Pharmacist" (WHO, 1997). According to Anthony Smith, the former dean and professor at the School of Pharmacy, University of London, UK, "Tomorrow's pharmacists will need to have the attributes of a professional, a practitioner, a scholar and a scientist, irrespective of the sector in which they work" (Alexander, 2010). Careful analysis of the current healthcare system has shown that the demand for patient care has moved the healthcare services closer to the patient (i.e., from tertiary care to secondary care to primary care). Thus, promotive care and public health have become more important than before (DiPietro Mager & Farris, 2016), which indicates that there are specific skills needed at each of the care levels and health sectors. The entire healthcare industry is changing and evolving to a value-based care model that pays for quality and performance (Tice, 2017). According to the Institute of Medicine, there are at least five competencies that all healthcare professionals should acquire when they are in college: "provide patient-centered care, work in interprofessional teams, employ evidence-based practice, apply quality improvement, and use informatics" (Burke, 2015; Institute of Medicines, 2003). The US Accreditation Council for Pharmacy Education (ACPE) in its revised standard of education has incorporated such recommendations from the Institute of Medicine. In addition, in the new standard of pharmacy educations (i.e., through the curriculum), the pharmacy graduates must be ever ready to directly contribute to patient care ("practice-ready") and work in collaboration with other healthcare professionals and providers ("team-ready") (ACPE, 2015). The American Pharmacy Association (APhA) stresses the importance of interprofessional education (IPE) (Bonner, 2014). This IPE component must be included in both the classroom as well as in the experiential learning environments. Pharmacy college is the primary setting where students could and should take advantage of the opportunity to develop their personal and professional attributes and it is the place that will assist the students to shape their future as a healthcare professional. Pharmacy

Pharmacy Education in the Twenty First Century and Beyond. https://doi.org/10.1016/B978-0-12-811909-9.00021-6

graduates are expected to have the qualities of leadership, professionalism, entrepreneurship, innovation, etc.

Thus, in relation to the call from various leaders and pharmacy organizations, this book presents important aspects related to pharmacy education for today and for the future. It also touches on the achievements and challenges experienced by the various stakeholders in pharmacy education. The book in your hand includes four sections: (1) Defining Pharmacy Education; (2) Basic Roles and Contributions of Pharmacy Education; (3) Features and Contributing Factors of Pharmacy Education; and (4) Special Issues in Pharmacy Education. Under each theme, there are several chapters, which can be summarized under the following topics: history of pharmacy education; theories, models and strategies in pharmacy education; relationship of pharmacy education and practice; contributions of pharmacy education toward pharmaceutical care and public health; pharmacy curriculum and degrees; teaching strategies and assessment methods; competency-based pharmacy education; and other significant issues related to pharmacy education, such as capacity building, continuing professional development (CPD), interprofessional education (IPE), quality and accreditation, regulation, and leadership. Finally, the book also presents "debatable issues and future directions" of pharmacy education. This final chapter summarizes and organizes the main ideas from all the sections and chapters.

DIFFERENT PERSPECTIVES, THEORIES, MODELS, AND STRATEGIES IN PHARMACY EDUCATION

History helps people understand and appreciate reasons and purposes of changes. The past causes the present and thus the future. There are several important factors, drivers, and enablers that caused the changes and advancement in Western pharmacy education. It is interesting to know how the pharmacy education development in the United States and Europe has not just influenced US and European pharmacy education, but also other parts of the world. To a certain extent, colonialism has impacted pharmacy education in many parts of the world (Harding & Taylor, 2016; Shizha & Kariwo, 2011). Accreditation, innovations, research, and policy have significantly caused transformational change in pharmacy education in the West. This is expected to continue and will place a great challenge before pharmacy educators and colleges in many ways.

The ancient past (i.e., antiquity) has greatly influenced pharmacy education in the East (e.g., the Arab, Chinese, and Indian era of civilization). For example, the use of medicinal plants and traditional medicines has a significant impact on pharmacy curriculum and practice. Great changes and improvements have occurred in Eastern pharmacy education over the years, especially with the influence of Western pharmacy education, advancement in practice, job opportunity abroad, and accreditation/quality standards.

The quality of pharmacists in the workforce relies heavily on the quality of pharmacy education obtained while in college, as well as during working (e.g., continuing education programs). Quality is value-based and explicitly is connected to accountability (Harvey & Green, 1993). Quality students will become quality pharmacists. Students' quality is shaped by various factors, such as the quality of the college and university in many aspects, the quality of the curriculum, and the effectiveness of the teaching styles and strategies. Hence, it is necessary for all pharmacy educators and trainers to be aware of different possible learning styles and to try to accommodate as many of them as possible when planning their instructional programs. Students' behavior and learning are significantly influenced by their preferred learning modes. The appropriate learning strategies should match the students' preferred learning modes.

CONTRIBUTIONS OF PHARMACY EDUCATION TOWARD PHARMACY PRACTICE, PHARMACEUTICAL CARE, AND PUBLIC HEALTH

The practice of pharmacy has moved from product-oriented and service-oriented to patient-centered care (i.e., traditional drug focus to an advanced patient focus). Hence the skill and knowledge of pharmacists has to be expanded and tailored to the present needs. Sound evidence-based information, evidence-based education, and evidence-based practice become so important when pharmacists focus more on patient-centered and pharmaceutical care for obtaining the best patient health outcomes. Research and education in schools of pharmacy will become ever more vital as the role and responsibility of pharmacists in healthcare diversifies. Pharmacy education needs to develop the educational outcomes, professional competencies, curricular content, and processes that are required to prepare competent graduates to assume an integrated and accountable role in the healthcare system, by having defined responsibilities for direct patient care. The advancement in the role of pharmacists also invites them to be part of the broader healthcare team working for providing better healthcare for the patients (i.e., interprofessional, collaborative patient-centered care) (Fox & Reeves, 2015). Future directions for both pharmacy practice and education will include: emphasis on interprofessional education and collaborative practice; expanding the role of the pharmacist in public or population health; and incorporating more intensive experiential education in teaching pharmaceutical care. While one perspective is on the individual patient's health, on the other end more focus is given to population or public health. Thus, pharmacy educators are encouraged to consider these two important perspectives on the healthcare system in order to improve the health of the society. Educators must be aware of the expansion and the diversification of the public health discipline. Online programs offer degrees and certificates in public health that pharmacists could opt for. In addition, pharmacy colleges should consider the following areas when revising and improving the curriculum: law and regulation; ethics; health policy; quality and outcomes; biostatistics; environmental health; epidemiology; development and disaster management; demography; and value for money.

THE IMPORTANCE OF QUALITY CURRICULUM, TEACHING STRATEGIES, ASSESSMENT METHODS, AND COMPETENCY-BASED EDUCATION IN PHARMACY EDUCATION

Over time, the traditional pharmacy education has been taken over by the modern pharmacy education. Today, many of the pharmacy colleges have adopted a clinically oriented curriculum. Education has evolved from being a product-oriented to a patient-focused approach. Many colleges are producing pharmacy graduates who will be clinically oriented and will be bridging the gaps between patients and physicians. We are in the era of a multidisciplinary healthcare system dealing with complex patients with complex therapy. We need to have pharmacy graduates who have sets of skills, knowledge, and competency to handle such situations. To achieve this, the pharmacy curriculum needs to be integrated between basic science and clinical science, between the two categories of sciences and administrative science, and between these three categories of sciences with practice.

Teaching and education in pharmacy colleges become more challenging with the transition and changes in pharmacy curricula. Curriculum change refers to "a whole set of concepts, including innovation, development, and adoption" (Leung, 2013).

In addition to the curricula changes, there are also significant changes and various options in pharmacy qualifications offered, the duration, and the number of programs. Pharmacy education systems in both the developed and developing countries are experiencing this. A great variation of entry-level degrees exists among different countries. The number of years it takes for full registration as a pharmacist also differs among countries. Countries also differ in terms of the practice/experiential training of pharmacists; some occurs after graduation while other training is part of the professional degree program. This book also explains that the duration, orientation, and structure of the first pharmacy professional degrees differ extensively among countries and also within some countries. Programs that offer postgraduate degrees also differ in terms of the objective, orientation, structure, and duration. In some countries, pharmacists have opportunities to join residencies, fellowships, and specialty training programs after completion of their professional degree. Pharmacists could also have an opportunity to pursue master's or doctoral degree programs if they are interested, and to obtain a PhD degree, especially if they would like to join the university as an academician.

In colleges, didactic lectures are commonly used in teaching and training for pharmacy students and pharmacists. Over the years, several other teaching styles and strategies, such as problem-based learning (PBL), team-based learning (TBL), self-directed learning (SDL), workshops, seminars, interactive learning, and blended modes have been introduced in pharmacy colleges. Pharmacy educators are encouraged to apply these methods, single or blended, as they are proven better and more effective at producing better student learning outcomes. There is a close relationship between learning and experience, which will significantly change the principles, behavior, values, and beliefs of the learners. Hence it is important for educators to build courses and educational programs that suit the needs of the learners and their environment.

In addition to having effective and appropriate learning models, styles, and strategies, pharmacy educators have to design a suitable method for student assessment. Assessment is an important component of the curriculum. It will influence what students eventually learn. There are three types of assessment: summative, formative, and diagnostic. Each is used for different reasons. Overall, the objective is to assess if the intended learning outcomes, knowledge, skills, and competencies are obtained. "One size fits all" does not work with course assessment. Different assessment methods need to be used for different learning outcomes; thus for a particular course pharmacy educators probably need to apply various methods of assessment, e.g., multiple choice questions, essay questions, short answer questions, objective structured clinical examinations (OSCE), oral examination, and/or field/laboratory work with report. Which assessment tools the educator decides to adopt—e.g., direct versus indirect, manual or automatic—will depend on several factors (i.e., the impact on education, feasibility, validity, reliability, acceptability, applicability, and cost of using the tool).

Another important aspect that is of growing interest in pharmacy education is competency-based education (CBE). CBE links theory to practice (Gervais, 2016). CBE is defined as "an outcome-based approach to education that incorporates modes of instructional delivery and assessment efforts designed to evaluate mastery of learning by students through their demonstration of the knowledge, attitudes, values, skills, and behaviors required for the degree sought" (Gervais, 2016). There are several advantages in transforming traditional pharmacy education into competency-based pharmacy education. It will allow pharmacy students to progress based on their capability to master a competency or a skill at their own pace regardless of the environment (Educause, 2017). CBE is "built around clearly defined competencies and measurable learning objectives that demonstrate mastery of those competencies" (Educause, 2014). CBE is significant in preparing for a trained and competent workforce, and there is great interest among pharmacy colleges nowadays to adopt CBE. This goes beyond colleges to pharmacy organizations for their members, e.g., pharmacy practitioners for their professional registration/licensure to practice pharmacy. The required competencies are determined by the healthcare needs of the society. Then the choice of curricular content, teaching and learning methods, assessment strategies, and educational environment will be determined by these competencies. Pharmacy colleges must ensure that their graduates are competent to enter practice.

CONTINUING PROFESSIONAL DEVELOPMENT, CAPACITY BUILDING, QUALITY, ACCREDITATION AND REGULATION ISSUES IN PHARMACY EDUCATION

After graduating from pharmacy colleges, continuing professional development (CPD) activities provide professionals with the opportunity to enhance their personal skills and proficiency throughout their careers. Professionals engage in activities that enable their learning to become proactive. CPD involves the "process of tracking and documenting the skills, knowledge and experience that they gained both formally and informally as they work, beyond any initial training" (Allen, 2009). The pharmacist is one of the healthcare professionals that needs lifelong learning to keep up with the changes in the healthcare system and patient demands. Participating in the CPD programs can fulfill these purposes. There are many countries in which CPD programs are regulated by the pharmacy regulatory body that mandates the pharmacy practitioners to participate as a aprerequisite for licensing and practice. The scope and implementation of CPD in pharmacy varies widely across countries and regions. Thus, accrediting the program becomes important as proof of quality.

Capacity building is critical in the pharmacy education sector. According to UNCED (1992), "capacity building encompasses the country's human, scientific, technological, organizational, institutional and resource capabilities" (UNCED, 1992). The capacity of the academic workforce to teach and train graduates is important to ensure having competent and capable pharmacy personnel in the pharmaceutical sector. Capacity building in the academic setting will include improving the abilities, skills, and competencies of pharmacy educators and, in addition, it will also comprise the development of infrastructure and infostructure. There is a worldwide shortage of pharmacy academics and practice-based preceptors or educators in the health institutional settings to train pharmacy students. There are several responses toward this problem and one of the approaches taken has been expanding the number of pharmacy colleges in the country. Many countries have created a cross appointment position in the colleges (i.e., practitioner-academic workforce), where individuals have a teaching workload in the college as well as practicing in the healthcare institutions. With this option, there must be a memorandum of understanding and agreement between the pharmacy colleges and the health institutions. Understanding the challenges and having the succession planning are crucial to develop academics for the future. What will be the focus areas of these future academicians: just a teaching focus or a research focus, or a blend of these?

According to Chitty (2002), education quality covers three main education goals, identified as human fulfilment, preparation for the world of work, and contributing to social progress and social change (Chitty, 2002). There are five dimensions of quality in education: effectiveness, efficiency, equality, relevance, and sustainability (Barrett et al., 2006). According to the European Commission (2018), "high quality and relevant higher education is able to equip students with the knowledge, skills and core transferable competences they need to succeed after graduation, within a high quality learning environment which recognizes and supports good teaching." The public becomes more confident and trusts the quality of higher education if it has quality assurance. Hence, every pharmacy education institution should have a rigorous system of internal quality assurance. Stakeholders are interested in quality education and they should be involved in the continuous quality improvement of the pharmacy education system. Further, many pharmacy colleges have gone through an accreditation process, a mechanism for the achievement and the recognition of quality of an academic program through adhering to a set of standards. It is one of the ways to achieve and sustain quality. Most of the evidence indicates that accreditation enhances procedures, processes, and outputs; however, no evidence is available on its positive effect on the actual outcomes of healthcare services or the academic programs. Cases in Latin America have shown that regulations also played an important role in maintaining the quality of pharmacy education. Government and pharmacy professional organizations were the driving forces and contributed to the establishment of higher education policies.

Globally, there is a shortage of pharmacy workforce. Due to several reasons, the pharmacy education sector has not been able to fulfill the demand for manpower in the pharmacy practice settings. This phenomena is more crucial in low- and middle-income countries. The International Pharmaceutical Federation (2012) reported that the number of pharmacists per 10,000 population ranges from as low as 0.02 in Somalia to 25.07 in Malta, while the mean number equates to 6.02 pharmacists per 10,000 population (FIP, 2012). Further, there is a mismatch between the need (e.g., disease burden), and supply of pharmacists in countries (e.g., in the African region) (FIP, 2015). In countries where there is a shortage of pharmacists, the pharmacies are operated by pharmacy technicians/assistants, at times with lack of quality and structured curricula. There is also an issue with gender distribution in the pharmacy workforce, where nowadays we have more female pharmacists. The focus areas in the pharmaceutical sector—e.g., hospital pharmacy, community pharmacy, and pharmaceutical industry—have also identified challenges that face the pharmacy education sector. For example, if a country is highly focused on the pharmaceutical industry and generic medicines are one of the main exported goods, are pharmacy colleges capable of producing competent graduates for the industry? There are challenges ahead for the pharmacy education sector: increasing the number of pharmacists; ensuring qualitative growth in the pharmacy profession; and catering to society's needs for specialized pharmacy services.

PHARMACY EDUCATION: DEBATABLE ISSUES AND FUTURE DIRECTIONS

With the complex healthcare system of today and the future, there are great challenges expected ahead. We are moving toward more clinical-oriented, patient-centered care and an integrated health service delivery model. The societal and healthcare environments are changing over time. There are plenty of opportunities for pharmacy professionals to play a collaborative and emerging role within the healthcare team in both institutional and community settings. Thus, we need leaders in the pharmacy education sector to lead and manage in a strategic direction. We are expecting the evolution of new expanded roles for pharmacists. The strategic direction must aligns with the global healthcare workforce development goals. If we are expecting new roles for pharmacists for new innovative services in the future, then we need pharmacy graduates with a special set of skills, knowledge, and competencies that fit with the future needs and expectations. Leading change in pharmacy education requires leading change in curriculum design and delivery. Leaders in the pharmacy education sector must be aware of the things happening in the practice environment (i.e., need to be connected to healthcare system at both local and international level). There is a need to make paradigmatic transformation in the curriculum design. We need leaders with a different mindset. In addition, there are numerous debatable issues and opportunities for future discussions regarding pharmacy as a profession, as well as pharmacy education in particular. What should be taught to the pharmacy students—teach for practice expectations today or for the future? Should we control the number of incoming students to match the expected workforce needs? Should we conduct strategic planning and marketing for the emerging concepts? Who should study pharmacy and what should they study? Who should own a pharmacy? What products should be sold in a pharmacy? What will be the impact and benefits of the use of automation and paraprofessionals on the future job market planning for pharmacists? Are there future opportunities for pharmacists? These are some of the issues that will challenge our mind and force us to think rationally (i.e., out-of-the-box thinking or divergent thinking).

FINAL REMARKS

Healthcare is a complex, uncentralized network, and its components are interdependent (Aronson, 2016). Alsharif (2012) pointed out that pharmacy education to a certain extent has been affected in this era of globalization. For pharmacy education to be successful, he recommended several major strategies: share expertise and resources; respect historic factors and ethical dilemmas that may have affected pharmacy education; consider local manpower needs; establish accreditation standards; engage stakeholders; empower students; and ensure the institution's accountability. According to Aronson (2016), healthcare professionals should focus and be attentive toward patient's needs, values, priorities, and preferences (Aronson, 2016). Porter (2010) argued that stakeholders in healthcare often differ in their goals and interest, including patient-centered access to services, cost containment, safety, satisfaction, high quality, convenience, and profitability. The predominant goal of healthcare delivery should be high value for patients. Thus, there are great challenges ahead in the pharmacy education sector. Colleges need to prepare graduates who are able to survive in the era of globalization, address stakeholder demands, and fulfill the patients' needs, providing satisfaction and health-related quality of life. Moreover, we need effective, competent, and experienced leaders and educators in the education sector who can lead in the present moment, keep in line with changes in pharmacy, read the future, and stay relevant.

ACKNOWLEDGMENT

We would like to thank all the contributors. Parts of the content in this chapter was obtained from the individual chapters.

REFERENCES

ACPE. (2015). *Accreditation standards and key elements for the professional program in pharmacy leading to the doctor of pharmacy degree*. Chicago, Illinois: ACPE. https://www.acpe-accredit.org/pdf/Standards2016FINAL.pdf (Accessed 25 October 2017).

Alexander, A. (2010). What are the attributes required to become tomorrow's pharmacists? *The Pharmaceutical Journal*, *284*, 458–459.

Allen, M. (2009). What is continuing professional development (CPD)? http://www.jobs.ac.uk/careers-advice/managing-your-career/1318/what-is-continuing-professional-development-cpd (Accessed 5 October 2017).

Alsharif, N. Z. (2012). Globalization of pharmacy education: What is needed? *American Journal of Pharmaceutical Education*, *76*(5)77.

Aronson, J. K. (2016). "Collaborative care" is preferable to "patient centred care". *BMJ*, *353*, i2926.

Barrett, A. M. et al. (2006). The concept of quality in education: a review of the 'international' literature on the concept of quality in education. EdQual Working Paper No. 3. http://www.edqual.org/publications/workingpaper/edqualwp3.pdf/at_download/file.pdf (Accessed 31 October 2017).

Bonner, L. (2014). Interprofessional education: Growing focus on preparing students for team-based care. Pharmacy Today. http://www.pharmacist.com/interprofessional-education-growing-focus-preparing-students-team-based-care (Accessed 25 October 2017).

Burke, R.M. (2015). Changes on the horizon for pharmacy education. http://www.pharmacist.com/changes-horizon-pharmacy-education (Accessed 1 November 2017).

Chitty, C. (2002). *Understanding schools and schooling*. London: Routledge Falme.

DiPietro Mager, N. A., & Farris, K. B. (2016). The importance of public health in pharmacy education and practice. American Journal of Pharmaceutical Education, 80(2), 18. doi: https://doi.org/10.5688/ajpe80218 (Accessed 1 November 2017).

Educause (2014). 7 things you should know about competency-based education. https://library.educause.edu/resources/2014/2/7-things-you-should-know-about-competencybased-education (Accessed 15 October 2017).

Educause (2017). Competency-based Education (CBE). https://library.educause.edu/topics/teaching-and-learning/competency-based-education-cbe.

European Commission (2018). Quality and relevance in higher education. http://ec.europa.eu/education/policy/higher-education/quality-relevance_en (Accessed 2 November 2017).

Fox, A., & Reeves, S. (2015). Interprofessional collaborative patient-centred care: A critical exploration of two related discourses. *Journal of Interprofessional Care*, *29*(2), 113–118. https://doi.org/10.3109/13561820.2014.954284.

Gervais, J. (2016). The operational definition of competency-based education. *The Journal of Competency-Based Education*, *1*(2), 98–106. https://doi.org/10.1002/cbe2.1011.

Harding, G., & Taylor, K. M. G. (2016). *Pharmacy practice* (2nd ed.). New York: CRC Press.

Harvey, L., & Green, D. (1993). Defining quality. *Assessment & Evaluation in Higher Education*, *18*(1), 9–34. https://doi.org/10.1080/0260293930180102.

Institute of Medicine (US) Committee on the Health Professions Education Summit. (2003). *Chapter 3, The Core Competencies Needed for Health Care Professionals. In A. C. Greiner & E. Knebel (Eds.), Health professions education: A bridge to quality*. Washington (DC): National Academies Press (US) Available from: https://www.ncbi.nlm.nih.gov/books/NBK221519/ (Accessed 20 October 2017).

International Pharmaceutical Federation (FIP) (2012). FIP Global pharmacy workforce report. Retrieved from Portugal: https://www.fip.org/humanresources (Accessed 30 September 2017).

International Pharmaceutical Federation (FIP) (2015). FIP Global pharmacy workforce intelligence: trends report. Retrieved from The Hague: http://fip.org/files/fip/PharmacyEducation/Trends/FIPEd_Trends_report_2015_web_v3.pdf (Accessed 25 October 2017).

Leung, A. W. L. (2013). *Strategies for change and curriculum implementation. In A. Yiu Chun Lo, K. T. Adamson, & J. T. S. Lam (Eds.), Curriculum change and innovation*. Hong Kong University Press https://doi.org/10.5790/hongkong/9789888139026.003.0007 (Accessed 31 October 2017).

Porter, M. E. (2010). What is value in health care? *The New England Journal of Medicine, 363*, 2477–2481. https://doi.org/10.1056/NEJMp1011024.

Shizha, E., & Kariwo, M. T. (2011). Impact of Colonialism on Education. In E. Shizha & M. T. Kariwo (Eds.), *Education and development in Zimbabwe*: Sense Publishers.

Tice, B. (2017). Evolving your pharmacy practice in an era of great change. Pharmacy Times. http://www.pharmacytimes.com/news/evolving-your-pharmacy-practice-in-an-era-of-great-change (Accessed 10 October 2017).

United Nations Conference on Environment and Development (UNCED) (1992). Chapter 37. Capacity Building—Agenda 21's definition http://www.gdrc.org/uem/capacity-define.html (Accessed 12 October 2017).

WHO (1997). The role of the pharmacist in the health care system. Preparing the future pharmacist: Curricular development. Report of a third WHO Consultative Group on the role of the pharmacist, Vancouver, Canada. Geneva: World Health Organization. WHO/PHARM/97/599. Available at: http://www.who.int/medicinedocs/ (Accessed 31 October 2017).

Index

Note: Page numbers followed by *f* indicate figures, *t* indicate tables, and *b* indicate boxes.

D

J

K

L

Q

R

S

T

U

Printed in the United States
By Bookmasters